Nutrition Recommendations

The Report of the Scientific Review Committee

1990

Published by the authority of the Minister of National Health and Welfare

Également disponible en français sous le titre:

Recommandations sur la nutrition

Rapport du comité scientifique de révision 1990

Available in Canada through

Associated Bookstores
and other booksellers

or by mail from

Canadian Government Publishing Centre
Supply and Services Canada
Ottawa, Canada K1A 0S9

Cat. No.: H49-42/1990E
ISBN: 0-660-13417-9

Preface

On October 1, 1987, the Honourable Jake Epp, Minister of National Health and Welfare, announced the appointment of two committees, jointly charged with "the review and revision of nutrition recommendations for a healthy Canadian population to ensure up-to-date nutrition recommendations for professionals and the public which will promote and maintain health and reduce the risk of nutrition-related diseases".

The Scientific Review Committee was made responsible for "reviewing scientific evidence from the public health perspective in order to revise the Nutrition Recommendations".

The Communications/Implementation Committee was "responsible for the expression of updated nutrition recommendations as dietary advice for the consumer and for the recommendation of implementation strategies".

The shared responsibility for revising nutrition recommendations is a unique and logical development. In the past this process has been completed by two or even three committees, operating independently. It is anticipated that the results of an integrated review will better meet the needs of all those who make use of it.

Separate reports will be produced relating to the respective responsibilities of the Committees.

This is the report of the Scientific Review Committee.

Committee Membership

T.K. Murray (Chairman)
K.K. Carroll
J. Davignon
H.H. Draper
S. Evers
C. Greenwood
E. Mongeau
S. Zlotkin
J. Beare-Rogers (Coordinator)
P. Fischer (Secretary)
D. Palin (CIC Coordinator, Liaison Member)

All members of the Committee and the following scientists drafted material for consideration in this report:

W. Behrens
B.A. Cooper
K. Dakshinamurti
G. Ferland
M. Gascon-Barré
S.G. Gilbert
T. Glanville
E. Gordon
K. Hoppner
M. L'Abbé
B.H. Lauer
A.G. Logan
B.E. McDonald
A. Miller
R. Mongeau
F.W. Scott
B.G. Shah
J.N. Thompson
E. Vavasour

In addition, the following scientists reviewed portions of the report:

J.V. Aranda
C.J. Bates
G.H. Beaton
W.J. Bettger
R.J. Boegman
E. Bright-See
R.C. Burgess
D.H. Calloway
A. Chan
J.D. Cook
J.M. Cooperman
F. Delange
A. Drewnowski
R. Elin
P.R. Flanagan
L. Fraher
S.W. French
R. Gibson
J. Greger
S.M. Grundy
C.H. Halsted
J.E. Harrison
B.E. Haskell
V. Herbert
M. Houde-Nadeau
G. Howe
A. Imbach
S.M. Innis
K.N. Jeejeebhoy
K.J. Jenkins
H. Johansen
J. Johnston
G. Jones
J.C. King
A. Kirksey
J.C. Laidlaw
L.A. Leiter
I. Macdonald
R. McLachlan
R. McPherson
R. Mendelson
F.H. Nielsen
R.E. Olson
J.A. Olson
G.A.J. Pitt
G.M. Reaven
H. Sauberlich
D. Shapcott
M. Spence
B. Stavric
J. Suttie
L.U. Thompson
B.A. Underwood
W.D. Woodward
V. Young

The Committee is indebted to the many contributors who assisted with this report.

Executive Summary

The Nutrition Recommendations for Canadians are a product of a review of the literature on nutrient requirements and on the various relationships linking nutrition and disease. They are intended to provide guidance in the selection of a dietary pattern that will supply recommended amounts of all essential nutrients, while reducing the risk of chronic diseases. Although the recommendations are presented as individual entities, it is stressed that they will be fully effective only when applied as a unit. It is also important to appreciate that the recommendations are not a prescription and they can be satisfied by many combinations of available foods without any general need of supplements.

Desired Characteristics of the Canadian Diet

The Canadian diet should provide energy consistent with the maintenance of body weight within the recommended range. Physical activity should be appropriate to circumstances and capabilities. Both longevity and the incidence of a number of chronic diseases are associated adversely with body weights above or below the recommended range. There is, thus, a health benefit to controlling weight, but a possible downside to control by energy intake alone; physical activity should also play a role. While the importance of maintaining some activity throughout life can be stressed, it is not possible to specify a level of physical activity appropriate for the whole population. As a general guideline it is desirable that adults, for as long as possible, maintain an activity level that permits an energy intake of at least 1800 kcal or 7.6 MJ/day while keeping weight within the recommended range.

The Canadian diet should include essential nutrients in amounts recommended in this report. One of the reasons for including physical activity as a desirable element in weight control is the increasing difficulty in meeting the recommended nutrient intake (RNI) as energy intake falls below about 1800 kcal or 7.6 MJ/day. While it is important that the diet provide the recommended amounts of nutrients, it should be understood that no evidence was found that intakes in excess of the RNIs confer any health benefit. There is no general need for supplements except for vitamin D for infants and folic acid during pregnancy. Vitamin D supplementation might be required for elderly persons not exposed to the sun, and iron for pregnant women with low iron stores. It should be noted that while the habitual intake of certain nutrients, eg. protein and vitamin C, greatly exceeds the RNI, there is no reason to suggest that present intakes be reduced.

The Canadian diet should include no more than 30% of energy as fat (33 g/1000 kcal or 39 g/5000 kJ) and no more than 10% as saturated fat (11 g/1000 kcal or 13 g/5000 kJ). Diets high in fat have been associated with a high incidence of heart disease and certain types of cancer, and a reduction in total fat intake is an important way to reduce the intake of saturated fat. The evidence linking saturated fat intake with elevated blood cholesterol and the risk of heart disease is among the most persuasive of all diet/disease relationships, and was an important factor in establishing the recommended dietary pattern. Dietary cholesterol, though not as influential in affecting levels of blood cholesterol, is not without importance. A reduction in cholesterol intake normally will accompany a reduction in total fat and saturated fat. The recommendation to reduce total fat intake does not apply to children under the age of two years.

The Canadian diet should provide 55% of energy as carbohydrate (138 g/1000 kcal or 165 g/5000 kJ) from a variety of sources. Sources should be selected that provide complex carbohydrates, a variety of dietary fibre and β-carotene.

Carbohydrate is the preferred replacement for fat as a source of energy, since protein intake already exceeds requirements. There are a number of reasons why the increased carbohydrate calories should be in the form of complex carbohydrates. Diets high in complex carbohydrates have been associated with a lower incidence of heart disease and cancer, and are sources of dietary fibre and of β–carotene.

The sodium content of the Canadian diet should be reduced. The present food supply provides sodium in an amount greatly exceeding requirements. While there is insufficient evidence to support a quantitative recommendation, potential benefit would be expected from a reduction in current sodium intake. Consumers are encouraged to reduce the use of salt (sodium chloride) in cooking and at the table, but individual efforts will be relatively ineffective unless the food industry makes a determined effort to reduce the sodium content of processed and prepared food. A diet rich in fruits and vegetables will ensure an adequate intake of potassium.

The Canadian diet should include no more than 5% of total energy as alcohol, or two drinks daily, whichever is less. There are many reasons to limit the use of alcohol. From the nutritional point of view alcohol dilutes the nutrient density of the diet and can undermine the consumption of RNIs. The deleterious influence of alcohol on blood pressure provides a more urgent reason for moderation. During pregnancy it is prudent to abstain from alcoholic beverages because a safe intake is not known with certainty.

The Canadian diet should contain no more caffeine than the equivalent of four regular cups of coffee per day. This is a prudent measure in view of the increased risk for cardiovascular disease associated with high intakes of caffeine.

Community water supplies containing less than 1 mg/litre should be fluoridated to that level. Fluoridation of community water supplies has proven to be a safe, effective and economical method of improving dental health.

Table of Contents

Part I

Nutritional Recommendations

Introduction

The importance of nutrition in the maintenance of good health is now more widely accepted than at any time within recollection. Nutritional advice generated from a variety of sources to meet the demand stimulated by this acceptance has been both good and bad, warranted and unwarranted.

In response to this situation, the Scientific Review Committee was established to "review scientific evidence from the public health perspective in order to revise the Nutrition Recommendations". In more closely defining this assignment a historic perspective may be helpful.

For more than forty years nutrition advice provided to Canadians (eg. Canada's Food Rules, more recently Canada's Food Guide) has been based on regularly up-dated compilations of nutrient requirements, now presented as Recommended Nutrient Intakes (RNIs). Not until the 1970s, when Nutrition Recommendations for Canadians, derived from the report of the Committee on Diet and Cardiovascular Disease, was integrated with Canada's Food Guide, did the influence of diet on a chronic disease become a part of advice to the public. Since that time there has been a striking change in emphasis in nutritional advice to the public; reduction in risk of chronic diseases has now become the primary focus, supplanting, in this respect, freedom from nutrient deficiency. Given the lesser threat posed by nutrient deficiency, as compared to heart disease, cancer etc., this development is understandable, but it should be remembered that reducing the risk of chronic diseases is not the prime reason for eating. Clearly a balanced approach is needed; our diet should meet the need for nutrients while providing maximum protection against chronic diseases.

To achieve this balance the Nutrition Recommendations presented in this report were based on a combined review of nutrient requirements and nutrient/disease relationships. This process provided, in addition to Nutrition Recommendations, a revision of Recommended Nutrient Intakes for Canadians, last issued in 1983. The updated RNIs appear in Part II.

The potential for confusion between the similarly titled Recommended Nutrient Intakes and Nutrition Recommendations may be reduced by introducing operational definitions. The RNIs deal with recommended intakes of essential nutrients; Nutrition Recommendations with dietary patterns that will provide nutrients in recommended amounts while minimizing the risk of chronic diseases.

The Review Process

Experts were enlisted to draft chapters for review, amendment and approval by the Scientific Review Committee. In addition, each chapter was subjected to at least two external reviews before final revision and committee approval. At this point in the process, consultation and collaboration with the committee charged with developing dietary advice for the consumer (The Communications and Implementation Committee) came into play. The decision to develop nutrition recommendations and recommended nutrient intakes from the same reviews made necessary an increased emphasis on nutrient/disease relationships in the development of RNIs, and consideration of an increased number of these relationships in the formulation of nutrition recommendations. It should be stressed that nutrient/disease relationships were considered only within the context of diet; pharmacological use of nutrients was not considered.

It is believed that this integrated approach to nutrition recommendations effectively combines the research/public health priorities in nutrition. An overriding consideration is the reality that the whole diet, not individual nutrients, is involved in the diet/health equation.

The subjects reviewed included alcohol, artificial sweeteners and caffeine. It was necessary, however, to draw the line at considering all of the non-nutrients that have been implicated in some way with ill health.

The chapters from which recommendations on nutrient intake and diet selection are taken appear in full in Part II. Recommendations arising from these chapters fall into the following categories:

- Energy intakes, presented as average requirements rather than the greatest or least needs of the population.
- The intake of nutrients, eg. vitamin, mineral, protein, believed to be sufficiently high to meet the requirements, including reducing the risk of chronic diseases, of almost all individuals in a group with specified characteristics (age, size, physiological state). Because these Recommended Nutrient Intakes are designed to meet the needs of all normal individuals (almost all), they must exceed the needs of most. No one method could be used to establish these recommended intakes because the available data varied from nutrient to nutrient. Where warranted by

the information available, the average requirement was increased by two standard deviations to take into account individual variability, assuming a normal distribution of requirements. This was not always possible and other methods were then applied, as described in the relevant chapters.

- Restriction on the intake of dietary components because of toxicity or association with an increased risk of chronic diseases.
- Dietary patterns associated with a low incidence of chronic diseases but without the clear cause/effect involvement of a specific nutrient or nutrients.

Factors to Consider

Target Population

The Nutrition Recommendations are intended for healthy individuals over the age of two years. The Recommended Nutrient Intakes apply to the entire healthy population.

Body Size

Nutrient requirement varies according to body size and, although it is customary to list the requirements of males and females separately, the differences, with a few obvious exceptions, are related to body size, not sex. The obvious exceptions include the effect of menstrual blood loss on iron requirements, the hormonal influence on calcium loss and the additional requirements imposed by pregnancy and lactation.

Age

As in previous reports, recommended intakes are arranged in age categories. This is a convenient way to take account of the physiological changes that mark our passage through life. In spite of increased interest in changes associated with old age there is still little evidence on this subject and hence only limited guidance specific to the later years.

Adaptation

In some cases our habitual diet influences the recommended intake. The most notable example is calcium, for which economy of utilization is determined by habitual intake. Many populations thrive on calcium intakes that would be considered grossly inadequate for Canadians, adapted as we are to a much more generous consumption.

Time Frame

Both Nutrition Recommendations and Recommended Nutrient Intakes should be thought of and applied in terms of usual practice or average intake over several days and not on a daily basis.

Use and Misuse of Nutrition Recommendations

The primary use of the Nutrition Recommendations is to form the basis for advice to the public on the choice of healthy diets. They should also be used by those responsible for planning and providing the national food supply, to facilitate public adherance to the guidelines by making appropriate foods available.

It would be a misuse of the Nutrition Recommendations to conclude that individuals who do not adhere to each part are doomed to suffer the associated chronic disease, or that embracing a specific recommendation will ensure avoidance of chronic diseases. As will be explained in the later section, the evidence upon which the recommendations are based does not support such a conclusion. It can, however, be expected that if Canadians adopt the dietary pattern recommended, the nutritional status of the population will improve and the incidence of chronic diseases will decline.

Use and Misuse of RNIs

The most immediate use of the Recommended Nutrient Intakes is to provide a basis for Nutrition Recommendations. They can, in addition, be used in planning diets and processing food supplies for individuals and groups, for estimating the total needs of the population for energy and nutrients, and for judging the need for public health interventions such as food fortification. In combination with the Nutrition Recommendations they can be used for planning and providing a food supply that is consistent with good health.

Compilations of Recommended Nutrient Intakes have been misused by describing intakes of less than that recommended as "deficient" or inadequate. As described earlier, the Recommended Nutrient Intakes are intended to meet the needs of almost all individuals and so exceed the actual requirements of almost all. It follows that an intake below that recommended cannot be described as inadequate, but it also follows that the more that intake falls below the RNI the greater the probability of inadequacy. Without additional information, however, all that can be concluded about low intakes is that they are less than those recommended. Most emphatically it is not possible to judge the nutritional status of an individual solely on the basis of dietary intake.

Nutrition and Disease

The concept of reducing the risk of disease by diet is relatively new and has been accompanied by considerable misunderstanding and a certain degree of both scepticism and over-optimism. In this part an attempt will be made to bring clarity and realism to these matters and to summarize the conclusions of the scientific review of nutrient/disease relationships.

Diet and Chronic Disease

The current public health emphasis on the prevention of the major chronic degenerative diseases is a direct response to changing patterns of morbidity and mortality in the past 50 years. There has been a shift from a dominance of acute, infectious diseases to chronic degenerative diseases. Advances in medical technology and changes in environmental conditions, such as improved nutritional status, are partly responsible for this alteration in disease patterns. In addition, the age composition of the Canadian population has changed dramatically over the past 50 years (Adler and Brusegard 1980). The proportion of the population aged 65 years and over has steadily increased while the age group 15 years and under has decreased. Successful control of infectious diseases has led to the survival of people who, in the early part of this century, would have died at a young age. For the most part, however, the change in age composition is due to the declining birth rate. The consequence is that an ever increasing proportion of Canadians are at risk of developing chronic degenerative diseases. The major causes of mortality among Canadians are heart disease and cancer (Ku *et al.* 1986); for both disease categories there is some evidence of a link with diet.

Cardiovascular disease continues to be the leading cause of death. In 1982, the Canadian age-standardized mortality rates (standardized to the 1976 world population) were 307.7 and 170.6 per 100 000 for men and women, respectively (Nicholls *et al.* 1986). On the other hand, however, Canada is one of the few countries to show a decrease in mortality rates for both sexes since 1950. The death rate for males has dropped by 32%. An even more substantial reduction, 50%, has occurred for females. The reasons for this decline have not been established (Klurfeld and Kritchevsky 1986). Medical treatment for heart disease has advanced at a rapid pace and behavioural factors such as a reduction in the prevalence of cigarette smoking, an increase in the level of physical fitness and improved dietary habits are believed to be partly responsible for this trend. Only a small proportion of the drop in heart disease mortality, however, has been directly attributed to a decrease in serum cholesterol, a decrease in diastolic blood pressure and a decline in cigarette smoking (Feinleib *et al.* 1982). At the population level, the potential for changes in dietary habits to reduce the incidence of heart disease is enormous (Hopkins and Williams 1986). For the individual, dietary changes cannot guarantee freedom from heart disease but will lower the risk. Obesity, for example, increases the risk of heart disease (Rabkin *et al.* 1977; Hubert *et al.* 1983). Weight loss alone could significantly lower susceptibility.

Cancer is the second leading cause of death among Canadians. Among males, total cancer incidence has increased by 1.8% annually since 1970 (Canadian Cancer Society 1988). Despite improvements in treatment and progress against some specific types of cancer, the mortality rate for males has also increased at 0.5% per year. The pattern for females is similar. The annual increase in cancer incidence since 1970 is 0.8%. The overall mortality rate has not changed. Cancer is not a single disease. Different factors will influence the initiation and development of tumors at different sites. As with heart disease, lifestyle factors are thought to affect cancer risk. While a reduction in cigarette smoking would have the greatest impact on the number of deaths due to cancer, it is estimated that approximately 35% of cancer mortality in the U.S. may be related to dietary factors (Doll and Peto 1981).

Establishing Causation

With the shift in the pattern of disease, the initial reaction to the increased incidence of chronic degenerative diseases was to accept this situation as a natural consequence of the successful treatment and control of infectious diseases. Only in the last few decades has there been evidence suggesting that environmental factors, such as diet, are related to these diseases. Furthermore, while some factors are immutable, others such as diet may be modified to reduce the risk.

In studies of chronic degenerative diseases it is difficult to identify a specific component of the diet and state with absolute certainty that an excess (or deficiency) will influence the incidence of the disease under investigation. A risk factor is simply an attribute or exposure that is associated with an increased probability of disease.

Unlike studies of nutrient deficiencies, investigations which seek to identify risk factors for chronic degenerative diseases are primarily epidemiological. The risk or likelihood of developing a specific disease is assigned to a population and not an individual. Thus, dietary recommendations based on the results of epidemiological studies should not be interpreted as a guarantee that following the recommendations will prevent disease in a particular individual. Rather, in a population following the recommendations there should be a reduction in the incidence of disease.

Most chronic degenerative diseases have a long latent period. For cardiovascular disease and cancer, the latent period between the initiation of the disease and the appearance of clinical signs can be 20 years or longer. The disease may be a consequence of continuous exposure to specific dietary factors over several decades. Thus, measurement of habitual intake over 20 or 30 years is important to our understanding of the relationship between diet and disease.

Yet another characteristic of chronic degenerative diseases makes study of the role of diet quite difficult. Most diseases are multifactorial. Not only are environmental and genetic factors involved, but their interaction can also influence the risk of disease. It is unlikely that a single nutrient acts alone to influence risk. It is more probable that interactions between nutrients and perhaps interactions between nutrient and non-nutrient components of the diet alter the likelihood of disease.

Proof of cause and effect relationships in studies of diet and chronic degenerative diseases is difficult to obtain. In simple terms, a cause is a risk factor whose reduction or elimination will result in a decline in the incidence of the disease under study. Unfortunately, the characteristics of chronic degenerative diseases preclude such a straightforward approach. Instead, a number of criteria should be met before an association between a certain factor and disease can be regarded as a cause and effect relationship (U.S. Surgeon General 1964).

1. Strength — this is indicated by the magnitude of the relative risk, not the size of the difference in risk. The relative risk is the ratio of disease incidence (number of new cases in a population at risk over a period of time) in the exposed group to the unexposed group. The larger the relative risk, the stronger the association.
2. Consistency — the association has been reported by different investigators in different populations, locations and times. There may be variations in the magnitude of the relative risk, but the association is consistent.
3. Logical time sequence — exposure to the factor (cause) must precede the onset of disease (effect). This criterion is essential to establish causation.
4. Specificity — the suspected causal factor is associated with a specific disease. The known risk factors for chronic degenerative diseases seldom have a single effect. Thus, lack of specificity does not rule out a causal relationship.
5. Coherence — the association must agree with known biologic facts or theory.

In studies of diet and chronic degenerative diseases, few (if any) associations will meet all the criteria necessary to firmly establish a cause and effect relationship. The evidence must be carefully evaluated, particularly when suspected associations between dietary factors and cancer are examined (Hebert and Miller 1988). Often there is little or no support for these associations in studies of human populations on the level of the individual.

Failure to observe a diet-disease association may be due to problems inherent in the methodology of such epidemiologic investigations. Some of the difficulty in establishing causation can be attributed to the lack of a clearly defined and accurate method for the assessment of long-term dietary intake. Much of the evidence has been obtained through descriptive epidemiology. The results of such studies are critical to the development of hypotheses for subsequent investigations, but do not determine whether a cause and effect relationship exists.

A valid and precise method for assessing the usual intake of an individual that is also easy to administer and not time-consuming has yet to be developed. The common techniques in dietary methodology (24-hour recall, food frequency questionnaires) yield variable results (Block 1982). Proper interpretation of epidemiologic studies of diet requires consideration of the limitations of such methods (Kushi *et al.* 1988). More accurate methods for collecting dietary intake data (weighed food intake, seven day and/or repeated dietary records) are often not suitable for epidemiological studies because of the characteristic low response rate.

In addition to the above limitations, studies of the long-term effects of diet are faced with other difficulties. Regardless of the method used, there is an assumption that current intake reflects past intake. Dietary habits, however, are a matter of choice. A variety of influences — cultural, economic, and social, as well as others — may alter food intake patterns over a lifetime. For studies including patients with chronic diseases, diagnosis and the onset of treatment are often followed by an alteration in food intake patterns. Thus, current intake may not reflect past intake. In investigations comparing the dietary intake of persons with a disease and healthy control subjects the intensity of recall can vary, particularly if an individual believes that certain foods caused the disease.

Biochemical and anthropometric measurements are important components of nutritional assessment studies. Such measurements, however, rarely reflect nutritional status for more than a few months. Animal experiments are critical to our understanding of the mechanisms of cause and effect relationships. Such effects must be confirmed in human populations before making recommendations for dietary changes; extrapolation from animal experiments is not sufficient.

Summary

Our knowledge of the cumulative effects of diet on the risk of chronic diseases, such as heart disease, has advanced considerably over the past 20 years. There is little doubt that diet is implicated in the etiology of these diseases; at present, however, we cannot quantify these relationships. It is difficult to assess long-term exposure to specific components of the diet. In addition, actual differences in levels of intake can be small, thereby impairing our ability to detect an association (Hebert and Miller 1988). Of all the suspected dietary risk factors for heart disease and cancer, obesity is perhaps most closely correlated with an increased risk (Lew and Garfinkel 1979). Thus, modification of energy intake and expenditure alone could bring about a reduction in disease frequency.

Dietary recommendations must be based on strong scientific evidence. Premature recommendations to the public can lead to confusion, especially if the public is faced with a reversal of advice as more evidence becomes available (Becker 1986). Thus, in general, to justify a recommendation to modify the Canadian diet, an increased risk of disease with exposure to certain levels of a nutrient or non-nutrient, or with interactions among dietary components, must be repeatedly observed in rigorous investigations conducted under different circumstances. In specific instances, however, changes in the diet have been recommended despite the inadequacy of scientific data, simply because there is little or no danger inherent in the change, and a strong likelihood that it may be beneficial. The recommendation to select a diet with a variety of fibre sources is representative of this category.

Nutrient/Disease Relationships

In the review of the evidence relating to diet and chronic diseases, many relationships were examined. The following identifies those judged important in the development of Nutrition Recommendations as well as those that did not stand up to critical examination.

Atherosclerotic Heart Disease

The first diet/disease relationship to markedly influence nutrition guidelines was the association between dietary lipids and heart disease. Over a 30-year period this relationship has stimulated a phenomenal amount of research, an impressive array of disagreement and commercial conflict. While this era is not yet behind us, there is a strong case for certain essential advice to the public.

The dominant dietary influence on serum cholesterol, and hence on heart disease, is saturated fat. Its reduction in the Canadian diet is a key factor in reducing the risk of heart disease. Although evidence linking total fat intake to the incidence of heart disease is not as powerful, it is impractical to reduce the intake of saturated fat without reducing total fat.

Polyunsaturated fatty acids, primarily of the n-6 series, have, over many years, been almost synonymous with control of serum cholesterol, but are now recognized as being of lesser importance in this regard than is saturated fat. Recently n-3 polyunsaturated fatty acids have been publicized as factors instrumental in reducing the risk of heart disease. These acids are not very effective in reducing serum cholesterol but they do lower elevated triglycerides and reduce blood clotting.

Monounsaturated fatty acids have been assigned a neutral role insofar as changes in serum cholesterol are concerned. This is probably an appropriate assignment in spite of recent publicity touting their cholesterol-lowering qualities.

Although dietary cholesterol does not rank as highly as saturated fat in its effect on serum cholesterol, it is not without influence. A worthwhile reduction in present intake can be achieved by reducing total fat or, more specifically, saturated fat consumption.

Dietary factors, in addition to lipids, are associated with heart disease. Energy imbalance leading to overweight increases the risk of heart disease, either directly, or through its undoubted influence on blood pressure, serum cholesterol, high density lipoprotein (HDL) and low density lipoprotein (LDL) levels and glucose tolerance.

Although diets high in complex carbohydrates have been associated with a low incidence of cardiovascular disease, there is no evidence that this is a direct effect of carbohydrate. More likely, the low fat content of these same diets is the important factor. It is also difficult to disassociate the metabolic effects of complex carbohydrates from those of dietary fibre, since diets high in one are usually high in the other.

Despite speculation to the contrary, simple sugars (glucose, fructose and sucrose) have not been found to be a risk factor for heart disease.

As is the case for complex carbohydrates, diets high in fibre have been associated with a low incidence of heart disease. Again, it is difficult to evaluate the importance of the fibre component as distinct from the low-fat content of these same diets. It is known that soluble fibre has an independent influence on serum cholesterol, though the amount required to achieve a measurable effect is very large.

A considerable body of evidence from animal experiments has associated a relative or absolute deficiency of copper with hypercholesterolemia. Confirmation of this association in humans is still pending and no action other than consumption of the RNI for copper is called for.

Evidence linking magnesium to heart disease has ranged from the higher incidence of ischemic heart disease in soft water areas to the lower concentration of myocardial magnesium in men dying of myocardial infarction. The difficulty of separating the effect of magnesium from that of other variables in hard water areas, and of eliminating the possibility that the redistribution of magnesium is a result of the disease rather than the cause, prevents any final conclusion on a magnesium/heart disease relationship. No action other than the consumption of the RNI for magnesium is called for.

Cancer

It has been estimated that the incidence of cancer can be reduced 35% by dietary means, but it has proven remarkably difficult to identify specific components of the diet that increase risk or provide protection in individuals. The tentative identification of candidates for these roles has received much media attention and kept consumers on edge.

There is no scarcity of epidemiological evidence linking the level of fat in the diet with the incidence of cancer at a variety of sites. Studies on experimental animals have tended to support this evidence but case-control and prospective studies have been inconclusive.

Similar evidence has linked diets high in fibre with a low incidence of colon cancer, while animal experiments have shown varying effects of different kinds of fibre.

Energy imbalances leading to either obesity or underweight correlates strongly with the incidence of certain cancers.

An association has been consistently observed between increased consumption of total vitamin A, carotene, green and yellow vegetables and a decreased risk of cancer in epithelial tissues. Recent evidence tends to negate the likelihood that preformed vitamin A is responsible for this association, and the possibility remains that carotene is only a marker for the active substance in protective diets. The evidence does not warrant a recommendation for a general increase in vitamin A intake but enhances the importance of sources of carotene (vegetables and fruits) in the diet.

Evidence that products of lipid peroxidation are mutagenic has prompted proposals that vitamin E in excess of present intakes might prevent cancer. Prospective studies have been inconclusive and vitamin E provides no protection against chemically-induced carcinogenesis. No change in dietary intake on the basis of cancer prevention is warranted. A correlation between vitamin C intake and cancer incidence has been observed in some epidemiological studies, but there has been no confirmation that vitamin C plays a specific role other than simply characterizing diets high in fruits and vegetables, low in fat and calories. Ascorbic acid reduces the formation of nitrosamines from nitrates in foods but is ineffective in reducing their oral carcinogenicity.

Prospective studies have indicated that serum selenium concentration in humans is inversely related to the risk of cancer in future years. The several intervention trials in progress are testing the effect of amounts of selenium already provided by typical Canadian diets. Because of this, and the narrow range of safe intakes of this element, no increase in present intakes is warranted.

Obesity

The negative influence of obesity on health is persuasive but often plays second fiddle to more glamorous, though less important, reasons to control weight. Long-term studies show that mortality rates from all causes are higher in those who are overweight, the risk increasing gradually with increases in weight. Overweight is a recognized risk factor for hypertension, hyperlipidemias, diabetes and as a result, cardiovascular disease. Both overweight and underweight are associated with an increased risk of cancer. A noteworthy exception to all of this is the increased survival of the moderately overweight elderly.

Hypertension

Casual observation suggests that one of the diet/disease relationships most readily acknowledged by the public is that between sodium and hypertension. This proposed relationship has also had an influence on the composition of some classes of processed foods, e.g. the removal of salt from baby food.

Evidence is insufficient to support a quantitative recommendation to reduce sodium intake. However, because a reduction in present intakes involves no risk and the possibility of benefit, it is recommended that present intakes of sodium be reduced. The public is encouraged to reduce the use of salt in cooking and at the table but since commercial processed and prepared foods provide most of our intake of sodium, the food industry must play a key role in reducing the sodium content of our food supply.

Osteoporosis

Of all nutrient/disease relationships none has seemed so obvious, nor so readily accepted by health professionals and the public alike, as that between dietary calcium and osteoporosis. As a result, women on both sides of menopause have been counselled to consume calcium in amounts exceeding the RNI. Many have done so. As is so often the case, reality is not bound by what seems obvious. Several recent studies have led to the conclusion that neither increased dietary calcium intake nor calcium supplementation has a significant influence on the rate of change in bone mineral around the time of menopause.

It is concluded that while no increase in the RNI for calcium is warranted, it is important to maintain intakes throughout life at present recommended levels. Special emphasis should be placed on an adequate intake during skeletal development.

While direct evidence is lacking that vitamin D deficiency is a factor in the development of osteoporosis, the observation that the level of active metabolites of vitamin D are low in some elderly Canadians, who also demonstrate a lower efficiency of calcium absorption, has led to an increase from 2.5 to 5 μg/day in the recommended intake of vitamin D for those over fifty years of age.

Inactivity is known to increase the loss of bone calcium, and consequently exercise is a positive factor in the maintenance of bone integrity.

The great importance of sunshine in meeting requirements for vitamin D must not be overlooked. Concern that exposure to the sun may increase the risk of skin cancer should not lead to complete avoidance of such exposure.

The high intakes by North Americans of phosphorus and protein have been cited as possibly contributing to osteoporosis. Human adults, however, seem able to maintain calcium balance at phosphorus intakes that are normal for this part of the world. Furthermore, the calciuric effect of dietary protein is counteracted, at least in part, by the hypocalciuric effect of excess dietary phosphorus.

Fluoride has been used therapeutically in the treatment of osteoporosis but with equivocal results; there has been no confirmation of a beneficial effect of fluoridated water on osteoporosis.

Dental Caries

The relationship between diet and dental caries has been known for many years and it is one case for which there is direct evidence of the benefit of corrective action.

The fluoridation of drinking water to a level of 1 mg/litre is a safe and most effective way of reducing tooth decay. The incidence of dental caries in children is reduced by 40-60% by this means, and the benefits continue into adulthood. In locations where fluoridated water is not available, fluoride tablets or topical application is an acceptable, though not equal, alternative.

Sugars are known to be involved in the development of dental caries. It is recommended that the use of sticky snacks, which tend to adhere to the teeth, be curtailed. Effective oral hygiene should be encouraged whatever the dietary practice.

Bowel Disease

The best evidence linking diet with the function and health of the large intestine is the effect of insoluble fibre on constipation. The relationship between diverticulosis and fibre intake has been studied without decisive result.

Conclusion

It is an important, though not unexpected finding, that a review of relevant literature reaffirmed the role of diet in reducing the incidence of chronic diseases but did not provide unequivocal evidence of cause and effect relationships between individual nutrients and specific diseases. Intakes of specific nutrients in excess of the

RNIs established by traditional means were not found to reduce the risk of chronic diseases. No magic bullets were identified.

This by no means negates or diminishes the importance of diet as a factor in the maintenance of health. It does reinforce the importance of the whole diet rather than the contribution of individual components.

References

Adler, H.J. and Brusegard, D.A., eds. 1980. Perspectives Canada III. Statistics Canada, Ottawa.

Becker, M.H. 1986. The tyranny of health promotion. Public Health Rev. 14:15-23.

Block, G. 1982. A review of validations of dietary assessment methods. Am. J. Epidemiol. 115:492-505.

Canadian Cancer Society. 1988. Canadian cancer statistics 1988. Toronto.

Doll, R. and Peto, R. 1981. The causes of cancer: quantitative estimates of avoidable risks of cancer in the United States today. J. Nat. Cancer Inst. 66:1191-1308.

Feinleib, M., Thom, T. and Havlik, R.J. 1982. Decline in coronary heart disease mortality in the United States. Atheroscler. Rev. 9:29-42.

Hebert, J.R. and Miller, D.R. 1988. Methodologic considerations for investigating the diet-cancer link. Am. J. Clin. Nutr. 47:1068-1077.

Hopkins, P.N. and Williams, R.R. 1986. Identification and relative weight of cardiovascular risk factors. Cardiology Clin. 4:3-31.

Hubert, H.B., Feinleib, M., McNamara, P.M. and Castelli, W.P. 1983. Obesity as an independent risk factor for cardiovascular disease: a 26-year follow-up of participants in the Framingham Heart Study. Circulation 67:968-977.

Klurfeld, D.M. and Kritchevsky, D. 1986. The Western diet: an examination of its relationship with chronic disease. J. Am. Coll. Nutr. 5:477-485.

Ku, P., Smith, E. and Mao, Y. 1986. Recent Canadian mortality trends. Chronic Dis. Can. 7:46-49.

Kushi, L.H., Samonds, K.W., Lacey, J.M., Brown, P.T., Bergan, J.G. and Sacks, F.M. 1988. The association of dietary fat with serum cholesterol in vegetarians: the effects of dietary assessment on the correlation coefficient. Am. J. Epidemiol. 128:1054-1064.

Lew, E.A. and Garfinkel, L. 1979. Variations in mortality by weight among 750,000 men and women. J. Chronic Dis. 32:563-576.

Nicholls, E., Nair, C., MacWilliam, L., Moen, J. and Mao, Y. 1986. Cardiovascular disease in Canada. Statistics Canada Cat. No. 82-544. Statistics Canada, Ottawa.

Rabkin, S.W., Mathewson, F.A.L. and Hsu, P.H. 1977. Relation of body weight to development of ischemic heart disease in a cohort of young North American men after a 26-year observation period. The Manitoba Study. Am. J. Cardiol. 39:452-458.

U.S. Surgeon General's Advisory Committee on Smoking and Health. 1964. Smoking and health: report of the Advisory Committee to the Surgeon General. Dept. of Health, Education and Welfare, U.S.G.P.O., Washington.

Part II

Recommended Nutrient Intakes

Energy

Carbohydrate

Fibre

Lipids

Cholesterol

Protein

Fat-soluble Vitamins

- Carotene and Vitamin A
- Vitamin D
- Vitamin E
- Vitamin K

Water-soluble Vitamins

- Vitamin C
- Thiamin
- Riboflavin
- Niacin
- Vitamin B_6
- Folate
- Vitamin B_{12}
- Biotin
- Pantothenic Acid

Minerals

- Calcium and Phosphorus
- Magnesium
- Iron
- Iodine
- Zinc
- Copper
- Fluoride
- Manganese
- Selenium
- Chromium
- Other Trace Elements

Electrolytes and Water

Energy

Function and Action

Energy is needed by the body for the maintenance of body composition and functions (basal metabolic rate), for physiological processes consecutive to the absorption of foods (thermic effect of food), for performing work, and for adapting to various environmental stresses such as changes in temperature, in food intake or in emotional tension (adaptive thermogenesis). In growing individuals and during pregnancy, additional energy is required for the synthesis of new tissues. In adults living in Western countries, resting metabolic rate is estimated to account for 60-70% of the caloric expenditure, the thermic effect of food for 10%, and physical activity for 20% to 30% (Katch and McArdle 1988).

Energy is supplied to the body in the form of chemical energy found in the organic molecules of foods, mostly in fats and carbohydrates. Once it has gone through the digestive and absorptive processes, the potential energy in foods is released gradually through various metabolic pathways that differ in efficiency, thus influencing energy requirements.

Energy can be stored in the body, and more precisely, in the adipocytes, principally as triacylglycerides. Through complex hormonally-controlled mechanisms, these stores are constantly used and rebuilt. Adipose tissue normally accounts for 15% of body mass in adult men, and 25% in adult women (Katch and McArdle 1988).

Energy Balance

Energy balance refers to the state of equilibrium between intake and output. This process is regulated by various physiological and metabolic mechanisms. Energy intake is influenced in the human by psychological and social factors. Energy utilization may be influenced by heredity (Canada. Health and Welfare 1988b).

Energy balance is achieved by adjusting intake when expenditure varies because of changes in activity, or by adjusting expenditure when underfeeding or overfeeding occurs. For example, it is now recognized that physical activity decreases in people subjected to marked chronic undernutrition (Beaton 1983). There are indications that there is a certain level of metabolic adaptation to under- or overfeeding (Sukhatme and Margen 1982), although the influence of this process on energy expenditure is believed to be small (FAO/WHO/UNU 1985). Regulatory mechanisms adjusting intake to output or vice versa do not operate on a day-to-day basis, but can be viewed as a long-term adaptation mechanism resulting in the maintenance of body weight and composition in most persons over a long period of time. The capacity to adapt is determined genetically and modulates the effect that energy imbalance may have on health. Some of the adaptation reactions themselves, eg. changes in body weight or composition, or decreases in activity or performance, are risk factors for the health or for the personal and social development of an individual, and are hence undesirable.

Effects on Health of Energy Imbalance

Underweight and overweight are recognized risk factors for many diseases, namely hypertension, diabetes, hyperlipidemias, and perhaps certain types of cancer. As noted by Roncari (1988) and by Pereira and White (1988) it is not possible to measure quantitatively the impact of obesity on the incidence of disease because: (1) the obese do not constitute a homogeneous group; (2) these diseases have a multifactorial etiology; and (3) the effect of obesity is probably mediated through various risk factors such as blood pressure, blood cholesterol, high density lipoprotein and low density lipoprotein levels, and glucose tolerance in the case of cardiovascular diseases. Strong correlations exist between indices of obesity or leanness, such as the body mass index (BMI)*, and the incidence of cardiovascular diseases, hypertension, type II diabetes and certain cancers. For example, in the Canada Fitness Survey, the probability of diastolic hypertension increases with the value of the BMI: it is about twice as high when the BMI is 27 or over than when it is 21 to 22, and it triples when the latter reaches a value of 30 (Pereira and White 1988). In a recent report from the Netherlands, the incidence of diabetes, gout, arteriosclerotic disease and arthrosis was higher among overweight men and women compared with a control group (Seidell *et al.*1986).

Long-term studies show that overall, mortality rates are higher among people who are overweight. At the 30-year follow-up of the Framingham Heart Study, survival rates were most favourable among male nonsmokers with a weight within 100% to 110% of ideal

* $\text{BMI} = \frac{\text{Weight (kg)}}{\text{Height (m)}^2}$

weight (Feinleib 1985). The risk of death increased gradually with increases in weight. In addition, there was greater mortality among thin men. Thus, the association between weight status and mortality seemed to follow a U-shaped curve. This relationship is quite complex. For example, mortality rates at all ages and categories of relative weight are higher for smokers compared with non-smokers.

Sidney *et al.*(1987) examined mortality patterns among thin and average weight persons aged 40-79 years. Thin smokers of both sexes were at increased risk of mortality compared with smokers of average weight. Among non-smokers, however, the risk of death was similar for thin and average weight groups.

Most studies of the health hazards associated with obesity show increased risk of mortality and morbidity with increasing weight. For the very elderly, however, moderate overweight may be associated with increased survival (Mattila *et al.*1986). In a five-year study of people aged 85 years and over, mortality decreased with increasing body mass index.

Since the body mass index was found to be the measure of body mass that best correlated with the risk of diseases, an Expert Group on Weight Standards, commissioned by Health and Welfare Canada (1988a) recommended the use of the body mass index as a measure of body weight and has proposed a range of BMIs associated with various degrees of risk (Table 1).

Table 1.
Chart of Weight-Health Standards, Age 20+

Zone 4	Zone 3	Zone 2	Zone 1
BMI	20	25	27
May be associated with health problems for some people	Good weight for most people	May lead to health problems in some people	Increasing risk of developing health problems
	← Generally acceptable range →		

Health and Welfare Canada: Promoting healthy weights: a discussion paper, 1988.

Table 2 shows the range of weights that will result in a BMI within the acceptable range (20-25) when heights are the average height of Canadians within each age/sex group.

Energy Requirements

Definitions

The concept of energy requirement is challenged by the fact that there is no fixed level of energy intake that is required by all individuals of the same age, sex and size rather there is a wide range of energy intakes that can be considered adequate, depending on the level of activity performed by an individual, or desirable in the society in which he lives, and on his degree of adaptation.

From a public health point of view, energy requirements should take into account the level of activity desirable in the social context in which the population lives, the risks of under- or overweight, and other effects on health of energy imbalance, such as the stress of adapting abruptly to very high or very low intakes. The FAO/WHO/UNU Report (1985) defines "energy requirement" as "...the amount of energy needed to maintain health, growth, and an appropriate level of physical activity". This amount may be above or below the observed intakes.

If one accepts this definition of energy requirement, the concept of appropriate or desirable level of activity has to be defined. Although there is evidence indicating that it is desirable to maintain a moderate degree of activity throughout life in order to prevent diseases such as cardiovascular diseases (Colt and Hashim 1986; Paffenbarger et al. 1986) and osteoporosis (Notelovitz 1986), the specific level of activity desirable in each age/sex group of the population cannot be defined with precision. In men aged 35 to 74 years and belonging to a high socio-economic group, Paffenbarger et al. (1986) found that death rates from cardiovascular and respiratory diseases declined as energy spent in various activities increased from 500 to 3500 kcal (2.1 to 14.7 MJ) per week. There are no comparable data on women, younger men or men with a different socio-economic status.

Table 2.
Range of Desirable Weights[a] Corresponding to Average Heights[b] of Canadians

	19-24 Years		25-49 Years		50-74 Years		75 +Years	
	M	F	M	F	M	F	M	F
Height (cm)	175	160	172	160	170	158	168	155
Weight range (kg)	61-77	51-64	59-74	51-64	58-72	50-62	56-71	48-60
Average desirable weight[c]	69	58	67	58	65	56	64	54

a. Corresponding to a BMI = 20-25.

b. Heights are those used in the 1983 ed. of RNIs (largely based on the results of Nutrition Canada Survey). A comparison with median heights derived from the Canada Health Survey revealed very small differences. Since Statistics Canada has important reservations about the use of these data (because of sample size), there appears to be no good reason for changing from Nutrition Canada Survey data to Canada Health Survey data.

c. Mid-point in the range of desirable weights rounded to the closest full figure.

On the other hand, it is generally accepted that a majority of Canadians have occupations that require little physical effort. The Canada Fitness Survey (1983) estimated at 13% the proportion of adults considered sedentary, 34% moderately active, and 53% active[1]. Although the young, 10 to 19 years, were more active than the adults, girls were considerably less active than boys and the latter showed a marked drop in activity around 18 to 19 years. These results, added to the fact that there is a high prevalence of obesity among Canadians, can be considered as an indication that the level of activity is probably less than desirable. But the difference, in terms of energy expenditure, between the actual and the desirable expenditure, can only be approximated.

Basis for Calculating Energy Requirements

Two approaches can be used to estimate the energy requirements of a population: a theoretical approach using a factorial method in which the energy needed for basal metabolism and other components of energy expenditure are estimated separately and then summed; and a "factual" approach based on the results of surveys of large samples of the population in which the energy intakes were evaluated. This latter approach assumes: (1) that data from dietary surveys are valid estimates of habitual intakes and (2) that subjects are in energy equilibrium, i.e. that their intake is equal to their output. This method was the basis for the average energy intakes defined in the Recommended Nutrient Intakes (RNIs) (Canada. Health and Welfare 1983). Since the latter were published, a limited number of studies on the dietary intakes of sub-groups of the Canadian population have been reported (Spady 1980; Martinez 1982; Richard and Roberge 1982; Sabry *et al.*1982; Yeung *et al.*1982; Seoane and Roberge 1983; Barr *et al.*1984; Gibson *et al.*1985). In general, the energy intakes observed in these surveys correspond fairly well to the RNIs in children up to 10 years, but tend to be 5% to 15% lower than the RNIs in adolescents and adults. Since the samples, in these surveys, were generally small and not representative of the Canadian population, and methodology varied from one study to another, it would be inappropriate to conclude from these data that the RNIs overestimate energy requirements.

The FAO/WHO/UNU Report on Energy and Protein Requirements (1985) uses a factorial method to determine energy requirements. Basal expenditure is calculated from equations based on weight, age, and sex (Table 3). Energy expenditure for occupational, discretionary (household and other tasks, exercise), and maintenance activities are evaluated as multiples of basal metabolic rate (BMR) and added to the latter to form the total energy requirement. Average factors, expressed as multiples of BMR, are suggested to determine the daily energy requirements of adults whose occupational work is classified as light, moderate, or heavy. In the case of individuals whose work is classified as light, the energy expenditure on which this factor is based includes, among discretionary activities, 20 minutes per day of physical exercise at about 60% of maximal work load (maximum work load = 6 × BMR), which is considered the minimum required to maintain fitness and promote cardiovascular health.

1. Active people were defined as those having an average of three hours or more of physical activities (including walking) per week for nine months or more per year.

Table 3.
Equations for Predicting Basal Metabolic Rate from Body Weight (W)[a]

Age Range (Years)	kcal/day	Correlation Coefficient	SD[b]	MJ/day	Correlation Coefficient	SD[b]
Males						
0-3	60.9 W - 54	0.97	53	0.255 W - 0.226	0.97	0.222
3-10	22.7 W + 495	0.86	62	0.0949 W + 2.07	0.86	0.259
10-18	17.5 W + 651	0.90	100	0.0732 W + 2.72	0.90	0.418
18-30	15.3 W + 679	0.65	151	0.0640 W + 2.84	0.65	0.632
30-60	11.6 W + 879	0.60	164	0.0485 W + 3.67	0.60	0.686
60	13.5 W + 487	0.79	148	0.0565 W + 2.04	0.79	0.619
Females						
0-3	61.0 W - 51	0.97	61	0.255 W - 0.214	0.97	0.255
3-10	22.5 W + 499	0.85	63	0.0941 W + 2.09	0.85	0.264
10-18	12.2 W + 746	0.75	117	0.0510 W + 3.12	0.75	0.489
18-30	14.7 W + 496	0.72	121	0.0615 W + 2.08	0.72	0.506
30-60	8.7 W + 829	0.70	108	0.0364 W + 3.47	0.70	0.452
60	10.5 W + 596	0.74	108	0.0439 W + 2.49	0.74	0.452

a. FAO/WHO/UNU 1985, p. 71.

b. Standard deviation of differences between actual BMRs and predicted estimates.

Table 4.
Daily Energy Requirements According to Age, Sex and Activity (kcal/day)[d]

	19-24 Years		25-49 Years		50-74 years		75 Years +	
	M	F	M	F	M	F	M	F
Weight	69	58	67	58	65	56	64	54
BMR	1735	1349	1654	1337	1472	1237	1351	1163
Light activity[a]	2700 (39/kg)	2100 (36/kg)	2600 (38/kg)	2100 (36/kg)	2300 (35/kg)	1900 (34/kg)	2100 (33/kg)	1800 (34/kg)
Moderate activity[b]	3100 (45/kg)	2200 (38/kg)	2900 (44/kg)	2200 (38/kg)	2600 (40/kg)	2000 (36/kg)	2400 (37.5/kg)	1900 (35/kg)
Heavy activity[c]	3600 (53/kg)	2500 (42/kg)	3500 (52/kg)	2400 (42/kg)	3100 (48/kg)	2300 (40/kg)	2800 (44/kg)	2100 (39/kg)

a. Calculated on the basis of average expenditure = 1.55 BMR for men and 1.56 BMR for women.

b. Calculated on the basis of average expenditure = 1.78 BMR for men and 1.64 BMR for women.

c. Calculated on the basis of average expenditure = 2.10 BMR for men and 1.82 BMR for women.

d. 1 kcal is equivalent to 4.184 KJ.

Table 5.
Average Energy Requirements

Age (Years)	Gender	Body Weight (kg)	BMI[a]	kcal/day	RNI[b] MJ/day	kcal/kg	MJ/kg
19-24	M	71	23.18	3000	12.6	42	0.18
	F	58	22.66	2100	8.8	36	0.15
25-49	M	74	25.01	2700	11.3	36	0.15
	F	59	23.05	1900	8.0	32	0.13
50-74	M	73	25.26	2300	9.7	31	0.13
	F	63	25.24	1800	7.6	29	0.12
75 +	M	69	24.45	2000	8.4	29	0.12
	F	64	26.64	1500	6.3	23	0.10

a. $\text{BMI} = \frac{\text{Weight (kg)}}{\text{Height (m)}^2}$

b. Canada. Health and Welfare. Health Protection Branch. Bureau of Nutritional Sciences. 1983. Recommended nutrient intakes for Canadians. Ottawa.

Theoretical estimates of average energy requirements using the procedure proposed by the FAO/WHO/UNU Report were calculated for the three levels of occupational activities (Table 4), using as desirable weights for each age/sex category the mid-point in the range of desirable weights presented in Table 2. Basal metabolism was estimated from the equations proposed by FAO/WHO/UNU (Table 3). Since the age categories in this series of equations did not correspond to that used in the present report, weighted values were estimated using two equations for each of the categories of 25 to 49 years and of 50 to 74 years.

When these estimates of energy requirements are compared with average energy requirements as determined in the RNIs (Table 5), it can be seen that the latter are fairly close to or lower than the theoretical estimates of groups having a light activity, except for the younger men category where the RNI is similar to the theoretical estimate of individuals with a moderate activity. It is to be noted that, in the absence of a strong basis for determining a desirable level of activity, the RNIs assumed that the current level was compatible with health. From the comparison of Tables 4 and 5, it appears that energy intakes are, in the case of women after age 25 and of older men, inferior to those considered minimal for health, according to the FAO/WHO/UNU Report.

Recommendations

The aim of recommended energy intakes, from a public health perspective, is to propose intakes that will maintain various categories of the population within the range of desirable body mass index (BMI) as presented in Table 1, or attain this objective when the BMI falls outside this range.

In spite of normal or low energy intakes, a large number of Canadians are overweight, presumably because they are too sedentary. Among people who participated in the Canada Fitness Study, 23.7% had a BMI greater than 27 (obesity), and 15.9% between 25 and 27 (overweight) (Canada. Health and Welfare 1988a). In such a situation, raising the level of activity would appear preferable to lowering the energy intake because: (1) a certain degree of physical activity is desirable for health, as previously indicated; (2) there are increasing risks of having insufficient intakes of nutrients, for example iron and calcium, when the diet provides less than a certain amount of energy (more or less 1800 kcal, or 7.6 MJ).

In spite of the high prevalence of obesity in the population, it is not recommended that the population in general lower their intake, but that they consume a diet corresponding to the minimum energy expenditure thought to be desirable for health and, if necessary, increase activity.

The recommended levels that appear in Table 4 for individuals with a light occupational activity correspond to this desirable level of intake. When expressed in relation to body weight, these estimates vary ±12.5% around the mean (FAO/WHO/UNO 1985). These recommended levels may be too high for those who need to lose weight in order to bring their BMI within the low-risk range. They can, however, serve as a guide, once normal weight has been attained, to indicate which level of activity should be maintained.

Requirements of groups of people having a moderate or high level of activity can be estimated using the coefficients (multiples of BMR) proposed by FAO/WHO/UNU and given in Table 4. Since the level of activity of any given individual cannot be estimated precisely with simple methods, the energy requirement of an individual can only be evaluated from observations of weight status over a long period of time.

Corrections for weight can be made to the figures given in Table 4 by using the estimate on a per kilogram basis. One has to remember, however, that the latter will tend to overestimate the requirement of the overweight, and to underestimate that of the underweight. Ideally, requirements should be expressed in terms of lean body mass, since this is the parameter of size that correlates best with resting metabolic rate, and the latter is responsible for the largest proportion of total energy expenditure in both normal and obese individuals (Ravussin *et al.*1982). Lean body mass is difficult to estimate either from anthropometric measurements such as skinfold thickness or with the use of a mathematical expression eg. Weight ($W^{0.73}$) kg. The practical value of expressing requirements in those terms is therefore questionable.

Since the figures in Table 4 take into account the lowering of the resting metabolic rate with age (2% to 3% per decade after age 25), no adjustment needs to be made for age except when aging is accompanied by a decrease in activity. McGandy *et al.*, cited by Munro (1984), have shown that a drop in activity accounts for about two-thirds of the decrease in energy expenditure with age. For the same reasons given for the population in general, older people should be encouraged to maintain a certain degree of physical activity as long as possible, rather than decreasing their energy intake.

Pregnancy and Lactation

The Recommended Nutrient Intakes for Canadians (Canada. Health and Welfare 1983) suggests a supplement of 100 kcal, or 0.42 MJ, per day during the first trimester of pregnancy and an additional 300 kcal, or 1.3 MJ, per day in the last two trimesters. These recommendations suppose that the women have a normal body weight when entering pregnancy and that their basic diet is adequate. The FAO/WHO/UNU Report (1985) recommends an addition of 285 kcal, or 1.2 MJ, per day for normal activity or of 200 kcal, or 0.8 MJ, per day for reduced activity throughout pregnancy, depending on whether or not the woman maintains or reduces her activity throughout this period. The RNIs fall between these two sets of recommendations. A variation of the same magnitude (±12.5%) as for basic energy requirements can be expected in the requirements for pregnancy when these are expressed in relation to body weight.

The RNIs for pregnant women represent a total supplementary energy intake of 65 000 kcal, or 273 KJ, during the 40 weeks of pregnancy. Theoretical requirements based on gain of various tissues are usually estimated at 80 000 kcal, or 336 KJ (Lederman 1985). Observed energy intakes of pregnant women, however, are much lower than most current recommendations. Durnin *et al.*(1985) recently reported that energy intake of pregnant women rose only by about 50 kcal, or 210 KJ, per day during the first 34 weeks of pregnancy and by 150 kcal, or 630 KJ, in the remaining weeks. The total extra energy consumed was thus less than 20 000 kcal (84 MJ) or one-quarter of theoretical estimates. This discrepancy was ascribed to a fall in BMR in the first stage of pregnancy (5th to 14th week approximately), that would be approximately equivalent to the rise in BMR that occurs after that period up to the 30th week. During the last 10 weeks, BMR was found to increase, but this would be at least partly compensated by a decrease in activity.

At the individual level, the best guideline for determining the adequacy of energy intakes during gestation is indeed a satisfactory weight gain at each stage of pregnancy. The Nutrition in Pregnancy National Guidelines, published recently (Canada. Health and Welfare 1987), recommend a weight gain of 10 to 14 kg throughout pregnancy, with a gain of 1 to 3 kg in the first trimester and a progressive gain throughout the remaining six months. Pre-pregnancy underweight and overweight are considered risk factors in pregnancy, as well as other factors that may increase energy requirements, such as multiple gestation, adolescent pregnancy, and stress (Canada. Health and Welfare 1987).

Since there appears to be no strong argument for modifying the current recommendations for pregnant women as formulated in the RNIs, the latter are maintained as recommendations in the present report.

During lactation, an increase of 450 kcal, or 1.9 MJ, per day was recommended (Canada. Health and Welfare 1983). This is based on a secretion of 750 mL of milk per day and an efficiency of 80% in the conversion to milk energy. It is also presumed that women have accumulated fat reserves during pregnancy and that these will be used, at least during the first months of lactation, to provide 200 to 300 kcal (0.8 to 1.3 MJ) per day. The FAO/WHO/UNU recommendation (1985) of an additional 500 kcal (2.1 MJ) per day is based on similar premises. This document, however, points out that milk production varies throughout lactation, reaching a maximum at about two to three months, and that maternal fat reserves cannot be expected to last more than six months. Consequently, mothers who would nurse their infant more than six months, and all those who would start lactation without energy reserves need to increase their energy intake by at least 200 kcal (0.8 MJ) over the 450 kcal (1.9 MJ) increase recommended. For the healthy woman living in the Western World who is presumably well fed and who will not nurse her child for more than six months, a supplement of 500 kcal (2.1 MJ) per day appears adequate and is recommended.

Infants and Children

The energy requirements of infants and children are usually estimated from the observed intakes of healthy children growing normally.

The average energy requirements of Canadian children varied from 120 kcal (0.5 MJ) per kilogram of body weight for newborns to 51 kcal (210 KJ) per kilogram for 16 to 18-year-old males and 40 kcal (170 KJ) per kilogram for females of similar ages (Table 6). (Canada. Health and Welfare 1983). There is no recognized desirable level of activity for children, but the sedentary lifestyles observed in industrialized countries, even in children, are considered undesirable in the FAO/WHO/UNU Report (1985), which sets their requirements 5% above observed intakes in those countries. Since the reported intakes (Seoane and Roberge 1983) and energy expenditure (Spady 1980) of school-age children and adolescents tend to be 5% to 15% lower than the RNIs, it is proposed that the RNIs be maintained as average energy intakes for children and adolescents.

Rate of growth is the best criterion for assessing the adequacy of the energy intake of children. Various charts are available for comparing the growth of a child with that of groups of healthy children, the most widely used in Canada being that of the National Center for Health Statistics in the U.S. (Hamill *et al.*1979).

Table 6.
Average Energy Requirements of Children and Adolescents[a]

Age	Sex	Average Height (cm)	Average Weight (kg)	Requirements					
				kcal/kg	MJ/kg	kcal/day	MJ/day	kcal/cm	MJ/cm
Months									
0-2	Both	55	4.5	120-100[b]	0.50-0.42	500	2.0	9	0.04
3-5	Both	63	7.0	100- 95	0.42-0.40	700	2.8	11	0.05
6-8	Both	69	8.5	95- 97	0.40-0.41	800	3.4	11.5	0.05
9-11	Both	73	9.5	97- 99	0.41	950	3.8	12.5	0.05
Years									
1	Both	82	11	101	0.42	1100	4.8	13.5	0.06
2-3	Both	95	14	94	0.39	1300	5.6	13.5	0.06
4-6	Both	107	18	100	0.42	1800	7.6	17	0.07
7-9	M	126	25	88	0.37	2200	9.2	17.5	0.07
	F	125	25	76	0.32	1900	8.0	15	0.06
10-12	M	141	34	73	0.30	2500	10.4	17.5	0.07
	F	143	36	61	0.25	2200	9.2	15.5	0.06
13-15	M	159	50	57	0.24	2800	12.0	17.5	0.07
	F	157	48	46	0.19	2200	9.2	14	0.06
16-18	M	172	62	510	.21	3200	13.2	18.50	.08
	F	160	53	40	0.17	2100	8.8	13	0.05

a. Canada. Health and Welfare 1983, p. 22.

b. First and second figures are averages at the beginning and at the end of the period.

There is still controversy over the relationship between infant feeding practices and subsequent obesity (U.S. Dept. of Health and Human Services 1984). Studies do not clearly indicate whether overweight in infancy persists into childhood and later years (Canada. Health and Welfare 1988b). There are indications that obesity which develops in later childhood and adolescence may be more likely to persist in adulthood (Canada. Health and Welfare 1988b). On the other hand, an overconcern about becoming obese might lead to undernutrition and anorexia nervosa (Anon. 1984). It is therefore particularly important that height and weight be monitored and kept within normal range at all stages of infancy and childhood by means of an adequate and well-balanced diet.

References

Anonymous. 1984. Unwarranted dieting retards growth and delays puberty. Nutr. Rev. 42:14-15.

Barr, S.I., Chrysomilides, S.A., Willis, E.J. and Beattie, B.L. 1984. Food intake of institutionalized women over 80 years of age. J. Can. Diet. Assoc. 45:42-51.

Beaton, G.H. 1983. Energy in human nutrition: perspectives and problems. Nutr. Rev. 41:325-340.

Canada. Fitness and Amateur Sport. Canada Fitness Survey. 1983. Fitness and lifestyle in Canada. Ottawa.

Canada. Health and Welfare. Health Protection Branch. Bureau of Nutritional Sciences. 1983. Recommended nutrient intakes for Canadians. Ottawa.

Canada. Health and Welfare. Federal-Provincial Subcommittee on Nutrition. 1987. Nutrition in pregnancy. National guidelines. Ottawa.

Canada. Health and Welfare. 1988a. Canadian guidelines for healthy weights. Report of an Expert Group convened by Health Promotion Directorate, Health Services and Promotion Branch. Ottawa.

Canada. Health and Welfare. Health Services and Promotion Branch. 1988b. Promoting healthy weights: a discussion paper. Ottawa.

Colt, E.W.D. and Hashim, S. 1986. Effect of exercise and diet on lipids and cardiovascular disease. *In* Current concepts in nutrition. Vol. 15. Nutrition and exercise. Winick, M., ed. Wiley, New York, pp. 117-143.

Durnin, J.V.G.A., Grant, S., McKillop, F.M. and Fitzgerald, G. 1985. Is nutritional status endangered by virtually no extra intake during pregnancy? Lancet 2:823-825.

FAO/WHO/UNU. 1985. Energy and protein requirements. Report of a Joint FAO/WHO/UNU Expert Consultation. W.H.O. Tech. Rep. Ser. 724.

Feinleib, M. 1985. Epidemiology of obesity in relation to health hazards. Ann. Intern. Med. 103:1019-1024.

Gibson, R.S., MacDonald, A.C. and Martinez, O.B. 1985. Dietary chromium and manganese intakes of a selected sample of Canadian elderly women. Hum. Nutr.: Appl. Nutr. 39A:43-52.

Hamill, P.V.V., Drizd, T.A., Johnson, C.L., Reed, R.B., Roche, A.F. and Moore, W.M. 1979. Physical growth: National Center for Health Statistics percentiles. Am. J. Clin. Nutr. 32:607-629.

Katch, F.I. and McArdle, W.D. 1988. Nutrition, weight control and exercise. 3rd ed. Lea & Febiger, Philadelphia.

Lederman, S.A. 1985. Physiological changes of pregnancy and their relation to nutrient needs. *In* Current concepts in nutrition. Vol. 14. Feeding the mother and infant. Winick, M., ed. Wiley, New York, pp. 13-43.

Martinez, O.B. 1982. Growth and dietary quality of young French Canadian school children. J. Can. Diet. Assoc. 43:28-35.

Mattila, K., Haavisto, M. and Rajala, S. 1986. Body mass index and mortality in the elderly. Br. Med. J. 292:867-868.

Munro, H.N. 1984. Nutrition and the elderly: a general overview. J. Am. Coll. Nutr. 3:341-350.

Notelovitz, M. 1986. Interrelations of exercise and diet on bone metabolism and osteoporosis. *In* Current concepts in nutrition. Vol. 15. Nutrition and exercise. Winick, M., ed. Wiley, New York, pp. 203-227.

Paffenbarger, R.S., Jr., Hyde, R.T., Wing, A.L. and Hsieh, C.-C. 1986. Physical activity, all-cause mortality and longevity of college alumni. N. Engl. J. Med. 314:605-613.

Pereira, L. and White, F. 1988. Epidemiological tabulation of the body mass index in association with selected morbidity and blood chemistry indicators, by age, sex and region. *In* Canadian guidelines for healthy weights. Health and Welfare, Ottawa, App. I and II.

Ravussin, E., Burnand, B., Schutz, Y. and Jequier, E. 1982. Twenty-four-hour energy expenditure and resting metabolic rate in obese, moderately obese, and control subjects. Am. J. Clin. Nutr. 35:566-573.

Richard, L. and Roberge, A.G. 1982. Comparison of caloric and nutrient intake of adults during week and week-end days. Nutr. Res. 2:661-668.

Roncari, D.A.K. 1988. Report on clinical-metabolic evidence for the impact of obesity on cardiovascular risk factors. *In* Canadian guidelines for healthy weights. Health and Welfare, Ottawa. App. III.

Sabry, J.H., Chorostecki, D.J. and Woolcott, D.M. 1982. Nutrient content of diets of businessmen: relation to body weight status, age, and education. J. Can. Diet. Assoc. 43:216-228.

Seidell, J.C., Bakx, K.C., Deurenberg, P., van den Hoogen, H.J., Hautvast, J.G. and Stijnen, T. 1986. Overweight and chronic illness - a retrospective cohort study, with a follow-up of 6-17 years, in men and women of initially 20-50 years of age. J. Chronic Dis. 39:585-593.

Seoane, N.A. and Roberge, A.G. 1983. Caloric and nutrient intake of adolescents in the Quebec city region. Can. J. Public Health 74:110-116.

Sidney, S., Friedman, G.D. and Siegelaub, A.B. 1987. Thinness and mortality. Am. J. Public Health 77:317-322.

Spady, D.W. 1980. Total daily energy expenditure of healthy, free ranging school children. Am. J. Clin. Nutr. 33:766-775.

Sukhatme, P.V. and Margen, S. 1982. Autoregulatory homestatic nature of energy balance. Am. J. Clin. Nutr. 35:355-365.

U.S. Dept. of Health and Human Services. 1984. Report of the Task Force on the Assessment of the Scientific Evidence Relating to Infant-Feeding Practices and Infant Health. Pediatrics 74 (Suppl.):579-762.

Yeung, D.L., Pennell, M.D., Hall, J. and Leung, M. 1982. Food and nutrient intake of infants during the first 18 months of life. Nutr. Res. 2:3-12.

Carbohydrate

Available carbohydrates in foods are those which can be digested, absorbed and metabolized. These include mono- and disaccharides such as glucose, fructose, sucrose, lactose and maltose as well as the glucose polymers: starch, dextrans and glycogen (Dahlqvist 1984). Sugar alcohols, added sweetener substitutes and certain polysaccharide bulking agents may also be present in small amounts. Unavailable carbohydrate is composed largely of nonstarch polysaccharides plus lignin (Bingham 1987) and will be discussed separately in the section on dietary fibre.

Function and Action

The main functions of dietary carbohydrate are to supply fuel in the form of glucose, particularly to the brain, spinal cord, peripheral nerves and red blood cells, and to permit the complete breakdown of fatty acids to water, carbon dioxide and energy (Cahill 1986). Approximately 180 g/day of glucose are needed for fat oxidation to go to completion, 130 g of which can be supplied from non-carbohydrate sources (Macdonald 1987). The remaining 50 g/day of carbohydrate must be obtained from the diet. If there is insufficient carbohydrate in the diet, ketone bodies will be formed and the functioning of the central nervous system, particularly the higher centres, can be impaired. Therefore, the equivalent of at least 50 g/day of glucose is required for the overall well-being of a healthy adult (Macdonald 1987). It has been suggested that from a metabolic viewpoint, there is no upper limit for dietary carbohydrate (Macdonald 1987), but this remains to be proven.

Estimates of Current Carbohydrate Intake

Food disappearance data (which overestimate actual food consumption) for the years 1963 to 1985 show that with some minor exceptions, the food calories available to Canadians remained relatively constant at approximately 3000 kcal or 12.6 MJ/person/day (Robbins 1987). During the same period, calories derived from carbohydrates decreased only slightly from 51% to 48%. However, the sources of carbohydrates in the Canadian diet appear to have changed. Recent data suggest that consumers have shifted their purchases away from staples such as flour, legumes and potatoes to more prepared baked goods, rice and pasta. Fruit and vegetable consumption by consumers has increased and demand for sugar and sugar-containing foods has changed relatively little. Approximately half of carbohydrate intake is in the form of complex carbohydrates (mainly starch) and most of this comes from vegetables and grains (Dahlqvist 1984; Glinsmann *et al.* 1986).

Carbohydrates and Disease

Sugars

An extensive report by the Sugars Task Force of the U.S. Food and Drug Administration (Glinsmann *et al.* 1986), provided estimates of current intake of sugars and reviewed the scientific literature on adverse health effects related to glucose, fructose and sucrose consumption. The committee examined several major health issues including: cardiovascular diseases, diabetes mellitus, lipidemias, glucose tolerance and dental caries, as well as obesity, malabsorption syndromes, food allergies, calciuria-induced renal disease, gallstones and carcinogenicity. Studies of carbohydrate-sensitive subgroups such as individuals with diabetes mellitus, Type IV hyperlipoproteinemia or genetic defects in metabolism of certain sugars were also included in the review.

The main conclusion of this task force was that with the exception of dental caries, no conclusive evidence existed that sugars (glucose, fructose and sucrose), when consumed at current levels, were hazardous to the health of the general public. However, they did concede there was evidence from both animal and human studies that when sugars were taken in very large doses (5-7 times normal amounts), many deleterious metabolic effects, including decreased insulin sensitivity, decreased glucose tolerance and increases in triglycerides and cholesterol, can be seen.

Since many of the studies showing ill effects of sugars on glucose tolerance or decreased sensitivity to insulin used high levels of sucrose or fructose, the committee concluded that at present levels of consumption, sugars were not an independent risk factor for development of impaired glucose tolerance (Glinsmann *et al.* 1986). As well, evidence for an independent association of dietary sugars to development of coronary artery disease was thought to be inconclusive, and there was little to support a role for sugars, as currently consumed, in obesity or behavioural changes in children.

However, the known involvement of sugars, particularly sucrose, in dental caries was recently confirmed (Lachapelle-Harvey and Sevigny 1985; Glinsmann *et al.* 1986; Scheinin and Odont 1987). It has been recommended that snacks containing sugars be avoided, as well as sticky foods which tend to adhere to enamel surfaces of teeth (Canada. Health and Welfare 1988).

Individuals with intolerances to certain sugars have been advised to avoid them. As well, persons predisposed to nephrolithiasis have also been counselled to avoid consuming high levels of sugars, since acute changes in excretion of calcium and magnesium can occur in them following ingestion of sugars (Glinsmann *et al.* 1986).

The main difficulty in trying to assess any relationship of sugars and health lies not only in the complexity of environment/disease interactions, but in trying to extrapolate short term exposure in experimental settings to development of chronic disease and in accurately determining consumer exposure. As well, many of the reports in the literature are of acute studies which do not take into account the effect of mixed meals as they are normally eaten. Resolving the role, if any, for sugars in chronic diseases other than caries may have to await new approaches.

Complex Carbohydrates

Canadians (Canada. Health and Welfare 1983) and other members of developed nations (Mann 1987) have been advised to increase their intake of complex carbohydrates at the expense of dietary fat. It is difficult to dissociate the metabolic effects of complex carbohydrates from fibre, since diets high in the one are often high in the other. Nevertheless, the focus of this discussion will be on the main complex carbohydrates in the diet, the starches.

It has generally been assumed that complex carbohydrates such as starches produce slower and more moderate increases in blood glucose and insulin compared to the simple carbohydrates such as the sugars: glucose, fructose and sucrose. However, it is becoming clear that biological responses to complex carbohydrates can vary greatly, and this variation may be due to the way the gut handles different starchy foods (Kolata 1983; Jenkins *et al.* 1988). The rate at which starchy foods are digested may vary considerably more than was previously appreciated and changes in this rate can occur through interaction with a variety of parameters (Kolata 1983; Jenkins *et al.* 1988).

Several factors must be considered when increasing the intake of starchy foods in the diet, such as the presence of "antinutrients" (Rea *et al.* 1985; Thompson *et al.* 1987), interactions with other nutrients and fibre (Reiser *et al.* 1985; Jenkins *et al.* 1986; Thorburn *et al.* 1986; Collier *et al.* 1987; Wood *et al.* 1987), the chemical form of starch and the food in which it is eaten (Jenkins *et al.* 1986; Olson *et al.* 1986), as well as the effects of storage, heating, cooking and chemical modification (Olson *et al.* 1986) on the handling of various carbohydrates by the gastrointestinal tract (Cummings *et al.* 1986; Mann 1987). The possibility that as much as 20% of starch from potatoes, bread, pasta and beans may be "resistant" to digestive enzymes and may be fermented in the colon in a fashion similar to dietary fibre has also been raised (Bjorck *et al.* 1987). In short, although increasing the amount of complex carbohydrates in the diet may be the only way to avoid the suspected detrimental effects of consuming a diet high in fat, it should be recognized that this manoeuver is not as simple a proposition as was previously thought. In order to achieve the desired beneficial effects of a high carbohydrate/low fat diet, it will be particularly important to take account of the level and type of dietary fibre in such a diet.

For certain groups such as the 5% of the Canadian population who have diabetes mellitus and the additional 4.6% of adults likely to have impaired glucose tolerance (Harlan *et al.* 1987), their dietary carbohydrate requirements should only be assessed on an individual basis. The finding that all complex carbohydrates do not produce the same rises in blood glucose and insulin may mean changes will be required in exchange diets for diabetics in which similar portions of various complex carbohydrates are considered to be interchangeable.

Recommendations

The two main reasons cited for recommending diets high in complex carbohydrates have been (i) to limit the intake of fat and (ii) to exploit the negative association of diets high in complex carbohydrates with cardiovascular disease (Mann 1987). Indeed, it has been pointed out that in four major epidemiological studies, the protective effect of high intakes of complex carbohydrates and fibre had a stronger negative association than the positive association between fat intake and coronary heart disease (Morris *et al.* 1977; Yano *et al.* 1978; Garcia-Palmieri *et al.* 1980; Kromhout *et al.* 1982).

Several experts in the field of carbohydrate nutrition have concluded that despite the "passenger" constituents and possible interactions from foods high in complex carbohydrates, the probable benefits of increasing dietary intake of complex carbohydrates outweigh the risks (Olson *et al.* 1986). Moreover, epidemiological data suggest that the increase in blood triglycerides seen when carbohydrate is substituted for fat is probably transient (Ahrens 1986). Considering previous recommendations (Canada. Health and Welfare 1983; Cahill 1986; Mann 1987), the putative benefits which may accrue, and the less tarnished reputation of complex carbohydrates compared to fats, it would seem appropriate to recommend that the amount of carbohydrate in the diet be increased at the expense of fat to between 50% and 60% of energy. It may be that increases in complex carbohydrates must be accompanied by substantial increases in dietary fibre to achieve the desired outcome (Jenkins *et al.* 1986; Coulston *et al.* 1987). Therefore, the recommended increase should come from foods high in complex carbohydrates and appropriate dietary fibres.

In future, research will be needed to more clearly define the biological responses to meals high in complex carbohydrates. The glycemic index (Jenkins *et al.* 1986) represents an attempt in this direction but remains controversial (Jenkins *et al.* 1988). It will be important to focus on chronic effects, particularly in sensitive subgroups in the population. It has been suggested that "advanced glycosylation end products" such as the non-enzymaticaly glycosylated hemoglobin (HbA_{1c}) seen in diabetes mellitus, may also play a role in the "normal" aging process (Cerami *et al.* 1987). These and other recent findings may focus renewed attention on the metabolic effects of various dietary carbohydrates.

References

Ahrens, E.H. 1986. Carbohydrates, plasma triglycerides and coronary heart disease. Nutr. Rev. 44:60-64.

Bingham, S. 1987. Definitions and intakes of dietary fiber. Am. J. Clin. Nutr. 45:1226-1231.

Bjorck, I., Nyman, M., Pedersen, B., Siljestrom, M., Asp, N-G. and Eggum, B.O. 1987. Formation of enzyme resistant starch during autoclaving of wheat starch: studies in vitro and in vivo. J. Cereal Sci. 6:159-172.

Cahill, G.F. 1986. The future of carbohydrates in human nutrition. Nutr. Rev. 44:40-43.

Canada. Health and Welfare. Health Protection Branch. Bureau of Nutritional Sciences. 1983. Carbohydrates and fibre. *In* Recommended nutrient intakes for Canadians. Ottawa, pp 28-30.

Canada. Health and Welfare. Health Services Directorate. 1988. Preventive dental services. 2nd ed. Ottawa.

Cerami, A., Vlassara, H. and Brownlee, M. 1987. Glucose and aging. Sci. Am. 256:90-96.

Collier, G.R., Wolever, T.M.S. and Jenkins, D.J.A. 1987. Concurrent ingestion of fat and reduction in starch content impairs carbohydrate tolerance to subsequent meals. Am. J. Clin. Nutr. 45:963-969.

Coulston, A.M., Hollenbeck, C.B., Swislocki, A.L.M., Ida Chen, Y-D. and Reaven, G.M. 1987. Deleterious metabolic effects of high-carbohydrate, sucrose-containing diets in patients with non-insulin-dependent diabetes mellitus. Am. J. Med. 82:213-220.

Cummings, J.H., Englyst, H.N. and Wiggins, H.S. 1986. The role of carbohydrates in lower gut function. Nutr. Rev. 44:50-54.

Dahlqvist, A. 1984. Carbohydrates. *In* Nutrition Reviews' Present knowledge in nutrition. 5th ed. Nutrition Foundation, Washington, pp. 116-130.

Garcia-Palmieri, M.R., Sorlie, P., Tillotson, J., Costas, R., Cordero, E. and Rodriguez, M. 1980. Relationship of dietary intake to subsequent coronary heart disease incidence: the Puerto Rico Heart Program. Am. J. Clin. Nutr. 33:1818-1827.

Glinsmann, W.H., Irausquin, H. and Park, Y.K. 1986. Evaluation of health aspects of sugars contained in carbohydrate sweeteners. Report of the Sugars Task Force. J. Nutr. 116(Suppl 11):S1-S216.

Harlan, L.C., Harlan, W.R., Landis, J.R. and Goldstein, N.G. 1987. Factors associated with glucose tolerance in adults in the United States. Am. J. Epidemiol. 126:674-684.

Jenkins, D.J.A., Jenkins, A.L., Wolever, T.M.S., Thompson, L.H. and Rao, A.V. 1986. Simple and complex carbohydrates. Nutr. Rev. 44:44-49.

Jenkins, D.J.A., Wolever, T.M.S. and Jenkins, A.L. 1988. Starchy foods and glycemic index. Diabetes Care 11:149-159.

Kolata, G. 1983. Dietary dogma disproved. Science 220:487-488.

Kromhout, D., Bosschieter, E.B. and De Lezenne Coulander, C. 1982. Dietary fibre and 10-year mortality from coronary heart disease, cancer and all causes. Lancet 2:518-522.

Lachapelle-Harvey, D. and Sevigny, J. 1985. Multiple regression analysis of dental status and related food behaviour of French Canadian adolescents. Community Dent. Oral Epidemiol. 13:226-229.

Macdonald, I. 1987. Metabolic requirements for dietary carbohydrates. Am. J. Clin. Nutr. 45:1193-1196.

Mann, J, 1987. Complex carbohydrates: replacement energy for fat or useful in their own right? Am. J. Clin. Nutr. 45:1202-1206.

Morris, J.N., Marr, J.W. and Clayton, D.G. 1977. Diet and heart: a postscript. Br. Med. J. 2:1307-1314.

Olson, R., James, P., Hockaday, D. and Werner, I. 1986. Summary [of the eleventh Marabou Symposium on The Nutritional Re-emergence of Starchy Foods]. Nutr. Rev. 44:89-91.

Rea, R.L., Thompson, L.U. and Jenkins, D.J.A. 1985. Lectins in foods and their relation to starch digestibility. Nutr. Res. 5:919-929.

Reiser, S., Smith, J.C., Mertz, W., Holbrook, J.T., Scholfield, D.J., Powell, A.S., Canfield, W.K. and Canary, J.J. 1985. Indices of copper status in humans consuming a typical American diet containing either fructose or starch. Am. J. Clin. Nutr. 42:242-251.

Robbins, L. 1987. The nutritive value of the Canadian food supply. Food Mark. Comment. 9:25-31.

Scheinin, A. and Odont, D. 1987. Dietary carbohydrates and dental disorders. Am. J. Clin. Nutr. 45:1218-1225.

Thompson, L.U., Button, C.L. and Jenkins, D.J.A. 1987. Phytic acid and calcium affect the in vitro rate of navy bean starch digestion and blood glucose response in humans. Am. J. Clin. Nutr. 46:467-473.

Thorburn, A.W., Brand, J.C. and Truswell, A.S. 1986. Salt and the glycemic response. Br. Med. J. 292:1697-1699.

Wood, R.J., Gerhardt, A. and Rosenberg, I.H. 1987. Effects of glucose and glucose polymers on calcium absorption in healthy subjects. Am. J. Clin. Nutr. 46:699-701.

Yano, K., Rhoads, G.G., Kagan, A. and Tillotson, J. 1978. Dietary intake and the risk of coronary heart disease in Japanese men living in Hawaii. Am. J. Clin. Nutr. 31:1270-1279.

Fibre

Dietary fibre is comprised of the endogenous components of plant material in the diet which are resistant to digestive secretions produced by humans. These components are predominantly nonstarch polysaccharides and lignin and may include, in addition, associated substances (Canada. Health and Welfare 1985). Some characteristics of carbohydrate-fibre fractions are shown in Table 7. Conventional dietary fibre is found mainly in whole grain cereals, legumes, vegetables, fruits and nuts. Most researchers believe that materials such as Maillard compounds, resistant starch, and man-made ingredients should not be considered components of dietary fibre because it is impractical to stretch the concept to include all such substances (Dreher 1987).

In the small intestine, food components are gradually digested and absorbed, but dietary fibre is concentrated during its progression towards the large intestine where bacterial fermentation occurs.

Methods for measuring dietary fibre are intended to simulate the enzymic and chemical treatments of food in the mouth, stomach and small intestine. Discrepancies in the published values for some processed foods can be partly explained by the characteristics of the enzymes used and, to some extent, by the principle of the method used (Paul and Southgate 1978; Baker and Holden 1981; Englyst *et al.* 1982; Mongeau and Brassard 1982).

Table 7.
Polysaccharidic Constituents of Fibre Fractions

	Constituents		
Name	Primary Chain	Secondary Chain	Characteristics
Cellulose	glucose		Unbranched A minor component of cereal fibres, a major component of vegetable and legume fibres Water soluble Fermentability: low in cereals moderate in legumes
Beta-Glucans	glucose		Unbranched A minor component of dietary fibre, highest concentration in barley and oat Water-soluble Fermentability: high
Hemicelluoses	xylose mannose galactose	arabinose galactose glucuronic acid	Main constituent of cereal fibre Partly water-insoluble Fermentability: Moderate-high, very low in raw corn bran
Pectin	galacturonic acid	rhamnose arabinose xylose fucose	Main source: citrus fruits Generally water-soluble Fermentability: high
Gums and Mucilages	galactose-mannose glucose-mannose arabinose-xylose galacturonic acid-mannose glucuronic acid-mannose galactose	galactose xylose fucose	Non-structural Water-soluble Fermentability: high eg. guar gum
Seaweed Extracts	mannose xylose glucuronic acid glucose	galactose	Non structural Water-soluble Fermentability: high eg. agar

Table 8 shows the fibre content of selected foods as measured by three representative methods.

Table 8
Dietary Fibre Content of Selected Foods
(% of fresh weight)

	Fibre Method[a]			
	HPB	AOAC	Englyst	Moisture
White bread	1.84	2.11	1.78	40.4
Whole wheat bread	5.43	5.18	3.89	40.8
White wheat flour	3.37	2.59	2.23	13.1
Oatmeal	9.82	9.25	7.29	11.1
Shredded wheat cereal	10.54	9.78	8.4	85.5
Rice	0.85	1.96	0.5	29.5
Corn kernels	2.08	2.06	1.57	73.4
Baked potatoes	2.07	2.56	1.54	72.3
Cabbage	1.57	1.77	1.60	92.4
Celery	1.46	1.67	1.52	94.3
Broccoli	2.21	2.57	2.25	91.8
Carrots	2.71	2.95	2.72	88.4
Onions	1.45	1.42	1.40	91.6
Rutabaga	2.22	2.50	2.29	89.2
Green beans	1.97	2.12	1.93	93.7
White baked beans	5.43	4.89	3.87	70.8
Peanuts	7.50	7.28	5.71	1.3
Orange	1.82	1.71	1.75	86.7
Grapefruit	1.79	1.58	1.30	87.9
Apple	1.77	1.83	1.67	87.5
Pears	2.06	2.17	1.66	82.1
Plums	1.54	1.44	1.09	84.8
Melon - cantaloupe	0.86	0.87	0.77	88.2
Blueberries	2.47	2.48	1.43	86.0

a. HPB method = soluble and insoluble dietary fibre, Mongeau et Brassard, In Press; AOAC = Total dietary fibre method according to the Association of Official Analytical Chemists, Prosky *et al.*, 1985; Englyst = non-starch polysaccharides, Englyst, 1985.

While there are small differences between methods, all the values in Table 8 are higher than the crude fibre values that would have been reported a few years ago and which included little but the cellulose fraction. There has been some debate whether "resistant starch", which is rapidly fermented in the colon, should be considered as dietary fibre. For the purposes of this review it is not.

Physiological Effects

Different kinds of dietary fibre vary in their physiological effects. Only a general account is possible in this presentation.

Small Intestine

The effect of dietary fibre is to slow and regulate digestion rather than induce a net decrease of intake and absorption. An example of the regulating effects of gel-forming fibres is the reduced rate of glucose absorption and the better control of blood glucose and insulin levels. Dietary fibre reduces "apparent protein digestibility" but the decrease is likely nutritionally insignificant (Staub *et al.* 1983; Dreher 1987). Also delayed, or marginally reduced, is the absorption of fat, carbohydrates, and certain minerals and vitamins (Dreher 1987).

Colligative properties of soluble fibre and surface properties of insoluble fibre influence viscosity, water-binding capacity, cation exchange and organic adsorption in the small intestinal lumen (Eastwood and Hamilton 1968; Kritchevsky and Story 1974; Eastwood and Mowbray 1976; Vahouny 1982; Dreher 1987).

Large Intestine

Dietary fibre is the major component of the material reaching the large intestine (Bijlani 1985) where the most significant of its action occurs. Generally, from 40-95% is fermented by the intestinal flora and serves as an often overlooked source of energy. Fermentation products account for part of its physiological effects. Coarse wheat bran provides a good example of the effect of dietary fibre on colonic function. The fermentable content provides substrates for bacterial growth, and bacterial cells form part of the fecal mass and provide moisture. The volatile fatty acids produced by the bacteria acidify the colonic content, act on the mucosa and, following absorption, modify the lipid metabolism. The fermentation of fibre may leave resistant structures; those from wheat bran represent about 50% of the ingested fibre. The large wheat bran particles take a curly shape on fermentation, constituting microenvironments in the distal colon, and providing a physical resistance against the removal of interstitial water and dispersed gases, thus counterbalancing the absorptive capacity of the colon. The resulting decrease in fecal density prevents impaction and constipation. The threshold volume is rapidly attained in the rectum and triggers the mechanisms of defecation, thus limiting the opportunity for reabsorption and hardening of the intestinal contents. Reducing the particle size eliminates this effect since small particles retain non-solid components less effectively. Coarse bran (from soft or hard wheat) reduces colon segmenting activity and intraluminal pressure, normalizes slow transit time (40-150 h) to about 20 h, and increases fecal weight (four times more than fine bran and seven times more than oat bran) (Smith 1979; Schneeman and Gallaher 1980; Smith *et al.* 1981; Dreher 1987). Fecal volume is responsible for triggering bowel movement, but this important parameter is not often measured because of technical problems (Phillips and Devroede 1979; Canada. Health and Welfare 1985).

Potential Adverse Effects

There are few reports of adverse effects on the gastrointestinal tract directly related to fibre. Particulate fibres are mostly cereal fibres. The mean particle size of fibre measured in ready-to-eat breakfast cereals varies from 350 µm to above 1 mm. The number of particles less than 150 µm is negligible. More finely ground fibre (even from wheat bran) may cause difficult or uncomfortable defecation. In addition, the gastrointestinal wall is not always a good barrier for particles smaller than 150 µm which, in minute amounts, may pass through the intestinal wall into the blood stream. The fibre particles are not degraded by blood enzymes and could impose a greater load of work on the kidneys and the macrophage-phagocytic system. The long term effect of ingestion of ultrafine, enzyme-resistant material is not known (Canada. Health and Welfare 1985).

Increasing the intake of dietary fibre may increase the risk of reducing the absorption of certain essential minerals, notably zinc, calcium and iron. These minerals bind to the dietary fibre itself or, more importantly, to the phytate commonly associated with it. Evidence of binding is unequivocal but it is doubtful whether such effects are of nutritional importance in the context of an adequate diet (i.e. a diet containing the current average levels of protein, vitamin C and minerals) (Sandstead *et al.* 1979; Staub *et al.* 1983; Southgate 1987). The quality of the diet is particularly important for certain population groups such as infants, post-menopausal women and the elderly. Higher calcium levels may be required for the latter group.

Disease Prevention

Much of the present interest in dietary fibre can be traced to the hypothesis of Trowell and Burkitt (1975): they stated that in their view, a low consumption of fibre was associated with an increased incidence of many diseases, including colon cancer, diverticular disease, appendicitis, constipation, hemorrhoids, hiatus hernia, varicose veins, diabetes, gallstones and obesity. Much research has since examined the sweeping claims of Trowell and Burkitt.

The beneficial effect of fibre on constipation was known long before Trowell and Burkitt formulated their hypothesis. Coarse wheat bran is particularly effective in correcting the low fecal output (<90 g/day) associated with constipation (Cummings *et al.* 1976; Spiller 1986; Guerre and Chaussade 1987). The addition of a source of wheat bran can prevent constipation in up to 60% of elderly patients (Hull *et al.* 1980) and in children (Becker and Rosskamp 1987). Wheat bran, added to the diet (4.2 g/day) prevented constipation and was well accepted by children aged six to 62 months. Blood levels of hemoglobin, calcium, phosphate, alkaline phosphatase, iron, transferrin, total protein, cholesterol and carotene were monitored at monthly intervals. The only changes noted in the wheat bran group were a slight decrease in carotene concentration and a small increase in alkaline phosphatase activity.

Thus there is general agreement that dietary fibre, especially from cereal and legumes, plays a useful role in the prevention of constipation. A low intake has been cited as the major cause of constipation (Cummings 1982).

Diverticular disease refers to several abnormalities of the colon characterized by the mucosa protruding through all muscle layers. It is difficult to determine the prevalence of this disorder because it is often asymptomatic.

Epidemiological studies, beginning with Trowell and Burkitt (1975), have demonstrated a relationship between the prevalence of diverticular disease and the fibre content of the diet (Ohi *et al.* 1983; Painter 1985). It has, however, been difficult to obtain supporting evidence by other means. Much of the related evidence deals with the treatment of diverticular disease and cannot automatically be equated with prevention (Painter *et al.* 1972; Findlay *et al.* 1974; Brodribb and Humphreys 1976; Brodribb 1979; Heaton 1981; Ornstein *et al.* 1981). Support for the epidemiological evidence has been provided by a lifespan experiment with rats (Fisher *et al.* 1985).

Most international epidemiological studies show an inverse relationship between colon cancer mortality and the fibre content of the diet (Jacobs 1986). Regional studies in Scandinavia (Jensen *et al.* 1982) and the United Kingdom (Bingham *et al.* 1985) reached a similar conclusion but studies in South Africa did not (Walker *et al.* 1986). These epidemiological studies suffer from an inability to disentangle the effect of the fibre content in the diet from the effect of fat and energy intake, which are also said to influence the development of colorectal cancer (Kolonel 1987). McKeown-Eyssen and Bright-See (1983) demonstrated a negative association between the availability of cereal fibre in different countries and the occurrence of colon cancer. This negative association persisted after adjustments were made for total meat, red meat, total fat or animal fat content of the diets. The details of this latter study have apparently not been published.

Case control studies have provided inconsistent results and, if anything, have shed doubt on the beneficial effects of fibre (Potter and McMichael 1986).

Animal experiments too have provided mixed results; some members of the fibre family (e.g. wheat bran) inhibit the induction of large bowel tumors in rodents, while others enhance the process (Jacobs 1986).

As is the case for a number of chronic diseases, epidemiological studies show an inverse relationship between fibre intake and heart disease (Liu *et al.* 1982; Anderson 1985). Some prospective studies have shown a greater consumption of foods containing dietary fibre to be associated with a lower risk of coronary heart disease (Morris *et al.* 1978; Kushi *et al.* 1985).

While these studies are not decisive because the diets in question differed in ways other than fibre content, there is evidence that fibre (e.g. from oat bran and legumes) can influence blood lipids in a beneficial way. Pectin and guar gum (12-30 grams daily) have been shown to lower serum cholesterol by 6-15% in normal volunteers (Keys *et al.* 1961; Kay and Truswell 1977). These gel-forming fibres have been shown to cause a decrease in low density lipoprotein cholesterol levels without raising serum triglyceride levels and thus may have an application in the treatment of hyperlipidemia (Jenkins *et al.* 1979). However, the effective intake is believed to be in the range of the estimated intake of total fibre by Canadians (Canada. Health and Welfare 1977) and much dietary fibre (e.g. wheat bran) gives inconsistent results (Miettinen 1987). In rats, the effectiveness of pectin has been shown to depend on the composition of the diet.

While a case can be made for substituting diets higher in complex carbohydrates and the accompanying dietary fibre for fat-rich, high energy diets, the evidence linking fibre directly to weight control is unconvincing (Van Itallie 1978; Heaton 1980; Ali *et al.* 1982; Kritchevsky 1982; Debry *et al.* 1983).

The evidence relating fibre intake (particularly from legumes) to the glycemic response has been summarized in the Report of the Expert Advisory Committee on Dietary Fibre (Canada. Health and Welfare 1985) and has led to significant changes in the dietary management of diabetes. Because this evidence deals with treatment rather than prevention, it will not be discussed further in this report.

Recommendations

The evidence confirms the widely held belief that dietary fibre plays an important role in regulating gastrointestinal function, and specifically aids in the prevention of constipation. This evidence is sufficient to support a qualitative, though not a quantitative recommendation to include fibre from cereal and legume sources in the diet.

A number of other diet/health relationships underline the merit of diets containing fibre, but are less successful in delineating the relative importance of fibre and other components of such diets. What evidence there is demonstrates that the various kinds of fibre perform different functions. This should come as no surprise considering their dissimilar natures, and provides a sound rationale for recommending that a variety of fibre-containing foods be included in the diet. The same evidence illustrates the folly of adding large amounts of a single source of purified fibre to the diet.

In formulating dietary advice it is impossible to deal independently with complex carbohydrates and fibre; one will accompany the other. The recommendation for carbohydrate is to increase intake to 55-60% of energy with the increase in the form of complex carbohydrates. The resulting dietary pattern will perforce increase present intakes of dietary fibre and should feature a variety of carbohydrate and fibre sources. Any dietary changes resulting in a substantial increase of dietary fibre intake should be gradual.

References

Ali, R., Staub, H., Leveille, G.A. and Boyle, P.C. 1982. Dietary fiber and obesity: a review. *In* Dietary fibre in health and disease. Vahouny, G.V. and Kritchevsky, D., eds. Plenum Press, New York, pp. 139-149.

Anderson, J.W. 1985. Health implications of wheat fiber. Am. J. Clin. Nutr. 41:1103-1112.

Baker, D. and Holden, J.M. 1981. Fiber in breakfast cereals. J. Food Sci. 46:396-398.

Becker, M. and Rosskamp, R. 1987. Therapie der Obstipation mit Weizenkleie im Sauglings - und Kleinkindesalter. [Therapy of constipation with wheat bran in infancy and early childhood]. Monatsschr. Kinderheilkd. 135:522-524.

Bijlani, R.L. 1985. Dietary fibre: consensus and controversy. Prog. Food Nutr. Sci. 9:343-393.

Bingham, S.A., Williams, D.R.R. and Cummings, J.H. 1985. Dietary fibre consumption in Britain: new estimates and their relation to large bowel cancer mortality. Br. J. Cancer 52:399-402.

Brodribb, A.J.M. 1979. The treatment of symptomatic diverticular disease with dietary fiber. *In* Dietary fiber: current developments of importance to health. Heaton, K.W., ed. Technomic Publishing, Westport, Ct, pp. 63-73.

Brodribb, A.J.M. and Humphreys, D.M. 1976. Diverticular disease: three studies. Part II. Treatment with bran. Br. Med. J. 1:425-428.

Canada. Health and Welfare. Nutrition Canada. Health Protection Branch. Bureau of Nutritional Sciences. 1977. Food consumption patterns report. Ottawa.

Canada. Health and Welfare. Health Protection Branch. 1985. Report of the Expert Advisory Committee on Dietary Fibre. Ottawa.

Cummings, J.H. 1982. Consequences of the metabolism of fiber in the human large intestine. *In* Dietary fiber in health and disease. Vahouny, G.V. and Kritchevsky, D., eds. Plenum Press, New York, pp. 9-22.

Cummings, J.H., Hill, M.J., Jenkins, D.J.A., Pearson, J.R. and Wiggins, H.S. 1976. Changes in fecal composition and colonic function due to cereal fiber. Am. J. Clin. Nutr. 29:1468-1473.

Debry, G., Garrel, D. and Karsenty, C. 1983. Fibres, overnutrition and obesity. *In* Biochemical pharmacology of obesity. Curtis-Prior, P.B., ed. Elsevier, New York, pp. 381-405.

Dreher, M.L. 1987. Handbook of dietary fiber. An applied approach. Dekker, New York.

Eastwood, M.A. and Hamilton, D. 1968. Studies on the adsorption of bile salts to non-absorbed components of diet. Biochim. Biophys. Acta 152:165-173.

Eastwood, M.A. and Mowbray, L. 1976. The binding of the components of mixed micelle to dietary fiber. Am. J. Clin. Nutr. 29:1461-1467.

Englyst, H. 1985. Englyst procedure for determination of dietary fibre as non-starch polysaccharides: measurement of constituent sugars by gas-liquid chromatography. (Bulletin No. 87). MAFF information bulletin for public analysts on EEC methods of analysis and sampling for foodstuffs. Ministry of Agriculture, Fisheries and Food, London.

Englyst, H., Wiggins, H.S. and Cummings, J.H. 1982. Determination of non-starch polysaccharides in plant foods by gas-liquid chromatography of constituent sugars as alditol acetates. Analyst 107:307-318.

Findlay, J.M., Smith, A.N., Mitchell, W.D., Anderson, A.J.B. and Eastwood, M.A. 1974. Effects of unprocessed bran on colon function in normal subjects and in diverticular disease. Lancet 1:146-149.

Fisher, N., Berry, C.S., Fearn, T., Gregory, J.A. and Hardy, J. 1985. Cereal dietary fiber consumption and diverticular disease: a lifespan study in rats. Am. J. Clin. Nutr. 42:788-804.

Guerre, J. and Chaussade, J. 1987. Constipation - nouvel abord. Ann. Gastroenterol. Hepatol. 23:201-205.

Heaton, K.W. 1980. Food intake regulation and fiber. *In* Medical aspects of dietary fiber. Spiller, G.A. and Kay, R.M., eds. Plenum Press, New York, pp. 223-238.

Heaton, K.W. 1981. Is bran useful in diverticular disease? Br Med. J. 283:1523-1524.

Hull, C., Greco, R.S. and Brooks, D.L. 1980. Alleviation of constipation in the elderly by dietary fiber supplementation. J. Am. Geriatr. Soc. 28:410-414.

Jacobs, L.R. 1986. Relationship between dietary fiber and cancer: metabolic, physiologic and cellular mechanisms. Proc. Soc. Exp. Biol. Med. 183:299-310.

Jenkins, D.J.A., Leeds, A.R., Slavin, B., Mann, J. and Jepson, E.M. 1979. Dietary fiber and blood lipids: reduction of serum cholesterol in type II hyperlipidemia by guar gum. Am. J. Clin. Nutr. 32:16-18.

Jensen, O.M., MacLennan, R. and Wahrendorf, J. 1982. Diet, bowel function, fecal characteristics, and large bowel cancer in Denmark and Finland. Nutr. Cancer 4:5-19.

Kay, R.M. and Truswell, A.S. 1977. Effect of citrus pectin on blood lipids and fecal steroid excretion in man. Am. J. Clin. Nutr. 30:171-175.

Keys, A., Grande, F. and Anderson, J.T. 1961. Fiber and pectin in the diet and serum cholesterol concentration in man. Proc. Soc. Exp. Biol. Med. 106:555-558.

Kolonel, L.N. 1987. Fat and colon cancer: how firm is the epidemiologic evidence? Am. J. Clin. Nutr. 45:336-341.

Kritchevsky, D. 1982. Fiber, obesity and diabetes. *In* Dietary fiber in health and disease. Vahouny, G.V. and Kritchevsky, D., eds. Plenum Press, New York, pp. 133-137.

Kritchevsky, D. and Story, J.A. 1974. Binding of bile salts in vitro by nonnutritive fiber. J. Nutr. 104:458-462.

Kushi, L.H., Lew, R.A., Stare, F.J., Ellison, C.R., el Lozy, M., Bourke, G., Daly, L., Graham, I., Hickey, N., Mulcahy, R. and Kevaney, J. 1985. Diet and 20-year mortality from coronary heart disease. N. Engl. J. Med. 312:811-818.

Liu, K., Stamler, J., Trevisan, M. and Moss, D. 1982. Dietary lipids, sugar, fiber and mortality from coronary heart disease. Arteriosclerosis 2:221-227.

McKeown-Eyssen, G. and Bright-See, E. 1983. Colon cancer mortality and fibre consumption: an international study. Fibre in human and animal nutrition (abst.). Bull.-R. Soc. N.Z. 20:35.

Miettinen, T.A. 1987. Dietary fiber and lipids. Am. J. Clin. Nutr. 45:1237-1242.

Mongeau, R. and Brassard, R. 1982. Determination of neutral detergent fiber in breakfast cereals: pentose, hemicellulose, cellulose and lignin content. J. Food Sci. 47:550-555.

Mongeau, R. and Brassard, R. In Press. A comparison of three methods for analyzing dietary fiber in 38 foods. J. Food Compos. Anal.

Morris, J.N., Marr, J.W. and Clayton, D.G. 1978. Dietary fibre from cereals and the incidence of coronary heart disease. J. Plant Food 3:45-56.

Ohi, G., Minowa, K., Oyama, T., Nagahashi, M., Yamazaki, N., Yamamoto, S., Nagasako, K., Hayakawa, K., Kimura, K. and Mori, B. 1983. Changes in dietary fiber intake among Japanese in the 20th century: a relationship to the prevalence of diverticular disease. Am. J. Clin. Nutr. 38:115-121.

Ornstein, M.H., Littlewood, E.R., McLear Baird, I., Fowler, J., North, W.R.S. and Cox, A.G. 1981. Are fibre supplements really necessary in diverticular disease of the colon? A controlled clinical trial. Br. Med. J. 282:1353-1356.

Painter, N. 1985. Diverticular disease of the colon. *In* Dietary Fibre, fibre-depleted foods and disease. Trowell, H., Burkitt, D. and Heaton, K., eds. Academic Press, New York, pp. 145-160.

Painter, N.S., Almeida, A.Z. and Colebourne, K.W. 1972. Unprocessed bran in treatment of diverticular disease of the colon. Br. Med. J. 2:137-140.

Paul, A.A. and Southgate, D.A.T. 1978. McCance and Widdowson's the composition of foods. Elsevier/North-Holland Biomedical, New York.

Phillips, S.F. and Devroede, G.J. 1979. Functions of the large intestine. Int. Rev. Physiol. 19:263-290.

Potter, J.D. and McMichael, A.J. 1986. Diet and cancer of the colon and rectum: a case-control study. J. Nat. Cancer Inst. 76:557-569.

Prosky, L., Asp, N.-G., Furda, I., DeVries, J.W., Schweizer, T.F. and Harland, B.F. 1985. Determination of total dietary fiber in foods and food products: collaborative study. J. Assoc. Off. Anal. Chem. 68:677-679.

Sandstead, H.H., Klevay, L.M., Jacob, R.A., Munoz, J.M., Logan, G.M., Reck, S.J., Dintzis, F.R., Inglett, G.E. and Shuey, W.C. 1979. Effects of dietary fiber and protein level on mineral element metabolism. *In* Dietary fibers: chemistry and nutrition. Inglett, G.E. and Falkehag, S.I., eds. Academic Press, New York, pp. 147-156.

Schneeman, B.O. and Gallaher, D. 1980. Changes in small intestinal digestive enzyme activity and bile acids with dietary cellulose in rats. J. Nutr. 110:584-590.

Smith, A.N. 1979. Effect of bulk additives on constipation and in diverticular disease. *In* Dietary fibre: current developments of importance to health. Heaton, K.W., ed. Technomic Publishing, Westport, Ct., pp. 97-104.

Smith, A.N., Drummond, E. and Eastwood, M.A. 1981. The effect of coarse and fine Canadian Red Spring Wheat and French Soft Wheat bran on colonic motility in patients with diverticular disease. Am. J. Clin. Nutr. 34:2460-2463.

Southgate, D.A.T. 1987. Minerals, trace elements and potential hazards. Am. J. Clin. Nutr. 45:1256-1266.

Spiller, G.A. 1986. CRC handbook of dietary fiber in human nutrition. CRC Press, Boca Raton, Fla.

Staub, H.W., Mardones, B. and Shah, N. 1983. Modern dietary fibre product development and nutrient bioavailability. *In* Dietary fibre. Birch, G.G. and Parker, K.J., eds. Applied Science, London, pp. 37-60.

Trowell, H. and Burkitt, D. 1975. Concluding considerations. *In* Refined carbohydrate foods and disease: some implications of dietary fibre. Burkitt, D.P. and Trowell, H.C., eds. Academic Press, London, pp. 333-345.

Vahouny, G.V. 1982. Dietary fibers and intestinal absorption of lipids. *In* Dietary fiber in health and disease. Vahouny, G.V. and Kritchevsky, D., eds. Plenum Press, New York, pp. 203-227.

Van Itallie, T.B. 1978. Dietary fiber and obesity. Am. J. Clin. Nutr. 31:S43-S52.

Walker, A.R.P., Walker, B.F. and Walker, A.J. 1986. Faecal pH, dietary fibre intake, and proneness to colon cancer in four South African populations. Br. J. Cancer 53:489-495.

Lipids

Function and Composition

Dietary lipids have a number of nutritional functions. They serve as a concentrated source of energy and as a source of essential fatty acids. They act as carriers of fat-soluble vitamins and affect the palatability of foods (Gurr and James 1980).

Dietary lipids are composed of mixtures of triacylglycerols (triglycerides), phospholipids, cholesterol and other sterols and fat-soluble vitamins. Since over 95% of the lipid in most diets is in the form of triacylglycerols, the characteristics of dietary lipids are determined largely by the nature and position of the fatty acids esterified to the glycerol. These consist mainly of straight-chain, even-numbered fatty acids which may be saturated, monounsaturated or polyunsaturated.

Monounsaturated fatty acids contain one double bond and polyunsaturated fatty acids contain two or more double bonds. The double bonds in naturally-occurring fatty acids have a *cis* configuration but can be isomerized to the *trans* form by ruminant animals or during partial hydrogenation in the industrial processing of oils and fats. The physical properties of *trans* fatty acids resemble those of saturated fatty acids. Fats are solid at room temperature and have a higher proportion of saturated and/or *trans* fatty acids whereas oils are liquid at room temperature and have higher proportions of mono- and polyunsaturated *cis* fatty acids.

The main saturated fatty acid in most fats and oils is palmitic acid which has a 16-carbon chain with no double bonds (16:0). Myristic acid (14:0) and stearic acid (18:0) are often present in substantial amounts and some fats such as butter and coconut oil may contain significant amounts of short-chain saturated acids. Oleic acid (18:1 n-9) is by far the most common monounsaturated fatty acid and is the major component of olive oil and canola oil. The n-9 designation means that the double bond is located 9 carbons from the methyl end of the chain.

The major polyunsaturated fatty acid in vegetable oils is linoleic acid (18:2 n-6). It can be converted in the body to other n-6 fatty acids, including arachidonic acid (20:4 n-6), by alternate chain elongation and desaturation reactions (Brenner 1987). Some vegetable oils, such as canola oil and soybean oil, also contain appreciable amounts of linolenic acid (18:3 n-3). This can be converted by a similar series of reactions to longer, more unsaturated fatty acids of the n-3 family, including eicosapentaenoic acid (20:5 n-3) and docosahexaenoic acid (22:6 n-3). Fish oils contain appreciable amounts of these n-3 fatty acids but relatively little of the n-6 fatty acids. It appears that long-chain, polyunsaturated n-3 fatty acids are digested, absorbed and transported in much the same way as other long-chain fatty acids (Nelson and Ackman 1988).

Essential Fatty Acids

The n-6 and n-3 families of polyunsaturated fatty acids (also known as omega-6 and omega-3 fatty acids) are not interconvertible. These fatty acids can be synthesized *de novo* by plants but not by animals, which are unable to insert double bonds at the n-6 and n-3 positions. Members of these families are important components of cell membranes and serve as precursors of a variety of biologically-active compounds, known as eicosanoids, which include prostaglandins, thromboxanes and leukotrienes (Oliw et al. 1983; Willis 1987). Since lack of these fatty acids leads to deficiency symptoms and they can be obtained only from the diet, they are essential dietary nutrients (Holman 1968, 1987; Budowski 1988).

Dietary linoleic acid is required by human infants for normal growth and development (Hansen *et al.* 1963). When linoleic acid is not available for conversion to arachidonic acid, the chain-elongating and desaturating enzymes convert oleic acid to eicosatrienoic acid (20:3 n-9). Thus a deficiency of n-6 fatty acids is characterized by an elevated ratio of eicosatrienoic acid to arachidonic acid in tissue lipids (Holman *et al.* 1964; Paulsrud *et al.* 1972). Data gathered from experimental animals and humans indicate that provision of linoleic acid at a level of 1% of food energy is sufficient to prevent deficiency symptoms (Holman 1977). However, since other dietary fatty acids compete for the chain-elongating and desaturating enzymes, a level of 3% of energy as essential fatty acids was proposed as a recommended intake for humans (FAO 1977). Although this recommendation did not distinguish between n-6 and n-3 fatty acids, the report did discuss them separately.

The initial difficulties in finding a role for the n-3 fatty acids stemmed from the lack of an effect on growth and reproduction of experimental animals receiving only trace amounts of n-3 fatty acids, present as a contaminant of casein (Tinoco *et al.* 1979). Capuchin monkeys, however, developed skin lesions when their dietary fat lacked n-3 fatty acids and recovered when an n-3 acid was supplied (Fiennes *et al.* 1973). Subsequently, skin lesions were cured in humans by n-3 fatty acid

(Bjerve *et al.* 1987). Docosahexaenoic acid (22:6 n-3), the last member of the n-3 series, is concentrated in the photoreceptor membranes of the retina and is present in substantial amounts in the brain lipids of various species (Anderson *et al.* 1974; Crawford *et al.* 1976). A deficiency of this n-3 fatty acid leads to loss of visual acuity in monkeys (Neuringer *et al.* 1984, 1988; Connor *et al.* 1984).

In humans, 22:6 n-3 accumulates in the brain during the rapid growth spurt which occurs between the third trimester of pregnancy and eighteen months post partum (Clandinin *et al.* 1980a,b). Red blood cells from human infants fed formula low in linolenic acid (n-3) had lower levels of docosahexaenoic acid than those from breast-fed infants (Putnam *et al.* 1982). The latter received about 0.3% of total fatty acids as C_{20} and C_{22} n-3 fatty acids as well as 0.6% as 18:3, n-3 acids (Carlson *et al.* 1986).

Without adequate information on infant requirements for polyunsaturated fatty acids, the best guide is the composition of human milk (Crawford 1987; Friedman 1987). Data from several countries indicate that the extra long-chain n-3 and n-6 fatty acids are present in milk in low concentrations and that the most prevalent n-3 fatty acid is linolenic acid at approximately 1% of total fatty acids (Sanders *et al.* 1978; Crawford 1980; Carlson *et al.* 1986). The level of linoleic acid in human milk varies with the intake of the mother, but is generally five to 10 times higher than in cow's milk, which contains some of the long-chain derivatives (Friedman 1980).

Feeding infant formula containing 0.6-0.9% fat as linolenic acid (18:3 n-3) reduced the amount of erythrocyte docosahexaenoic acid (22:6 n-3) in preterm infants (Carlson *et al.* 1986), and the amount of 22:6 in the brain of piglets (Hrboticky *et al.* In Press a,b). When preterm infants received a formula containing 1% of energy (2% fat) as 18:3 n-3 and no other n-3 fatty acids during the first two months of life, their level of erythrocyte 22:6 was similar to that of infants receiving breast milk (Innis *et al.* In Press). Desaturation and elongation therefore appear to progress and to lead to normal amounts of 22:6 with about 1% energy from n-3 linolenic acid in the diet.

The ratio of n-6 to n-3 fatty acids is an important consideration because of the competition between these two families of fatty acids for enzymes involved in their metabolism and their incorporation into tissue lipids. Thus, n-3 and n-6 fatty acids may have a restraining effect on each other. Neuringer and Connor (1986) suggested that the ratio of n-6 to n-3 should be between 4:1 to 10:1, particularly during pregnancy, lactation, and infancy.

Effects of Dietary Lipids on Chronic Disease

Cardiovascular Disease

Dietary fat has been implicated in the etiology of cardiovascular disease by a large body of evidence from epidemiologic, clinical and animal research. Many population studies have revealed an association between dietary fat, serum cholesterol levels and coronary heart disease (Keys 1980; Stallones 1983; Stamler 1983). It is widely recognized that an elevated level of serum cholesterol (hypercholesterolemia) is a major risk factor for a heart attack (Kannel *et al.* 1971; Pooling Project Research Group 1978; Stamler *et al.* 1986; Kannel 1988). Much emphasis has therefore been focussed on the effect of dietary fat on serum cholesterol levels (Grundy 1986, 1987; American Heart Association 1988; Kris-Etherton *et al.* 1988; Canadian Consensus Conference on Cholesterol 1988; Schonfeld 1988; Connor and Connor 1989)

The cholesterol in serum is associated with various classes of lipoproteins, which differ in their effects on atherosclerosis and coronary heart disease. Thus, whereas early studies dealt mainly with the effect of dietary fat on total serum cholesterol, there has been increasing interest in its effects on the distribution of cholesterol in the different lipoprotein classes. These include chylomicrons, very low density lipoproteins (VLDL), intermediate density lipoproteins (IDL), low density lipoproteins (LDL) and high density lipoproteins (HDL). The origins, structure, metabolism and function of the plasma lipoproteins have been studied intensively in recent years (Gotto 1987; Havel 1987; Brewer *et al.* 1988), and are described in detail in the chapter on cholesterol.

Effects of Dietary Fat on Serum Lipids and Lipoproteins

Interest in the effects of dietary fat on serum cholesterol levels was stimulated by the work of Kinsell *et al.* (1952), Ahrens *et al.* (1954) and Beveridge *et al.* (1955), indicating that polyunsaturated fats reduced the level of serum cholesterol relative to other types of dietary fat. Further studies by Keys and his associates (1965) led to development of the following formula:

$$\Delta C = 1.35\ (2\Delta S - \Delta P) + 1.5Z$$

where ΔC represents the change in mg/dL of serum cholesterol, ΔS the change in dietary saturated fatty acids as percent of total energy,: ΔP the change in dietary polyunsaturated fatty acids and Z the square root of the change in dietary cholesterol intake in mg/kcal. This equation indicates that saturated fatty acids raise serum cholesterol twice as much as polyunsaturated fatty acids decrease it. Similar equations have been developed by Hegsted *et al.* and Thomasson *et al.* and reviewed by McGandy and Hegsted 1975; Keys 1980; Hegsted and Ausman 1988.

These equations provide a useful summary of the effects of dietary fat on serum cholesterol levels but have some limitations. They were developed largely from studies on middle-aged men consuming high-fat diets, and are not necessarily valid for other segments of the population or for other dietary conditions. Furthermore, since there is considerable individual variation in the effects of dietary fats on the level of serum cholesterol, the equations are more applicable to groups than individuals (Grundy and Vega 1988; Katan *et al.* 1988). No distinction is made between different types of saturated and polyunsaturated fat, although individual fatty acids differ in their biological effects. For example, the hypercholesterolemic effects of saturated fats are due to lauric (C12:0), myristic (C14:0) and palmitic acids (C16:0). The longer-chain stearic acid (18:0) and saturated fatty acids with 10 or fewer carbon atoms do not share these hypercholesterolemic properties (Keys *et al.* 1965; Bonanome and Grundy 1988).

A reduction in saturated fat is the most effective dietary means of decreasing blood cholesterol (Keys *et al.* 1965; Brown 1971; McGandy and Hegsted 1975; Mattson and Grundy 1985). The response of blood lipids to dietary cholesterol also depends upon the level of saturated fat (Schonfeld *et al.* 1982).

The main polyunsaturated fatty acid in the dietary fats and oils used in developing the above equations is the n-6 fatty acid, linoleic acid. Fish oils, whose major polyunsaturated fatty acids belong to the n-3 family, are not particularly effective in lowering serum cholesterol levels, but produce a marked reduction in serum triacylglycerols in hypertriglyceridemic subjects (Phillipson *et al.* 1985; Carroll 1986; Herold and Kinsella 1986; Budowski 1988; Harris 1989).

The formulas developed by Keys and others contained no term for monounsaturated fatty acids, which were considered to be "neutral" in terms of their effects on serum cholesterol levels. While replacement of dietary saturated fatty acids by monounsaturated fatty acids (mainly oleic acid) lowers blood cholesterol levels (Mensink and Katan 1987; Grundy *et al.* 1988; Grundy 1989; Mensink *et al.* 1989), this effect is probably due primarily to removal of the hypercholesterolemic saturated fatty acids.

Monounsaturated fatty acids with a *trans* double bond resemble saturated fatty acids in their physical properties. Studies on the effects of these fatty acids on serum cholesterol levels have given inconclusive results, but there is little reason to think that they increase the risk of cardiovascular disease at current levels of intake (Beare-Rogers 1983; Senti 1985; Hunter and Applewhite 1986).

The influence of dietary cholesterol on serum cholesterol levels is generally less important than that of dietary fat (McNamara 1987a; Bowman *et al.* 1988) and this was recognized in developing the predictive equations. An indication of the relative effects of dietary cholesterol and saturated fat is also provided by the cholesterol-saturated fat index (CSI), designed as a measure of the plasma cholesterol elevating effect of different foods (Connor *et al.* 1986):

$$\text{CSI} = 1.01 \times \text{g saturated fat} + 0.05 \times \text{mg cholesterol}$$

However, the effect of any particular food has to be considered in the context of the entire diet (Tunstall-Pedoe *et al.* 1986).

The response of serum cholesterol to dietary saturated fats and to cholesterol is affected by genetic factors and may vary among individuals (Katan *et al.* 1986; McNamara *et al.* 1987; Grundy and Vega 1988). The response of an individual may also vary with time (Katan *et al.* 1988). Responsiveness to saturated fat and dietary cholesterol tends to go together in people of normal cholesterol intake (Katan *et al.* 1988).

The increases in serum cholesterol produced by dietary saturated fats and the decreases produced by polyunsaturated fats are due largely to changes in the level of LDL cholesterol (Gordon *et al.* 1982). Although high levels of dietary polyunsaturated fat have been found to lower HDL cholesterol (Mattson and Grundy 1985), this has not usually been observed (Becker *et al.* 1983; Weisweiler *et al.* 1985; Malmendier and Lontie 1987).

The reduction of serum triacylglycerols by dietary fish oils containing n-3 polyunsaturated fatty acids is associated with a corresponding decrease in VLDL (Phillipson *et al.* 1985; Sanders *et al.* 1985; Harris *et al.* 1988). LDL cholesterol may be increased by dietary fish oil (Sullivan *et al.* 1986). Reported effects on HDL have varied from decreases to no effect to increases (Von Schacky 1987). Under experimental conditions, replacement of saturated fat by carbohydrate led to a decrease in both LDL and HDL cholesterol and an increase in triacylglycerols (Mensink and Katan 1987; Grundy *et al.* 1988; Grundy 1989). This effect of high-carbohydrate diets on plasma lipids was transient (Cominacini *et al.* 1988).

Decreasing dietary fat from 39% to 23% of energy reduced the levels of both LDL and HDL (Kuusi *et al.* 1985). In diets containing 25% of calories from fat, increasing the polyunsaturated/saturated (P/S) ratios from 0.3 to 1.0 lowered total and LDL cholesterol but did not affect HDL cholesterol (Judd *et al.* 1988).

In the studies of Denke and Breslow (1988) on normal young adults of both sexes, replacing a diet high in fat (42% of energy) with a diet of lower fat content (30% of energy) significantly reduced total LDL cholesterol levels. A further reduction of dietary fat to 25% of energy significantly lowered HDL cholesterol as well. The LDL/HDL cholesterol ratio, which is thought to be a better predictor of disease incidence than either LDL or HDL alone, was similar with either 30% or 25% energy from fat.

Epidemiological data on boys and men from 20 different countries indicated that there are three dietary factors that influence serum lipids: the saturated fat, which raises total cholesterol; total fat, which raises HDL cholesterol; and excess energy leading to obesity, which lowers HDL cholesterol (Knuiman *et al.* 1987). In another study, changes in body weight were positively related to serum total cholesterol and inversely related to changes in HDL cholesterol (Kromhout *et al.* 1987). In this long-term intervention study, a diet enriched in linoleic acid (P/S ratio of 2) was found to lower total cholesterol without affecting HDL cholesterol. Fehily *et al.* (1988) detected statistically significant positive associations between saturated fat intake and both total and LDL cholesterol, and negative associations between carbohydrate intake and both total and HDL cholesterol. In an overview of many studies, Pietinen and Huttunen (1987) concluded that diets having a P/S ratio between 0.2 and 1.5 generally produced no change in HDL.

Effects of dietary fat and cholesterol on serum cholesterol have been studied much less extensively in women than in men, although cardiovascular disease is a leading cause of death in both sexes (Bush *et al.* 1988). Reducing the level of dietary fat from 40% to 20% of total energy produced an increase in triacylglycerols and no significant change in plasma total cholesterol in a group of premenopausal women (Jones *et al.* 1987a). Ingram *et al.* (1987), however, reported a decrease in serum cholesterol in women who reduced their dietary fat intake. In summary, reducing the intake of saturated fatty acids of chain-length C_{12} to C_{16} appears to be the most effective way of lowering total and LDL cholesterol in the blood serum.

Effects of Dietary Fat on Thrombosis

Dietary fat may alter the risk of cardiovascular disease by its effects on blood clotting. In epidemiologic studies in Great Britain and France, the clotting activity of platelets and their response to thrombin-induced aggregation showed a close relationship to the intake of saturated fatty acids, including stearic acid (Renaud *et al.* 1986a,b, 1987; Renaud 1987). These effects were associated with the appearance in platelet phospholipids of small amounts of eicosatrienoic acid (20:3 n-9), a potent platelet-aggregating substance (Lagarde *et al.* 1983, 1985). Whereas the hyperlipemic effects of saturated fatty acids in humans appear to be confined mainly to lauric, myristic and palmitic acids, experiments have indicated that palmitic and stearic acids are the most thrombogenic in rats (McGregor *et al.* 1980).

Dietary monounsaturated fats have generally been considered to have little effect on thrombogenesis (Hornstra 1985), but platelet aggregation induced by collagen was reduced in healthy subjects on a moderate intake of fat with high monounsaturated fatty acid content, compared to that in subjects on a similar intake of fat with a high content of polyunsaturated n-6 fatty acids (Sirtori *et al.* 1986). Effects of dietary polyunsaturated fatty acids on blood clotting are thought to be related to their conversion to various biologically active eicosanoids (Dyerberg *et al.* 1978; Goodnight *et al.* 1982; Bunting *et al.* 1983; Carroll 1986; Holub 1988). Arachidonic acid (20:4, n-6) can be converted by platelets to thromboxane A_2 which causes vasoconstriction and platelet aggregation and promotes blood clotting, and in the walls of blood vessels to prostacyclin (PGI_2) which counteracts these effects. Since thromboxane A_2 and prostacyclin are both formed from arachidonic acid, there is uncertainty about the optimum level of dietary n-6 fatty acids required to minimize the risk of thrombosis.

Eicosapentaenoic acid (EPA, 20:5 n-3) competes with arachidonic acid for the cyclooxygenase enzyme that initiates the formation of eicosanoids. This acid may be converted to thromboxane A_3 (TXA_3) and prostacyclin (PGI_3). TXA_3 is produced in smaller amounts and lacks the platelet-aggregating and vasoconstrictive effects of TXA_2, whereas PGI_3 has effects similar to those of PGI_2 (Von Schacky 1987; Leaf and Weber 1988).

Arachidonic acid is normally present in the diet only in small amounts but can be formed in the body by desaturation and chain elongation of linoleic acid (Brenner 1987). EPA may be ingested in substantial amounts as a component of fish oils and oils of other marine animals, and may be formed from linolenic acid (18:3 n-3) by a series of reactions analogous to those involved in the formation of arachidonic acid from linoleic acid. In fact, n-3 fatty acids compete with n-6 fatty acids for the enzymes involved in these transformations, so dietary linolenic acid can inhibit the conversion of linoleic acid to arachidonic acid. Furthermore, EPA competes with arachidonic acid for incorporation into tissue phospholipids (Leaf and Weber 1988).

Studies by Renaud *et al.* (1986a, 1987) showed that increasing the intake of polyunsaturated vegetable oil in place of saturated fat decreased the clotting activity of platelets and their aggregation by thrombin, in both men and women. Multivariate analysis indicated that these effects on platelet function were inversely correlated with dietary linolenate (n-3) but not with linoleate (n-6).

The studies of Dyerberg and Bang (1979) showed that the bleeding time of Eskimos was longer than that of Danes and that their platelet lipids were enriched in n-3 fatty acids at the expense of n-6 fatty acids. Subsequent studies on human diets indicated that platelet aggregation could be inhibited and bleeding time prolonged by ingestion of fish, fish oil or fish oil concentrates (Siess *et al.* 1980; Brox *et al.* 1981; Thorngren and Gustafson 1981; Sanders *et al.* 1981; Ahmed and Holub 1984; Dyerberg 1986; Von Schacky 1987; Holub 1988). However, a reduction in platelet aggregation was not found consistently (Mortensen *et al.* 1983; Sanders and Roshanai 1983; Hirai *et al.* 1987). These effects are presumably a result of altered eicosanoid production (Bunting *et al.* 1983; Von Schacky and Weber 1985).

Dietary fish oil increases the ratio of n-3 to n-6 fatty acids in platelet phospholipids (Goodnight *et al.* 1981). EPA is selectively incorporated into phosphatidylcholine and phosphatidylethanolamine fractions (Ahmed and Holub 1984; Galloway *et al.* 1985) and into an ether-linked, ethanolamine-containing phospholipid (Holub *et al.* 1988). Ethanolamine- and choline-containing phospholipids are the main sources of EPA released by platelet stimulation (Mahadevappa and Holub 1987).

Other changes observed following ingestion of fish, fish oil or fish oil concentrates include a reduction in blood pressure, a decrease in blood viscosity, an increase in erythrocyte deformability and an increase in the velocity of capillary blood flow (Dyerberg 1986; Von Schacky 1987; Holub 1988). These changes may contribute to the observed low mortality rate from cardiovascular disease in coastal Greenland Eskimos (Kromann and Green 1980) and in Japanese whose diet includes a relatively high proportion of fish (Hirai *et al.* 1987). A recent study of West Coast Canadian Inuit revealed higher levels of long-chain, n-3 polyunsaturated fatty acids in erythrocyte phospholipid than in Vancouver residents, but the serum cholesterol levels were not significantly different (Innis *et al.* 1988). Consumption of fish is preferred to ingestion of concentrates of n-3 polyunsaturated fatty acids which may have pharmacological action.

Cancer

As for cardiovascular disease, epidemiological data on cancer incidence and mortality show large geographical differences. From studies on migrating populations and on time trends within countries, it appears that these differences are related to environmental and life style factors rather than to genetic factors. Dietary fat has been implicated as a factor because it shows a strong positive correlation with cancer mortality and incidence at sites such as breast, colon and prostate, and to a lesser extent, with cancer at other sites including the ovary, pancreas and rectum. Studies on experimental models of mammary, colon and pancreatic cancer have also shown consistently that animals fed high-fat diets *ad libitum* develop cancer at these sites more readily than animals fed low-fat diets (Armstrong and Doll 1975; Carroll and Khor 1975; Reddy *et al.* 1980; Ip *et al.* 1986; Reddy and Cohen 1986).

Case-control and prospective studies on dietary fat and breast cancer have given more variable results, ranging from positive associations to no relationship or in some cases to negative correlations (Miller *et al.* 1978; Howe 1985; Hislop *et al.* 1986; Katsouyanni *et al.* 1986; Lubin *et al.* 1986; Hirohata *et al.* 1987; Jones *et al.* 1987b; Willett *et al.* 1987; Rohan *et al.* 1988; Verrault *et al.* 1988; Toniolo *et al.* 1989). Such studies have provided more consistent evidence relating dietary fat to colorectal cancer (Miller *et al.* 1983; Stemmermann *et al.* 1984; Howe *et al.* 1986; Macquart-Moulin *et al.* 1986; Kolonel 1987; Kune *et al.* 1987; Graham *et al.* 1988; Tuyns *et al.* 1988). Several case-control studies have also yielded evidence of a positive association between dietary fat and prostatic cancer (Graham *et al.* 1983; Heshmat *et al.* 1985; Kolonel *et al.* 1988).

The inconclusive nature of the evidence regarding an association of dietary fat with breast cancer and colorectal cancer may be related to methodological problems. These may be compounded by the fact that differences in fat intake between diseased and non-diseased groups are usually small (Goodwin and Boyd 1987; Freudenheim and Marshall 1988; Prentice *et al.* 1988). Even in animal studies, the effects of dietary fat on mammary tumorigenesis are not apparent at all times of the experiment (Jacobson *et al.* 1988).

Intercountry comparisons have shown that total dietary fat correlates with mortality from cancer of the breast, colon and prostate as well as or better than does any particular type of fat (Carroll 1983; Carroll *et al.* 1986). Caution is required in drawing conclusions from such intercountry comparisons, however, since estimates of cancer incidence and mortality, and of food consumption based on disappearance data are subject to many sources of error (Carroll and Khor 1975). All that can be concluded with confidence is that the incidence of cancer at certain sites is lower in populations with a low-fat diet.

In experimental animals given a chemical carcinogen a high fat diet appears to act primarily as a promoter of carcinogenesis (Carroll and Khor 1975; Reddy and Cohen 1986; Welsch 1987). There is evidence that changing to a low-fat diet decreases the level of estrogens in serum (Rose *et al.* 1987a). Ingram *et al.* (1987) observed a decrease in non-protein-bound estradiol in women following a change to a low-fat diet. Rose *et al.* (1987b) reported a decrease in prolactin levels on a low-fat diet. The relief of symptoms of cyclical mastopathy observed by Boyd *et al.* (1988) in women who reduced their fat intake to 15% of energy may be due to alterations in hormonal patterns, although other explanations are possible.

It is known that carcinogenesis can be inhibited in animals by caloric restriction (Tannenbaum and Silverstone 1953; Pariza and Boutwell 1987; Pariza 1988) and this can occur even with high-fat diets (Klurfeld *et al.* 1987), but these experiments often involve rather severe restriction. Voluntary exercise has also been shown to have an inhibitory effect on mammary carcinogenesis in rats (Cohen *et al.* 1988) and in humans (Frisch *et al.* 1987). The balance between energy intake and expenditure may be more important than intake alone.

Hypertension

There is controversy about a role of dietary fat in hypertension. Puska *et al.* (1985) reported that decreasing the level of dietary fat from 30% of energy to 23%, while increasing the P/S ratio from 0.2 to approximately 1.0 led to a reduction in blood pressure. However, after evaluating the literature, Weinsier and Norris (1985) concluded that reduction of total fat alone had no effect in either normotensive or borderline hypertensives. They cited evidence that increasing the linoleate content of the diet is associated with a reduction in blood pressure of mildly as well as overtly hypertensive patients. Reductions in blood pressure and blood viscosity have been observed in subjects fed fish oil or fish oil concentrates (Holub 1988).

Obesity

An excess of energy intake over energy expenditure can lead to obesity. High-fat diets have a higher caloric density than low-fat diets and deposition of dietary fat in body tissues requires less energy expenditure than deposition of fat derived from dietary carbohydrate or protein, since energy is required to convert the carbohydrate and protein to fat. These considerations have led to the conclusion that the true energy content of fat relative to carbohydrate and protein in terms of potential for storage is higher than that indicated by the familiar Atwater values of 9, 4 and 4 kcal (37, 17, 17 kJ) per g (Donato and Hegsted 1985; Anon. 1988). The type of dietary fat may influence its storage potential, since there is evidence that polyunsaturated fatty acids are oxidized more readily than saturated fatty acids (Jones and Schoeller 1988; Anon. 1988). It has been suggested that high-fat diets may encourage overeating because satiety is reached at a higher level of energy intake on high-fat diets than on low-fat, fibre-rich diets (Duncan *et al.* 1983). It should be emphasized, however, that energy balance depends on expenditure as well as input, and a sedentary lifestyle may contribute significantly to obesity.

Recommendations

The n-6 fatty acids should be at least 3% of energy and the n-3 fatty acids at least 0.5% of energy with a ratio of n-6 to n-3 fatty acids in the range of 4:1 to 10:1. When the diet of infants contains no n-3 C_{20} and C_{22} fatty acids, 1% energy should be provided by n-3 linolenic acid.

The present level of total fat, and particularly of saturated fat, in the Canadian diet constitutes a risk factor for cardiovascular disease and possibly for certain other diseases including some forms of cancer. Consequently, it is recommended that the fat content of the diet be reduced to 30% of total energy (33 g/1000 kcal or 40 g/5000 kJ). The intake of saturated fat should not exceed 10% of total energy (11 g/1000 kcal or 13 g/5000 kJ). Current levels of *trans* fatty acids in the diet should not be increased.

The optimal amount of lipid in the diet is related to the stage of development and the requirement for energy. During infancy, when growth is rapid and gastrointestinal capacity limited, a high-fat diet helps to ensure an adequate intake of energy. Dietary fat supplies about half of the energy in human milk but less in the diet of the child after weaning. It is stressed that the recommendation to reduce dietary fat does not apply to children under two years of age.

References

Ahmed, A.A. and Holub, B.J. 1984. Alteration and recovery of bleeding times, platelet aggregation and fatty acid compostion of individual phospholipids in platelets of human subjects receiving a supplement of cod-liver oil. Lipids 19:617-624.

Ahrens, E.H., Jr., Blankenhorn, D.H. and Tsaltas, T.T. 1954. Effect on human serum lipids of substituting plant for animal fat in diet. Proc. Soc. Exp. Biol. Med. 86:872-878.

American Heart Association. 1988. Dietary guidelines for healthy American adults: a statement for physicians and health professionals by the Nutrition Committee. Circulation 77:721A-724A.

Anderson, R.E., Benolken, R.M., Dudley, P.A., Landis, D.J. and Wheeler, T.G. 1974. Polyunsaturated fatty acids of photoreceptor membranes. Exp. Eye Res. 18: 205-213.

Anonymous. 1988. Role of fat and fatty acids in modulation of energy exchange. Nutr. Rev. 46:382-384.

Armstrong, B. and Doll, R. 1975. Environmental factors and cancer incidence and mortality in different countries, with special reference to dietary practices. Int. J. Cancer 15:617-631.

Beare-Rogers, J.L. 1983. *trans-* and positional isomers of common fatty acids. Adv. Nutr. Res. 5:171-200.

Becker, N., Illingworth, D.R., Alaupovic, P., Connor, W.E. and Sundberg, E.E. 1983. Effects of saturated, monounsaturated, and ω-6 polyunsaturated fatty acids on plasma lipids, lipoproteins, and apoproteins in humans. Am. J. Clin. Nutr. 37:355-360.

Beveridge, J.M.R., Connell, W.F., Mayer, G.A., Firstbrook, J.B. and DeWolfe, M.S. 1955. The effects of certain vegetable and animal fats on the plasma lipids of humans. J. Nutr. 56:311-320.

Bjerve, K.S., Fischer, S. and Alme, K. 1987. Alpha-linolenic acid deficiency in man: effect of ethyl linolenate on plasma and erythrocyte composition and biosynthesis of prostanoids. Am. J. Clin. Nutr. 46:570-576.

Bonanome, A. and Grundy, S.M. 1988. Effect of dietary stearic acid on plasma cholesterol and lipoprotein levels. N. Engl. J. Med. 318:1244-1248.

Bowman, M.P., VanDoren, J., Taper, L.J., Thye, F.W. and Ritchey, S.J. 1988. Effect of dietary fat and cholesterol on plasma lipids and lipoprotein fractions in normolipidemic men. J. Nutr. 118:555-560.

Boyd, N.F., Shannon, P., Kriukov, V., Fish, E., Lockwood, G., McGuire, V., Cousins, M., Mahoney, L., Lickley, L. and Tritchler, D. 1988. Effect of a low-fat, high-carbohydrate diet on symptoms of cyclical mastopathy. Lancet 2:128-132.

Brenner, R.R. 1987. Biosynthesis and interconversion of the essential fatty acids. *In* CRC handbook of eicosanoids: prostaglandins and related lipids. Vol. 1. Chemical and biophysical aspects, Part A. Willis, A.L. ed., CRC Press, Boca Raton, Fla., pp. 99-118.

Brewer, H.B., Jr., Gregg, R.E., Hoeg, J.M. and Fojo, S.S. 1988. Apolipoproteins and lipoproteins in human plasma: an overview. Clin. Chem. 34 (Suppl. 8B):B4-B8.

Brown, H.B. 1971. Food patterns that lower blood lipids in man. J. Am. Diet. Assoc. 58:303-311.

Brox, J.H., Killie, J.-E., Gunnes, S. and Nordoy, A. 1981. The effect of cod liver oil and corn oil on platelets and vessel wall in man. Thromb. Haemostasis 46:604-611.

Budowski, P. 1988. ω3 Fatty acids in health and disease. World Rev. Nutr. Diet. 57:214-274.

Bunting, S., Moncada, S. and Vane, J.R. 1983. The prostacyclin-thromboxane A_2 balance: pathophysiological and therapeutic implications. Br. Med. Bull. 39:271-276.

Bush, T.L., Fried, L.P. and Barrett-Connor, E. 1988. Cholesterol, lipoproteins, and coronary heart disease in women. Clin. Chem. 34 (Suppl. 8B):B60-B70.

Canadian Consensus Conference on the Prevention of Heart and Vascular Disease by Altering Serum Cholesterol and Lipoprotein Risk Factors. 1988. Canadian Consensus Conference on Cholesterol: final report. Can. Med. Assoc. J. 139 (Suppl.):1-8.

Carlson, S.E., Rhodes, P.G. and Ferguson, M.G. 1986. Docosahexaenoic acid status of preterm infants at birth and following feeding with human milk or formula. Am. J. Clin. Nutr. 44:798-804.

Carroll, K.K. 1983. Diet and carcinogenesis. *In* Atherosclerosis VI: proceedings of the sixth international symposium. Shettler, G., Gotto, A.M., Middelhoff, G., Habenicht, A.J.R. and Jrutka, K.R., eds. Springer-Verlag, Berlin, pp. 223-227.

Carroll, K.K. 1986. Biological effects of fish oils in relation to chronic diseases. Lipids 21:731-732.

Carroll, K.K., Braden, L.M., Bell, J.A. and Kalamegham, R. 1986. Fat and cancer. Cancer 58:1818-1825.

Carroll, K.K. and Khor, H.T. 1975. Dietary fat in relation to tumorigenesis. Prog. Biochem. Pharmacol. 10:308-353.

Clandinin, M.T., Chappell, J.E., Leong, S., Heim, T., Swyer, P.R. and Chance, G.W. 1980a. Intrauterine fatty acid accretion rates in human brain: implications for fatty acid requirements. Early Hum. Dev. 4:121-129.

Clandinin, M.T., Chappell, J.E., Leong, S., Heim, T., Swyer, P.R. and Chance, G.W. 1980b. Extrauterine fatty acid accretion in infant brain: implications for fatty acid requirements. Early Hum. Dev. 4:131-138.

Cohen, L.A., Choi, K. and Wang, C-X. 1988. Influence of dietary fat, caloric restriction, and voluntary exercise on N-nitrosomethylurea-induced mammary tumorigenesis in rats. Cancer Res. 48:4276-4283.

Cominacini, L., Zocca, I., Garbin, U., Davoli, A., Compri, R., Brunetti, L. and Bosello, O. 1988. Long-term effects of a low-fat, high-carbohydrate diet on plasma lipids of patients affected by familial endogenous hypertriglyceridemia. Am. J. Clin. Nutr. 48:57-65.

Connor, S.L. and Connor, W.E. 1989. Coronary heart disease: prevention and treatment by nutritional change. *In* Diet, nutrition and health. Carroll, K.K., ed. McGill-Queen's University Press, Kingston.

Connor, S.L., Artaud-Wild, S.M., Classick-Kohn, C.J., Gustafson, J.R., Flaveil, D.P., Hatcher, L.F. and Connor, W.E. 1986. The cholesterol saturated fat index: an indication of the hypercholesterolaemic and atherogenic potential of food. Lancet 1:1229-1232.

Connor, W.E., Neuringer, M., Barstad, L. and Lin, D.S. 1984. Dietary deprivation of linolenic acid in rhesus monkeys: effects on plasma and tissue fatty acid composition and on visual function. Trans. Assoc. Am. Physicians 97:1-9.

Crawford, M.A. 1980. Estimation of essential fatty acid requirements in pregnancy and lactation. Prog. Food Nutr. Sci. 4:75-80.

Crawford, M.A. 1987. Essential fatty acids and brain development. *In* Nestlé nutrition workshop series. Vol. 13. Lipids in modern nutrition. Horisberger, M. and Bracco, U., eds. Raven Press, New York, pp. 67-78.

Crawford, M.A., Hassam, A.G. and Williams, G. 1976. Essential fatty acids and fetal brain growth. Lancet 1:452-453.

Denke, M.A. and Breslow, J.L. 1988. Effects of a low fat diet with and without intermittent saturated fat and cholesterol ingestion on plasma lipid, lipoprotein, and apolipoprotein levels in normal volunteers. J. Lipid Res. 29:963-969.

Donato, K. and Hegsted, D.M. 1985. Efficiency of utilization of various sources of energy for growth. Proc. Nat. Acad. Sci. U.S.A. 82:4866-4870.

Dougherty, R.M., Fong, A.K.H. and Iacono, J.M. 1988. Nutrient content of the diet when the fat is reduced. Am. J. Clin. Nutr. 48:970-979.

Duncan, K.H., Bacon, J.A. and Weinsier, R.L. 1983. The effects of high and low energy density diets on satiety, energy intake, and eating time of obese and nonobese subjects. Am. J. Clin. Nutr. 37:763-767.

Dyerberg, J. 1986. Linolenate-derived polyunsaturated fatty acids and prevention of atherosclerosis. Nutr. Rev. 44:125-137.

Dyerberg, J. and Bang, H.O. 1979. Haemostatic function and platelet polyunsaturated fatty acids in Eskimos. Lancet 2:433-435.

Dyerberg, J., Bang, H.O., Stoffersen, E., Moncada, S. and Vane, J.R. 1978. Eicosapentaenoic acid and prevention of thrombosis and atherosclerosis? Lancet 2:117-119.

FAO/WHO. 1977. Dietary fats and oils in human nutrition: report of an expert consultation. Rome.

FAO. 1980. Food balance sheets 1975-77 average and per caput food supplies 1961-65 average 1967 to 1977. Rome.

Fehily, A.M., Yarnell, J.W.G., Bolton, C.H. and Butland, B.K. 1988. Dietary determinants of plasma lipids and lipoproteins: the Caerphilly study. Eur. J. Clin. Nutr. 42:405-413.

Fiennes, R.N., Sinclair, A.J. and Crawford, M.A. 1973. Essential fatty acid studies in primates. Linolenic acid requirements of capuchins. J. Med. Primatol. 2:155-169.

Freudenheim, J.L. and Marshall, J.R. 1988. The problem of profound mismeasurement and the power of epidemiological studies of diet and cancer. Nutr. Cancer 11:243-250.

Friedman, Z. 1980. Essential fatty acids revisited. Am. J. Dis. Child. 134:397-408.

Friedman, Z. 1987. Essential fatty acid requirements for term and preterm infants. *In* Nestlé nutrition workshop series. Vol. 13. Lipids in modern nutrition. Horisberger, M. and Bracco, U., eds., Raven Press, New York, pp. 79-92.

Frisch, R.E., Wyshak, G., Albright, N.L., Albright, T.E., Schiff, I., Witschi, J. and Marguglio, M. 1987. Lower lifetime occurrence of breast cancer and cancers of the reproductive system among former college athletes. Am. J. Clin. Nutr. 45:328-335.

Galloway, J.H., Cartwright, I.J., Woodcock, B.E., Greaves, M., Russell, R.G. and Preston, F.E. 1985. Effects of dietary fish oil supplementation on the fatty acid composition of the human platelet membrane: demonstration of selectivity in the incorporation of eicosapentaenoic acid into membrane phospholipid pools. Clin. Sci. 68:449-454.

Goodnight, S.H., Jr., Harris, W.S. and Connor, W.E. 1981. The effects of dietary ω3 fatty acids on platelet composition and function in man: a prospective, controlled study. Blood 58:880-885.

Goodnight, S.H., Jr., Harris, W.S., Connor, W.E. and Illingworth, D.R. 1982. Polyunsaturated fatty acids, hyperlipidemia, and thrombosis. Arteriosclerosis 2:87-113.

Goodwin, P.J. and Boyd, N.F. 1987. Critical appraisal of the evidence that dietary fat intake is related to breast cancer risk in humans. J. Nat. Cancer Inst. 79:473-485.

Gordon, D.J., Salz, K.M., Roggenkamp, K.J. and Franklin, F.A., Jr. 1982. Dietary determinants of plasma cholesterol change in the recruitment phase of the Lipid Research Clinics Coronary Primary Prevention Trial. Arteriosclerosis 2:537-548.

Gotto, A.M., Jr., ed. 1987. New comprehensive biochemistry. Vol. 14. Plasma lipoproteins. Elsevier, Amsterdam.

Graham, S., Haughey, B., Marshall, J., Priore, R., Byers, T., Rzepka, T., Mettlin, C. and Pontes, J.E. 1983. Diet in the epidemiology of carcinoma of the prostate gland. J. Nat. Cancer Inst. 70:687-692.

Graham, S., Marshall, J., Haughey, B., Mittelman, A., Swanson, M., Zielezny, M., Byers, T., Wilkinson, G. and West, D. 1988. Dietary epidemiology of cancer of the colon in Western New York. Am. J. Epidemiol. 128:490-503.

Grundy, S.M. 1986. Cholesterol and coronary heart disease: a new era. J. Am. Med. Assoc. 256:2849-2858.

Grundy, S.M. 1987. Dietary treatment of hyperlipidemia. *In* Hypercholesterolemia and atherosclerosis. Pathogenesis and prevention. Steinberg, D. and Olefsky, J.M., eds. Churchill Livingstone, New York, pp. 169-193.

Grundy, S.M. 1989. Monounsaturated fatty acids and cholesterol metabolism: implications for dietary recommendations. J. Nutr. 119:529-533.

Grundy, S.M. and Vega, G.L. 1988. Plasma cholesterol responsiveness to saturated fatty acids. Am. J. Clin. Nutr. 47:822-824.

Grundy, S.M., Florentin, L., Nix, D. and Whelan, M.F. 1988. Comparison of monounsaturated fatty acids and carbohydrates for reducing raised levels of plasma cholesterol in man. Am. J. Clin. Nutr. 47:965-969.

Gurr, M.I. and James, A.T. 1980. Lipid biochemistry: an introduction. 3rd ed. Chapman and Hall, London.

Hansen, A.E., Wiese, H.F., Boelsche, A.N., Haggard, M.E., Adam, D.J.D. and Davis, H. 1963. Role of linoleic acid in infant nutrition. Clinical and chemical study of 428 infants fed on milk mixtures varying in kind and amount of fat. Pediatrics 31:171-192.

Harris, W.S. 1989. Fish oils and plasma lipid and lipoprotein metabolism in humans: a critical review. J. Lipid Res. 30:785-807.

Harris, W.S., Connor, W.E., Alam, N. and Illingworth, D.R. 1988. Reduction of postprandial triglyceridemia in humans by dietary n-3 fatty acids. J. Lipid Res. 29:1451-1460.

Havel, R.J. 1987. Origin, metabolic fate, and metabolic function of plasma lipoproteins. *In* Hypercholesterolemia and atherosclerosis. Pathogenesis and prevention. Steinberg, D. and Olefsky, J.M., eds. Churchill Livingstone, New York, pp. 117-141.

Hegsted, D.M. and Ausman, L.M. 1988. Diet, alcohol and coronary heart disease in men. J. Nutr. 118:1184-1189.

Herold, P.M. and Kinsella, J.E. 1986. Fish oil consumption and decreased risk of cardiovascular disease: a comparison of findings from animal and human feeding trials. Am. J. Clin. Nutr. 43:566-598.

Heshmat, M.Y., Kaul, L., Kovi, J., Jackson, M.A., Jackson, A.G., Jones, G.W., Edson, M., Enterline, J.P., Worrell, R.G. and Perry, S.L. 1985. Nutrition and prostate cancer: a case-control study. Prostate 6:7-17.

Hirai, A., Terano, T., Saito, H., Tamura, Y. and Yoshida, S. 1987. Clinical and epidemiological studies of eicosapentaenoic acid in Japan. *In* Proceedings of the AOCS short course on polyunsaturated fatty acids and eicosanoids. Lands, W.E.M., ed. American Oil Chemists' Society, Champaign, Il, pp. 9-24.

Hirohata, T., Nomura, A.M.Y., Hankin, J.H., Kolonel, L.N. and Lee, J. 1987. An epidemiologic study on the association between diet and breast cancer. J. Nat. Cancer Inst. 78:595-600.

Hislop, T.G., Coldman, A.J., Elwood, J.M., Brauer, G. and Kan, L. 1986. Childhood and recent eating patterns and risk of breast cancer. Cancer Detect. Prev. 9:47-58.

Holman, R.T. 1968. Essential fatty acid deficiency. Prog. Chem. Fats Other Lipids 9:275-348.

Holman, R.T. 1977. The deficiency of essential fatty acids. *In* Polyunsaturated fatty acids. Kunau, W.H. and Holman, R.T., eds. Am. Oil Chem. Soc., Champaign, Il, pp. 163-191.

Holman, R.T. 1987. Essential fatty acids and nutritional disorders. *In* Nestlé nutrition workshop series. Vol. 13. Lipids in modern nutrition. Horisberger, M. and Bracco, U., eds. Raven Press, New York, pp. 157-171.

Holman, R.T., Caster, W.O. and Wiese, H.F. 1964. The essential fatty acid requirement of infants and the assessment of their dietary intake of linoleate by serum fatty acid analysis. Am. J. Clin. Nutr. 14:70-75.

Holub, B.J. 1988. Dietary fish oils containing eicosapentaenoic acid and the prevention of atherosclerosis and thrombosis. Can. Med. Assoc. J. 139:377-381.

Holub, B.J., Celi, B. and Skeaff, C.M. 1988. The alkenylacyl class of ethanolamine phospholipid represents a major form of eicosapentaenoic acid (EPA)-containing phospholipid in the platelets of human subjects consuming a fish oil concentrate. Thromb. Res. 50:135-143.

Hornstra, G. 1985. Dietary lipids, platelet function and arterial thrombosis in animals and man. Proc. Nutr. Soc. 44:371-378.

Howe, G.R. 1985. The use of polytomous dual response data to increase power in case-control studies: an application to the association between dietary fat and breast cancer. J. Chronic Dis. 38:663-670.

Howe, G.R., Miller, A.B. and Jain, M. 1986. Re: "Total energy intake: implications for epidemiologic analysis". Am. J. Epidemiol. 124:157-159.

Hrboticky, N., MacKinnon, M.J. and Innis, S.M. In Press a. Effect of a linoleic acid rich vegetable oil infant formula on tissue fatty acid accretion in the newborn piglet: correspondence between brain, liver, plasma and erythrocytes. Am. J. Clin. Nutr. 50.

Hrboticky, N., MacKinnon, M.J., Puterman, M.L. and Innis, S.M. In Press b. Effect of linoleic acid rich formula feeding on brain synaptosomal lipid accretion and enzyme thermotropic behaviour in the piglet. J. Lipid Res. 30:1173-1184.

Hunter, J.E. and Applewhite, T.H. 1986. Isomeric fatty acids in the U.S. diet: levels and health perspectives. Am. J. Clin. Nutr. 44:707-717.

Ingram, D.M., Bennett, F.C., Willcox, D. and deKlerk, N. 1987. Effect of low-fat diet on female sex hormone levels. J. Nat. Cancer Inst. 79:1225-1229.

Innis, S.M., Foote, K.D., MacKinnon, M.J. and King, D.J. In Press. Plasma and red blood cell fatty acids of low birthweight infants fed their mother's expressed breast milk or preterm infant formula. Am. J. Clin. Nutr. 50.

Innis, S.M., Kuhnlein, H.V. and Kinloch, D. 1988. The composition of red cell membrane phospholipids in Canadian Inuit consuming a diet high in marine mammals. Lipids 23:1064-1068.

Ip, C., Birt, D.F., Rogers, A.E. and Mettlin, C., eds. 1986. Dietary fat and cancer. Vol. 222. Progress in clinical and biological research. A. R. Liss, New York.

Jacobson, E.A., James, K.A., Frei, J.V. and Carroll, K.K. 1988. Effects of dietary fat on long-term growth and mammary tumorigenesis in female Sprague-Dawley rats given a low dose of DMBA. Nutr. Cancer 11:221-227.

Jones, D.Y., Judd, J.T., Taylor, P.R., Campbell, W.S. and Nair, P.P. 1987a. Influence of caloric contribution and saturation of dietary fat on plasma lipids of premenopausal women. Am. J. Clin. Nutr. 45:1451-1456.

Jones, D.Y., Schatzkin, A., Green, S.B., Block, G., Brinton, L.A., Ziegler, R.G., Hoover, R. and Taylor, P.R. 1987b. Dietary fat and breast cancer in the National Health and Nutrition Examination Survey. Epidemiologic Follow-up Study. J. Nat. Cancer Inst. 79:465-471.

Jones, P.J.H. and Schoeller, D.A. 1988. Polyunsaturated: saturated ratio of diet fat influences energy substrate utilization in the human. Metababolism 37:145-151.

Judd, J.T., Oh, S.Y., Hennig, B., Dupont, J. and Marshall, M.W. 1988. Effects of low fat diets differing in degree of fat unsaturation on plasma lipids, lipoproteins, and apolipoproteins in adult men. J. Am. Coll. Nutr. 7:223-234.

Kannel, W.B. 1988. Cholesterol and risk of coronary heart disease and mortality in men. Clin. Chem. 34 (Suppl. 8B):B53-B59.

Kannel, W.B., Castelli, W.P., Gordon, T. and McNamara, P.M. 1971. Serum cholesterol, lipoproteins, and the risk of coronary heart disease. The Framinghman study. Ann. Intern. Med. 74:1-12.

Katan, M.B., Beynen, A.C., De Vries, J.H.M. and Nobels, A. 1986. Existence of consistent hypo- and hyperresponders to dietary cholesterol in man. Am. J. Epidemiol. 123:221-234.

Katan, M.B., Berns, A.M., Glatz, J.F.C., Knuiman, J.T., Nobels, A. and deVries, J.H.M. 1988. Congruence of individual responsiveness to dietary cholesterol and to saturated fat in humans. J. Lipid Res. 29:883-892.

Katsouyanni, K., Trichopoulos, D., Boyle, P., Xirouchaki, E., Trichopoulou, A., Lisseos, B., Vasilaros, S. and MacMahon, B. 1986. Diet and breast cancer: a case-control study in Greece. Int. J. Cancer 38:815-820.

Keys, A. 1980. Seven countries. A multivariate analysis of death and coronary heart disease. Harvard University Press, Cambridge, MA.

Keys, A., Anderson, J.T. and Grande, F. 1965. Serum cholesterol response to changes in the diet. IV. Particular saturated fatty acids in the diet. Metabolism 13:776-787.

Knuiman, J.T., West, C.E., Katan, M.B. and Hautvast, J.G.A.J. 1987. Total cholesterol and high density lipoprotein cholesterol levels in populations differing in fat and carbohydrate intake. Arteriosclerosis 7:612-619.

Kinsell, L.W., Partridge, J., Boling, L., Margen, S. and Michaels, G. 1952. Dietary modification of serum cholesterol and phospholipid levels. J. Clin. Endocrinol. 12:909-913.

Klurfeld, D.M., Weber, M.M. and Kritchevsky, D. 1987. Inhibition of chemically induced mammary and colon tumor promotion by caloric restriction in rats fed increased dietary fat. Cancer Res. 47:2759-2762.

Kolonel, L.N. 1987. Fat and colon cancer: how firm is the epidemiologic evidence? Am. J. Clin. Nutr. 45:336-341.

Kolonel, L.N., Yoshizawa, C.N. and Hankin, J.H. 1988. Diet and prostatic cancer: a case-control study in Hawaii. Am. J. Epidemiol. 127:999-1012.

Kris-Etherton, P.M., Krummel, D., Russell, M.E., Dreon, D., Mackey, S., Borchers, J. and Wood, P.D. 1988. The effect of diet on plasma lipids, lipoproteins, and coronary heart disease. J. Am. Diet. Assoc. 88:1373-1400.

Kromhout, D., Arntzenius, A.C., Kempen-Voogd, N., Kempen, H.J., Barth, J.D., van der Voort, H.A. and van der Velde, E.A. 1987. Long-term effects of a linoleic acid-enriched diet, changes in body weight and alcohol consumption on serum total and HDL-cholesterol. Atherosclerosis 66:99-105.

Kromann, N. and Green, A. 1980. Epidemiological studies in the Upernavik district, Greenland. Acta Med. Scand. 208:401-406.

Kune, S., Kune, G.A. and Watson, L.F. 1987. Case-control study of dietary etiological factors: the Melbourne Colorectal Cancer Study. Nutr. Cancer 9:21-42.

Kuusi, T., Ehnholm, C., Huttunen, J.K., Kostiainen, E., Pietinen, P., Leino, U., Uusitalo, U., Nikkari, T., Iacono, J.M. and Puska, P. 1985. Concentration and composition of serum lipoproteins during a low-fat diet at two levels of polyunsaturated fat. J. Lipid Res. 26:360-367.

Lagarde, M., Burtin, M., Sprecher, H. Dechavanne, M. and Renaud, S. 1983. Potentiating effect of 5,8,11-eicosatrienoic acid on human platelet aggregation. Lipids 18:291-294.

Lagarde, M., Burtin, M., Rigaud, M., Sprecher, H., Dechavanne, M. and Renaud, S. 1985. Prostaglandin E_2-like activity of 20:3n-9 platelet lipoxygenase end-product. FEBS Lett. 181:53-6.

Leaf, A. and Weber, P.C. 1988. Cardiovascular effects of n-3 fatty acids. N. Engl. J. Med. 318:549-557.

Lubin, F., Wax, Y. and Modan, B. 1986. Role of fat, animal protein, and dietary fiber in breast cancer etiology: a case-control study. J. Nat. Cancer Inst. 77:605-612.

Macquart-Moulin, G., Riboli, E., Cornée, J., Charnay, B., Berthezene, P. and Day, N. 1986. Case-control study on colorectal cancer and diet in Marseilles. Int. J. Cancer 38:183-191.

Mahadevappa, V.G. and Holub, B.J. 1987. Quantitative loss of individual eicosapentaenoyl- relative to arachidonoyl-containing phospholipids in thrombin-stimulated human platelets. J. Lipid Res. 28:1275-1280.

Malmendier, C.L. and Lontie, J.F. 1987. Effects of dietary fat modifications on plasma lipid and apolipoprotein metabolism in humans. Adv. Exp. Med. Biol. 210:153-158.

Mattson, F.H. and Grundy, S.M. 1985. Comparison of effects of dietary saturated, monounsaturated, and polyunsaturated fatty acids on plasma lipids and lipoproteins in man. J. Lipid Res. 26:194-202.

McGandy, R.B. and Hegsted, D.M. 1975. Quantitative effects of dietary fat and cholesterol on serum cholesterol in man. *In* The role of fats in human nutrition. Vergroesen, A.J., ed. Academic Press, New York, pp. 211-230.

McGregor, L., Morazain, R. and Renaud, S. 1980. A comparison of the effects of dietary short and long chain saturated fatty acids on platelet functions, platelet phospholipids, and blood coagulation in rats. Lab Invest. 43:438-442.

McNamara, D.J. 1987. Diet and heart disease: the role of cholesterol and fat. JAOCS, J. Am. Oil Chem. Soc. 64:1565-1574.

McNamara, D.J., Kolb, R., Parker, T.S., Batwin, H., Samuel, P., Brown, C.D. and Ahrens, E.H., Jr. 1987. Heterogeneity of cholesterol homeostasis in man. Response to changes in dietary fat quality and cholesterol quantity. J. Clin. Invest. 79:1729-1739.

Mensink, R.P. and Katan, M.B. 1987. Effect of monounsaturated fatty acids versus complex carbohydrates on high-density lipoproteins in healthy men and women. Lancet 1: 122-124.

Mensink, R.P., de Groot, M.J.M., van den Broeke, L.T., Severijnen-Nobels, A.P., Demacker, P.N.M. and Katan, M.B. 1989. Effects of monounsaturated fatty acids v complex carbohydrates on serum lipoproteins and apoproteins in healthy men and women. Metabolism 38:172-178.

Miller, A.B., Kelly, A., Choi, N.W. Matthews, V., Morgan, R.W., Munan, L., Burch, J.D., Feather, J., Howe, G.R. and Jain, M. 1978. A study of diet and breast cancer. Am. J. Epidemiol. 107: 499-509.

Miller, A.B., Howe, G.R., Jain, M., Craib, K.J.P. and Harrison, L. 1983. Food items and food groups as risk factors in a case-control study of diet and colorectal cancer. Int. J. Cancer 32:155-161.

Mortensen, J.Z., Schmidt, E.B., Nielsen, A.H. and Dyerberg, J. 1983. The effect of N-6 and N-3 polyunsaturated fatty acids on hemostasis, blood lipids and blood pressure. Thromb. Haemostasis 50:543-546.

Nelson, G.J. and Ackman, R.G. 1988. Absorption and transport of fat in mammals with emphasis on n-3 polyunsaturated fatty acids. Lipids 23:1005-1014.

Neuringer, M. and Connor, W.E. 1986. n-3 Fatty acids in the brain and retina: evidence for their essentiality. Nutr. Rev. 44:285-294.

Neuringer, M., Connor, W.E., Van Petten, C. and Barstad, L. 1984. Dietary omega-3 fatty acid deficiency and visual loss in infant rhesus monkeys. J. Clin. Invest. 73:272-276.

Neuringer, M., Anderson, G.J. and Connor, W.E. 1988. The essentiality of n-3 fatty acids for the development and function of the retina and brain. Annu. Rev. Nutr. 8:517-541.

Oliw, E., Granstrom, E. and Anggard, E. 1983. The prostaglandins and essential fatty acids. *In* New comprehensive biochemistry. Vol. 5. Prostaglandins and related substances. Pace-Asciak, C. and Granstrom, E., eds. Elsevier, Amsterdam, pp. 1-44.

Pariza, M.W. 1988. Dietary fat and cancer risk: evidence and research needs. Annu. Rev. Nutr. 8:167-183.

Pariza, M.W. and Boutwell, R.K. 1987. Historical perspective: calories and energy expenditure in carcinogenesis. Am. J. Clin. Nutr. 45:151-156.

Paulsrud, J.R., Pensler, L., Whitten, C.F., Stewart, S. and Holman, R.T. 1972. Essential fatty acid deficiency in infants induced by fat-free intravenous feeding. Am. J. Clin. Nutr. 25:897-904.

Phillipson, B.E., Rothrock, D.W., Connor, W.E., Harris, W.S. and Illingworth, D.R. 1985. Reduction of plasma lipids, lipoproteins, and apoproteins by dietary fish oils in patients with hypertriglyceridemia. N. Engl. J. Med. 312: 1210-1216.

Pietinen, P. and Huttunen, J.K. 1987. Dietary determinants of plasma high-density lipoprotein cholesterol. Am. Heart J. 113:620-625.

Pooling Project Research Group. 1978. Relationship of blood pressure, serum cholesterol, smoking habit, relative weight and ECG abnormalities to incidence of major coronary events. Final report of the Pooling Project. J. Chronic Dis. 31:201-306.

Prentice, R.L., Kakar, F., Hursting, S., Sheppard, L., Klein, R. and Kushi, L.H. 1988. Aspects of the rationale for the Women's Health Trial. J. Nat. Cancer Inst. 80:802-814.

Puska, P., Iacono, J.M., Nissinen, A., Vartiainen, E., Dougherty, R., Pietinen, P., Leino, U., Uusitalo, U., Kuusi, T., Kostiainen, E., Nikkari, T., Seppala, E., Vapaatalo, H. and Huttunen, J.K. 1985. Dietary fat and blood pressure: an intervention study on the effects of a low-fat diet with two levels of polyunsaturated fat. Prev. Med. 14:573-584.

Putnam, J.C., Carleson, S.E., DeVoe, P.W. and Barness, L.A. 1982. The effect of variations in dietary fatty acids on the fatty acid composition of erythrocyte phosphatidylcholine and phosphatidylethanolamine in human infants. Am. J. Clin. Nutr. 36:105-114.

Reddy, B.S. and Cohen, L.A. eds., 1986. Diet, nutrition and cancer: a critical evaluation. Vol. I. Macronutrients and cancer. CRC Press, Boca Raton, Fla.

Reddy, B.S., Cohen, L.A., McCoy, G.D., Hill, P., Weisburger, J.H. and Wynder, E.L. 1980. Nutrition and its relationship to cancer. Adv. Cancer Res. 32:237-345.

Renaud, S. 1987. Nutrients, platelet functions and coronary heart disease. *In* Emerging problems in human nutrition. Vol. 40. Bibliotheca nutritio et dieta. Somogyi, J.C., Renaud, S. and Astier-Dumas, M., eds. Karger, Basel, pp. 1-17.

Renaud, S., Morazain, R., Godsey, F., Dumont, E., Thevenon, C., Martin, J.L. and Mendy, F. 1986a. Nutrients, platelet function and composition in nine groups of French and British farmers. Atherosclerosis 60:37-48.

Renaud, S., Godsey, F., Dumont, E., Thevenon, C., Ortchanian, E. and Martin, J.L. 1986b. Influence of long-term diet modification on platelet function and composition in Moselle farmers. Am. J. Clin. Nutr. 43:136-150.

Renaud, S., Martin, J.L. and Thevenon, C. 1987. Long-term effects of dietary linoleic and linolenic acids on platelet functions and lipemia in man and woman. *In* Proceedings of the AOCS short course on polyunsaturated fatty acids and eicosanoids. Lands, W.E.M., ed. American Oil Chemists' Society, Champaign, I1, pp. 56-61.

Rohan, T.E., McMichael, A.J. and Baghurst, P.A. 1988. A population-based case-control study of diet and breast cancer in Australia. Am. J. Epidemiol. 128: 478-489.

Rose, D.P., Boyar, A.P., Cohen, C. and Strong, L.E. 1987a. Effect of a low-fat diet on hormone levels in women with cystic breast disease. I. Serum steroids and gonadotropins. J. Nat. Cancer Inst. 78:623-626.

Rose, D.P., Cohen, L.A., Berke, B. and Boyar, A.P. 1987b. Effect of a low-fat diet on hormone levels in women with cystic breast disease II. Serum radioimmunoassayable prolactin and growth hormone and bioactive lactogenic hormones. J. Nat. Cancer Inst. 78:627-631.

Sanders, T.A.B. and Roshanai, F. 1983. The influence of different types of ω-3 polyunsaturated fatty acids on blood lipids and platelet function in healthy volunteers. Clin. Sci. 64:91-99.

Sanders, T.A.B., Ellis, F.R. and Dickerson, J.W.T. 1978. Studies of vegans: the fatty acid composition of plasma choline phosphoglycerides, erythrocytes, adipose tissue, and breast milk, and some indicators of susceptibility to ischemic heart disease in vegans and omnivore controls. Am. J. Clin. Nutr. 31:805-813.

Sanders, T.A.B., Vickers, M. and Haines, A.P. 1981. Effect on blood lipids and hemostasis of a supplement of cod-liver oil, rich in eicosapentaenoic and docosahexaenoic acids, in healthy young men. Clin. Sci. 61:317-324.

Sanders, T.A.B., Sullivan, D.R., Reeve, J. and Thompson, G.R. 1985. Triglyceride-lowering effect of marine polyunsaturates in patients with hypertriglyceridemia. Arteriosclerosis 5:459-465.

Schonfeld, G. 1988. Dietary treatment of hyperlipidemia. Clin. Chem. 34(Suppl. 8B):B111-B114.

Schonfeld, G., Patsch, W., Rudel, L.L., Nelson, C., Epstein, M. and Olson, R.E. 1982. Effects of dietary cholesterol and fatty acids on plasma lipoproteins. J. Clin. Invest. 69:1072-1080.

Senti, F.R., ed. 1985. Health aspects of dietary trans fatty acids. Life Sciences Research Office, Federation of American Societies for Experimental Biology, Bethesda, Md.

Siess, W., Roth, P., Scherer, B., Kurzmann, I., Bohlig, B. and Weber, P.C. 1980. Platelet-membrane fatty acids, platelet aggregation, and thromboxane formation during a mackerel diet. Lancet 1:441-444.

Sirtori, C.R., Tremoli, E., Gatti, E., Montanari, G., Sirtori, M., Colli, S., Gianfranceschi, G., Maderna, P., Dentone, C.A., Testolin, G. and Galli, C. 1986. Controlled evaluation of fat intake in the Mediterranean diet: comparative activities of olive oil and corn oil on plasma lipids and platelets in high-risk patients. Am. J. Clin. Nutr. 44:635-642.

Stallones, R.A. 1983. Ischemic heart disease and lipids in blood and diet. Annu. Rev. Nutr. 3:155-185.

Stamler, J. 1983. Nutrition-related risk factors for the atherosclerotic diseases - present status. Prog. Biochem. Pharmacol. 19:245-308.

Stamler, J., Wentworth, D. and Neaton, J.D. 1986. Is relationship between serum cholesterol and risk of premature death from coronary heart disease continuous and graded? J. Am. Med. Assoc. 256:2823-2828.

Stemmermann, G.N., Nomura, A.M.Y. and Heilbrun, L.K. 1984. Dietary fat and the risk of colorectal cancer. Cancer Res. 44:4633-4637.

Sullivan, D.R., Sanders, T.A.B., Trayner, I.M. and Thompson, G.R. 1986. Paradoxical elevation of LDL apoprotein B levels in hypertriglyceridaemic patients and normal subjects ingesting fish oil. Atherosclerosis 61:129-134.

Tannenbaum, A. and Silverstone, H. 1953. Nutrition in relation to cancer. Adv. Cancer Res. 1:451-501.

Thorngren, M. and Gustafson, A. 1981. Effects of 11-week increase in dietary eicosapentaenoic acid on bleeding time, lipids and platelet aggregation. Lancet 2:1190-1193.

Tinoco, J., Babcock, R., Hincenbergs, I., Medwadowski, B., Miljanich, P. and Williams, M.A. 1979. Linolenic acid deficiency. Lipids 14:166-173.

Toniolo, P., Riboli, E., Protta, F., Charrel, M. and Cappa, A.P.M. 1989. Calorie-providing nutrients and risk of breast cancer. J. Nat. Cancer Inst. 81:278-286.

Tunstall-Pedoe, H., Smith, W.C.S., Crombie, I.K. and Thomson, M. 1986. Polyunsaturated fat and coronary heart disease. Lancet 2:344-345.

Tuyns, A.J., Kaaks, R. and Haelterman, M. 1988. Colorectal cancer and the consumption of foods: a case-control study in Belgium. Nutr. Cancer 11:189-204.

U.S. National Research Council. Assembly of Life Sciences. Committee on Diet, Nutrition and Cancer. 1982. Diet, nutrition and cancer. National Academy Press, Washington, D.C.

Verrault, R., Brisson, J., Deschenes, L., Naud, F., Meyer, F. and Belanger, L. 1988. Dietary fat in relation to prognostic indicators in breast cancer. J. Nat. Cancer Inst. 80:819-825.

Von Schacky, C. 1987. Prophylaxis of atherosclerosis with marine omega-3 fatty acids. A comprehensive strategy. Ann. Intern. Med. 107:890-899.

Von Schacky, C. and Weber, P.C. 1985. Metabolism and effects on platelet function of the purified eicosapentaenoic and docosahexaenoic acids in humans. J. Clin. Invest. 76:2446-2450.

Weinsier, R.L. and Norris, D. 1985. Recent developments in the etiology and treatment of hypertension: dietary calcium, fat and magnesium. Am. J. Clin. Nutr. 42:1331-1338.

Weisweiler, P., Janetschek, P. and Schwandt, P. 1985. Influence of polyunsaturated fats and fat restriction on serum lipoproteins in humans. Metabolism 34:83-87.

Welsch, C.W. 1987. Enhancement of mammary tumorigenesis by dietary fat: review of potential mechanisms. Am. J. Clin. Nutr. 45:192-202.

Willett, W.C., Stampfer, M.J., Colditz, G.A., Rosner, B.A., Hennekens, C.H. and Speizer, F.E. 1987. Dietary fat and the risk of breast cancer. N. Engl. J. Med. 316:22-28.

Willis, A.L., ed. 1987. CRC handbook of eicosanoids: prostaglandins and related lipids. Vol. 1. Chemical and biochemical aspects. Part A. CRC Press, Boca Raton, Fla.

Cholesterol

Cholesterol: Function, Metabolism

Cholesterol is a fatty substance with an ubiquitous distribution in animals, in which it is a major structural component of cellular membranes (Myant 1981).

This 27-carbon steroid is synthesized from acetate and built up from the assembly of isoprene units through numerous metabolic steps in virtually all animal cells (Bloch 1965; Myant 1981). The reduction of hydroxy-methyl-glutarate (HMG) to mevalonate by HMG-Coenzyme A reductase is a critical step, being the major site of inhibition of cholesterol synthesis via negative feedback. Another critical step is the 7-alpha-hydroxylation of cholesterol by cholesterol-7-alpha-hydroxylase, the rate-limiting step in bile acid synthesis (bile acids are hydroxylated derivatives of the 24-carbon cholane nucleus with strong detergent properties). Liver and intestine are the most active tissues for the synthesis of cholesterol. The endogenous sources of cholesterol may represent as much as 70% to 80% of the total cholesterol. Cholesterol synthesis averages 11 mg per kg body weight per day or 770 mg for a 70 kg man on a low cholesterol diet (i.e. less than 300 mg/day) (McNamara 1987) but has ranged from 730 to 1700 mg (Nestel *et al.* 1969). The total cholesterol content of the body is roughly 1 g/kg, with 23 g in the plasma pool and 43 g in a slowly exchangeable pool that includes adipose tissue and skeletal muscle (Nestel *et al.* 1969; Myant 1981). The cholesterol distribution in the bulk tissues of man tends to increase with age (Crouse *et al.* 1972).

Cholesterol is an important precursor to key biological substances. In the liver, it is converted to bile acids which are necessary for fat absorption. In the adrenals, it yields the anti-inflammatory glucocorticoids, cortisone and hydrocortisone, the sodium-regulating aldosterone and desoxycorticosterone, as well as progesterone (also synthesized by all steroid-producing glands including ovaries, placenta and corpus luteum). In the ovaries and testes cholesterol is also a precursor for estrogens and androgens essential for normal sexual function. In the skin a precursor of cholesterol, 7 dehydro-cholesterol, is converted to vitamin D_3 necessary for the homeostasis of calcium-phosphate metabolism in the body. These metabolic pathways are minor in terms of total cholesterol economy. Several cholesterol precursors also branch off to contribute to various metabolic pathways leading to acetyl Co A, fatty acids, ubiquinones, dolichol, etc.

Cholesterol is in the free form in membranes, myelin and bile. In liver, adrenals, plasma and other organs, the functional hydroxyl group in the three position may be esterified with fatty acids of various chain length and saturation to yield the less polar cholesteryl esters. The major enzyme responsible for cholesterol esterification in plasma is lecithin:cholesterol acyl transferase (LCAT) which transfers a fatty acid (usually an unsaturated acid) from the two position of phospholipids to cholesterol. Cholesteryl esters (CE) represent a transport form as well as a storage form of cholesterol. The more polar sulfated esters of cholesterol have a role in membrane stabilization, sperm physiology and steroid hormone synthesis by the adrenals (Roberts *et al.* 1964; Huang *et al.* 1981; Langlais *et al.* 1981).

An understanding of cholesterol absorption, transport and metabolism is necessary to appreciate the relationships between dietary cholesterol, plasma cholesterol and the pathogenesis of atherosclerosis (Mahley 1979; Davignon *et al.* 1983; Mahley and Innerarity 1983; Grundy 1986). The average North American adult ingests 400 to 500 mg/day of cholesterol (range 200-2000 mg/d) and another 800 to 1200 mg/day enters the intestine in bile. The absorption of cholesterol ranges from 30% to 60% of that entering the intestine. Newly absorbed cholesterol, which is insoluble in the aqueous plasma phase, must be transported by lipoproteins, an association of amphipathic surface components (phospholipids, free cholesterol and proteins) and a non-polar lipid core (triacylglycerols and cholesteryl esters).

Cholesterol (free and esterified) is incorporated into chylomicrons in the intestinal mucosa for transport through the lymph into the circulation. These particles, rich in exogenous triacylglycerols, have apolipoprotein (apo) B-48 and apo Cs as their major surface protein components when they are formed. Apo B is essential for their passage into the lymph and apo CII is an activator of lipoprotein lipase (LPL), the enzyme responsible for their clearance from plasma at the surface of capillary endothelium. The triacylglycerols are gradually hydrolyzed to fatty acids and glycerol, while most of the cholesterol remains with the resulting chylomicron remnants. These smaller lipoprotein particles, after losing their apo C and acquiring apo E in plasma, are cleared by liver apo E receptors (remnant receptor) (and probably by the B,E or low density lipoprotein (LDL)-receptor also). An atherogenic potential has been ascribed to these remnant particles (Zilversmit 1973; Chung *et al.* 1987).

Very low density lipoproteins (VLDL) are the major carriers of endogenous triacylglycerols synthesized in the liver. VLDL with apo B 100, apo Cs and apo E on their surface undergo gradual lipolysis in plasma under the action of LPL and hepatic triacylglycerol lipase to yield VLDL remnants, some associated with IDL (intermediate density lipoproteins). The latter, also potentially atherogenic, have only apo E and apo B 100 as their surface apolipoproteins. They may be removed directly by the liver via the apo E or the apo B,E receptor (one way to return cholesterol to the liver) or degraded further to smaller low density lipoproteins, the major cholesterol-carrying lipoproteins of plasma. Hepatic triacylglycerol lipase is apparently involved more actively in this last stage of the VLDL catabolic cascade.

Low density lipoproteins constitute the catabolic endpoint of VLDL, although a small amount may also be directly produced by the liver. Their only surface protein is apo B 100, the ligand for interaction with the apo B,E (or LDL) receptor, necessary for their removal from circulation (Brown and Goldstein 1986). The liver, rich in high affinity LDL-receptors, plays the major role in LDL removal, but about one-third may be cleared by a non-receptor-mediated pathway in a variety of tissues. Altered or "modified" LDL may be taken up by macrophages either via the "acetyl LDL receptor" or via an LDL-receptor when it is turned on (Goldstein *et al.* 1979; Gianturco *et al.* 1985). LDL transport over two-thirds of plasma cholesterol and are considered to be the most atherogenic lipoprotein fraction.

Cholesterol transported to peripheral tissues with LDL must be returned to the liver for excretion as bile acids or free cholesterol. This "reverse cholesterol transport" is ascribed to high density lipoproteins (HDL), and confers an antiatherogenic role to these particles (Miller and Miller 1975; Miller *et al.* 1981). Free cholesterol, on the surfaces of cells or lipoproteins, may be transferred to HDL where it is esterified by LCAT (activated by apo AI) and moves to the core of the lipoprotein. CE may be transferred to other lipoproteins, especially VLDL, in exchange for triacylglycerols with the help of a cholesterol-ester transfer protein (Hesler *et al.* 1988).

Cholesterol metabolism is finely regulated, and in the steady state the input (dietary plus endogenous production) is equal to the output (essentially fecal excretion as acidic and neutral sterols). Regulation occurs at many sites (absorption, synthesis, transport, catabolism) but cell surface receptors play a major role in this process. Cholesterol entering the liver through a still ill-defined "unregulated" apo E receptor (remnant receptor) may down-regulate the activity of the LDL-receptor on the liver cell surface, leading to a reduced catabolism of LDL particles and an increase in plasma LDL-cholesterol. Hepatic cholesterol may also inhibit endogenous synthesis of cholesterol to keep hepatic concentrations at optimum levels through a direct effect on HMG CoA reductase.

It may be partially converted into bile acids (stimulation of 7-alpha-hydroxylase activity), be secreted into bile as free cholesterol, be stored in situ as cholesteryl esters (mostly oleate) by enhancing the activity of Acyl-CoA:Cholesterol-Acyltransferase (ACAT), or be incorporated into VLDL. The cellular cholesterol balance is finely tuned by the LDL-receptor. The binding of LDL to the LDL-receptors in the coated pits of the cell plasma membrane is the first step in the cellular cholesterol pathway described by Brown and Goldstein (1986). In the absence of exogenous cholesterol, cells continue to thrive, relying more heavily on endogenous synthesis. In the absence of LDL-receptors, only scavenger pathways are operative to clear LDL from the plasma. In the normal situation there is an enterohepatic recirculation of bile acids, which are 95% reabsorbed in the distal third of the small intestine. Some drugs, as well as dietary constituents, may interfere with the reabsorption of bile salts.

Plasma Cholesterol and Atherosclerosis, a Causal Relationship?

Atherosclerosis is a multifactorial disorder resulting from a complex interplay between environment, genes and the arterial wall (Davignon 1977; Ross 1981; Davignon *et al.* 1983; Steinberg 1983). Three key elements are necessary for its pathogenesis:

- Injury to the endothelium
- Proliferative intimal response of the arterial wall (blood monocyte derived macrophages and smooth muscle cells migrating from the media)
- Lipid infiltration (mostly cholesterol derived from circulating plasma LDL).

A large number of factors promote or enhance the susceptibility to atherosclerosis. In an exhaustive survey of the literature, Hopkins and Williams (1981) identified 246 such "risk factors", new ones being added to the list every year (Hopkins and Williams 1986). Their relative impact on atherogenesis, however, differs widely and some are operative only in rare clinical or ecological contexts. The classical risk factors derived from a wide range of case control, cross-sectional and prospective epidemiological studies remain the major determinants to contend with in practical terms: hyperlipidemia, hypertension, cigarette smoking, and diabetes. An excess in dietary saturated fats and cholesterol, the male sex and aging are also major contributors.

Plasma cholesterol has been closely linked to the atherogenic process and considered to be etiologically related on the following basis (Davignon *et al.* 1983):

1. Cholesterol which accumulates in the atheromatous lesions is derived mainly from plasma LDL. This has been shown both in experimental animals and in man.
2. Measures that increase plasma cholesterol levels can induce atherosclerotic lesions in animals — not only in herbivorous and susceptible species (rabbits) but also in omnivorous animals (pigs) and in non-human primates. A high dietary intake of cholesterol and saturated fat has been uniformly used to produce atherosclerosis in animals (Stehbens 1986). The human species, with the highest prevalence of "spontaneous" atherosclerosis, and inordinately high levels of plasma cholesterol early in life, is not an exception. Interestingly, like man, susceptible species transport most of their plasma cholesterol in the form of LDL-cholesterol (pigs, monkeys) whereas in the resistant species (rats, dogs) cholesterol is mostly associated with the HDL fraction.
3. In experiments carried out with pigs (Lee *et al.* 1974) cholesterol itself was found to affect the endothelium (mitotic activity, increased permeability) as early as three days after initiation of cholesterol feeding.
4. Measures aimed at reducing plasma cholesterol levels in experimental hypercholesterolemia and atherosclerosis, especially in primates, have been shown to reduce the size of arterial lesions (Armstrong and Megan 1972; Kokatnur *et al.* 1975; Armstrong 1976; DePalma *et al.* 1979; Srinivasan *et al.* 1980; Clarkson *et al.* 1981; Wissler and Vesselinovitch 1983).
5. Whatever the experimental model, even endothelial injury from repeated trauma by an indwelling catheter in the artery of a normolipidemic rabbit (Moore 1973), it is cholesterol which accumulates in the intima.
6. Prospective and comparative epidemiologic studies have strikingly related the occurrence of atherosclerotic vascular disease to serum cholesterol levels (Gordon 1970; Kannel *et al.* 1971, 1979, 1986; Nichols *et al.* 1976; Pooling Project Research Group 1978; Mahley 1979; Goldbourt *et al.* 1985; Stamler *et al.* 1986; Stamler 1987; Stamler and Shekelle 1988). The risk of developing coronary artery disease is an exponential function of the plasma cholesterol (or LDL-cholesterol levels) and the steepness of the slope of this exponential is greatly accentuated by the combination of other risk factors.
7. Patients with familial hyperlipoproteinemias, and especially with hereditary forms of hypercholesterolemia, are more likely to develop atherosclerosis and its complications. The severity and prematurity of atherosclerotic vascular disease is a function of the plasma levels of cholesterol and LDL-cholesterol (Brown and Goldstein 1986). Homozygous familial hypercholesterolemia in man with no LDL-receptor for the normal catabolism of LDL-cholesterol is a dramatic illustration of this relationship. An inbred rabbit with virtually no LDL-receptors on the cell surface (Watanabe 1980) has provided an experimental model reproducing faithfully this human disease (Goldstein *et al.* 1983).
8. A direct relationship between LDL-cholesterol levels and the extensiveness of fatty streak formation has now been demonstrated in children and young adults from autopsy studies carried out in subjects participating in the Bogalusa Heart Study who eventually died accidentally (Newman *et al.* 1986). This relationship was found to exist from the lowest levels of LDL-cholesterol. Not all fatty streaks, however, evolve to become plaques (Strong and McGill 1969).
9. Similarly, in man, reduction of plasma cholesterol by diet (Miettinen *et al.* 1972; Hjermann *et al.* 1981) and drugs (Coronary Drug Project Research Group 1975; Lipid Research Clinics Program 1984; Nikkila *et al.* 1984; Blankenhorn *et al.* 1987; Frick *et al.* 1987) decreases the risk of symptomatic coronary artery disease. No effect on total mortality was observed but these studies were not designed to test this effect. In a follow-up study of patients treated with niacin in the Coronary Drug Project, Canner *et al.* (1986) did find an effect on total mortality after 15 years. Meta-analysis of pooled clinical trials has emphasized the benefits of cholesterol lowering on coronary artery disease mortality (Peto *et al.* 1985).

There is now direct evidence that reducing plasma cholesterol can retard the progression or induce regression of atherosclerosis in peripheral arteries (Ost and Stenson 1967; Zelis *et al.* 1970; Basta *et al.* 1976; Barndt *et al.* 1977; Olsson *et al.* 1982; Duffield *et al.* 1983), coronary arteries (Kuo *et al.* 1979; Buchwald *et al.* 1983; Nash *et al.* 1983; Nikkila *et al.* 1984; Brenksike *et al.* 1984; Levy *et al.* 1984; Arntzenius *et al.* 1985; Blankenhorn *et al.* 1987) and coronary artery bypass grafts (Blankenhorn *et al.* 1987). The evidence is derived from both anecdotal (Ost and Stenson 1967; Basta *et al.* 1976; Buchwald *et al.* 1983; Nash *et al.* 1983) and controlled (Kuo *et al.* 1979; Duffield *et al.* 1983; Brensike *et al.* 1984; Nikkila *et al.* 1984; Arntzenius *et al.* 1985; Blankenhorn *et al.* 1987) studies. Several other trials are still in progress: partial ileal bypass trial (Buchwald *et al.* 1982), probucol-cholestyramine trial (PQRST) (Walldius *et al.* 1988), lovastatin trial etc.

Attention should also be given to the reduction in the incidence of coronary artery disease over the past 20 years in the USA, which constitutes a "natural experiment". Goldman and Cook (1984) have identified and assessed the relative contributions of the factors that determined this decrease. They calculated that of the 21% reduction in coronary artery disease mortality occurring between 1968 and 1976, 30% was attributable to the lowering of plasma cholesterol, and 24% to the cessation of cigarette smoking, whereas the control of high blood pressure accounted only for 7% of the decline. The hypothesis that this decrease in coronary artery disease mortality is related to a reduction in coronary atherosclerosis is supported by data derived from autopsy studies in New Orleans, conducted during the same time span. Solberg and Strong (1983) found that among white men in New Orleans, who had died of an accident, the percentage of raised lesions in the coronary tree at autopsy was lower between 1969 and 1972 than the percentage found in patients of comparable age and studied between 1960 and 1964. Between these periods there were major changes in dietary habits in the USA: a major decline in the consumption of butter, eggs and animal fat, and an increase in the consumption of vegetable fat (Stephen 1988). Similar trends for the decline of coronary artery disease mortality have been observed in Canada (Nicholls *et al.* 1981, 1986; Davies *et al.* 1988) with concomitant dietary changes (Robbins and Robichon-Hunt 1986). In summary, the major arguments in support of the causal relationship of plasma cholesterol (and more accurately LDL-cholesterol) to atherosclerosis come from the fact that cholesterol is a major component of the lesion, that raising cholesterol increases arterial wall involvement with atherosclerosis, and that lowering cholesterol has the opposite effect. Thus the lipid hypothesis appears to be proven (Simons 1984).

Caveats

Given the current state of knowledge, it is an over-simplification to focus entirely on cholesterol. Myocardial infarction and coronary artery disease occur in the absence of hyperlipidemia in about 40% of subjects (Davignon *et al.* 1977) and if plasma cholesterol is a good discriminant for risk of coronary artery disease across populations (Keys 1970), it is a poor one within a given population (Kannel *et al.* 1979; Davignon *et al.* 1980). Lipoproteins are the natural vehicle for the transport of cholesterol in the circulation. Although cholesterol remains a central element in atherogenesis, the composition and nature of its carrier lipoprotein is as much a determinant of its atherogenic potential as its concentration in plasma. Thus, large cholesterol-enriched VLDL (Gianturco *et al.* 1985; Eisenberg 1987), LDL with a high triacylglycerol content (Kakis *et al.* 1983) or HDL with phospholipids rich in saturated fatty acids (Miettinen *et al.* 1982) have been ascribed an atherogenic potential and are considered new indicators of coronary artery disease risk.

In recent years, the protective role of HDL (Miller and Miller 1975; Davignon *et al.* 1983) and the value of the LDL/HDL ratio as an atherogenic index (Castelli 1977) have been emphasized. LDL are instrumental in delivering cholesterol to the tissues and HDL in retrieving it. Hypoalphalipoproteinemia (low HDL levels) has been recognized as a condition often (Vergani and Bettale 1981; Davignon *et al.* 1983), but not always (Davignon *et al.* 1986), associated with an increased coronary artery disease risk, and HDL subfractions differ in terms of the relative protection they afford (Miller *et al.* 1981; Fielding and Fielding 1982; Puchois *et al.* 1985; Barbaras *et al.* 1987; Koren *et al.* 1987).

Much attention is now given to the role of apolipoproteins in mediating coronary artery disease risk (Brunzell *et al.* 1984; Thompson 1984). The apolipoproteins on the surface of the lipoproteins not only play a role in maintaining the lipids in "solution" in the aqueous plasma, but determine the metabolic fate of the lipoproteins (Mahley *et al.* 1984). Apo B is considered an independent coronary artery disease risk factor from studies on total plasma apo B and LDL-apo B (Sniderman 1988). The protective role of HDL has been attributed to apo AI (Fruchart *et al.* 1982; Norum *et al.* 1982; Schaefer *et al.* 1982; Maciejko *et al.* 1983; Noma *et al.* 1983) and the apo B/apo AI ratio has been considered a good predictor of risk, especially in individuals with normal or near normal LDL-cholesterol (Avogaro *et al.* 1979; Fruchart *et al.* 1982; Noma *et al.* 1983). There is increasing evidence that apolipoprotein E, a polymorphic apolipoprotein determining six phenotypes in the population and coded by three alleles, modulates the expression of hyperlipidemia (Davignon *et al.* 1988). The epsilon 2 allele is associated with lower and the epsilon 4 allele with higher plasma LDL-cholesterol concentrations (Sing and Davignon 1985) and many arguments are currently raised in support of the hypothesis that the presence of the epsilon 4 allele constitutes another coronary artery disease risk factor (Davignon *et al.* 1987; Davignon *et al.* 1988). Lp(a) is another polymorphic lipoprotein that is an important risk factor when present in excess (Rhoads *et al.* 1986).

Finally, altered lipoproteins are known to be taken up more readily by the macrophage "acetyl-LDL-receptor" (Goldstein *et al.* 1979; Steinberg 1983; Gianturco *et al.* 1985). Accumulation of cholesterol in the phagocytic cells of the intima (whether monocyte-derived or smooth muscle cell-derived) is the basis for the formation of foam cells and fatty streaks, perhaps the earliest precursor of the atheromatous plaque. We know now that oxidized LDL (Parthasarathy *et al.* 1987) and glycosylated LDL (Witztum *et al.* 1981) are preferentially taken up by the macrophage receptors rather than by the LDL-receptors. These modified lipoproteins might be a key factor in the atherogenic process as proposed by Steinberg and co-workers (Witztum *et al.* 1981; Steinberg 1983; Carew *et al.* 1987; Parthasarathy *et al.* 1987). Recent evidence that probucol, a potent antioxidant, can dramatically reduce atheroma formation in the Watanabe rabbit in spite of high LDL-cholesterol levels, strongly supports this hypothesis (Carew *et al.* 1987; Kita *et al.* 1987).

From the foregoing, it would appear that it is now more accurate to speak of the "lipoprotein hypothesis" rather than of the "lipid hypothesis". More than cholesterol is involved in getting cholesterol to accumulate in the arterial wall. Focusing on the central role of cholesterol is important, but it would be naive to neglect the complex interactions that lead to its accumulation.

Dietary Cholesterol

Incorporation of cholesterol into the diet has been a universal means of producing experimental atherosclerosis. There is a large body of evidence in man that plasma cholesterol levels are closely associated with the risk of developing coronary artery disease, and this risk may be reduced by lowering plasma cholesterol. Both dietary saturated fats and cholesterol are capable of increasing plasma cholesterol levels in man but the impact of cholesterol alone is less impressive and subject to marked individual variability (McGill 1979). Adaptive mechanisms are used to prevent accumulation of cholesterol in the body, but their effectiveness also varies greatly from person to person. The atherogenic effect of dietary cholesterol may not be solely linked with its ability to raise plasma cholesterol levels. Alterations of lipoprotein composition and some triacylglycerol-rich lipoproteins occurring in plasma after cholesterol absorption may have an atherogenic potential. In this section we will review the aspects of dietary cholesterol pertinent to the understanding of its role as a risk factor for coronary artery disease, considering in turn dietary sources, impact on plasma cholesterol and lipoproteins, adaptive mechanisms and relation to coronary artery disease in humans.

Dietary Sources

Because of its ubiquitous distribution in animal tissues, dietary sources of cholesterol are numerous and plentiful. Due to the ability of the body to produce its own cholesterol, no nutritional deficiencies attributable to a lack of this substance have been reported. Indeed the Tarahumara Indians, a tribe of the Sierra Madre Occidental Mountains of Mexico, thrive on a diet that averages 75 mg/day (33 mg/day in children) intake of cholesterol, with a mean plasma level of about 137 mg/dL (Connor *et al.* 1978). About half of the world population consumes less that 300 mg of cholesterol per day without obvious adverse effects. Diseases associated with low plasma cholesterol levels, such as chronic debilitating diseases, cancer, or abnormalities of lipoprotein transport, such as abetalipoproteinemia (Malloy and Kane 1982) are not improved by cholesterol supplementation.

On the other hand, diets high in cholesterol have been closely linked with atherogenesis and coronary artery disease incidence (Connor *et al.* 1961, 1964; Nichols *et al.* 1976; Mahley 1979; Shekelle *et al.* 1981). It is thus reasonable to consider lowering dietary cholesterol in countries where dietary overindulgence is a contributing factor to this major cause of mortality. Since cholesterol is closely associated with animal fat, it has been difficult to dissociate the atherogenic effect of cholesterol from that of saturated fats in the diet.

Cholesterol in the diet comes from animal products. The major sources are egg yolk, organ meats (liver, sweetbreads and brain), animal flesh (beef, veal, pork, lamb, chicken, fish), milk and milk products (cheese, cream, ice cream, butter...). Muscle and adipose tissue have approximately the same concentration on a wet-weight basis. Animal fat is also rich in saturated fatty acids, but fish, and other seafoods, though relatively rich in cholesterol, contain polyunsaturated fatty acids of the n-3 series.

A medium size egg contains 250 mg of cholesterol. Egg consumption may contribute from 18% (Grundy *et al.* 1988) to 39% of the daily dietary cholesterol intake (McGill 1979). It differs from certain other animal products in that it adds few calories (3%) and little saturated fat (2%) to the diet of the Western developed countries (McGill 1979).

There have been controversies in the past regarding inclusion of shellfish in a cholesterol-lowering diet. Sterols other than cholesterol are present in shellfish such as clams, oysters and scallops, and their cholesterol content is considerably lower than previously believed (Connor and Lin 1982; Mondeika 1985; Gregg *et al.* 1986). Shellfish are relatively low in calories and fat. The only sterol found in shrimps, lobster and crab, however, is cholesterol.

Cholesterol consumption varies between 350 to 600 mg/day in industrialized countries and has been changing over the years in many different populations. In Japan it went from 93 mg/day to 381 mg/day from 1950 to 1968 (Wen and Gershoff 1973) and was 464 mg/day on average in the Ni-Hon-San study (Marmot *et al.* 1975). In the U.S. it has been steadily declining over the last 30 years (Grundy *et al.* 1988) and men consume more cholesterol than women (Gordon 1970; Nichols *et al.* 1976). In Canada the average cholesterol intake was 442 mg/day in 1986 and averaged 456 for men and 328 for women in studies carried out within the last 10 years (Lloyd LE, personal communication). The average weekly egg consumption is 4.6 eggs per capita.

Dietary Cholesterol and Plasma Cholesterol in Humans

Many short-term experiments have been conducted to evaluate the effect of cholesterol intake on plasma cholesterol levels in man. Although excessive egg consumption has been anecdotally associated with the development of severe hypercholesterolemia and xanthomatosis (Rhomberg and Braunsteiner 1976), the effect of cholesterol feeding on plasma cholesterol has been rather moderate, variable, and a matter of controversy (Wells and Bronte-Stewart 1963; McGill 1979; Myant 1981; Roberts *et al.* 1981; Grundy *et al.* 1988). It appears that carefully controlled studies carried out under metabolic ward conditions (Beveridge *et al.* 1960; Connor 1961; Connor *et al.* 1961, 1964; Steiner *et al.* 1962; Erickson *et al.* 1964; Hegsted *et al.* 1965; Keys *et al.* 1965; Quintao *et al.* 1971; Mattson *et al.* 1972) or using a double-blind crossover design (Roberts *et al.* 1981) leave little doubt that increasing dietary cholesterol raises plasma total cholesterol in most people. A review of 26 experiments from 10 studies involving 193 subjects with a wide range of dietary cholesterol comparisons (0 to 4800 mg/d) showed an average increase of 33 mg/dL or 19% in plasma cholesterol for intakes from 0-116 mg to 241-4800 mg/day of cholesterol (Roberts *et al.* 1981). The lack of such an effect in some (Slater *et al.* 1976; Porter *et al.* 1977; Flynn *et al.* 1979) but not all (Sacks *et al.* 1984) outpatient studies or in hospitalized patients not in metabolic ward conditions (Kummerow *et al.* 1977) may be related to the variability in response among individuals, the lack of sensitivity of the design to detect a small effect, failure to achieve a steady state on a given regimen, the lack of control on the behavior of the free-living test subjects, the diminishing response at higher intakes of cholesterol, too short a duration of the period of exposure, or interference from variation in amounts and types of concomitant fat intake.

There is evidence from several studies that the effect of cholesterol may be dissociated from that of other fats (Mattson *et al.* 1972; Anderson *et al.* 1976; Roberts *et al.* 1981; Applebaum-Bowden *et al.* 1984). Mattson *et al.* (1972) concluded that, in normal men, an increase of 100 mg of cholesterol per 1000 dietary calories caused, on average, a rise in plasma cholesterol concentration of 12 mg/dL. One key experiment performed on six subjects with four diets showed that the effect of adding 725 mg of cholesterol per day was much greater than the effect of type of fat. All subjects responded to dietary cholesterol by an increase in plasma cholesterol of 21 to 49 mg/dL (Connor *et al.* 1964) and an analysis of variance (McGill 1979) showed an independent significant effect of cholesterol (p.<005) but no significant effect of type of fat and no interaction. The lack of interaction between dietary fat and dietary cholesterol on plasma cholesterol (Connor *et al.* 1964; Hegsted *et al.* 1965; Anderson *et al.* 1976) was not consistently found. In one experiment, cholesterol added to butter fat produced a higher elevation in plasma cholesterol than if added to medium chain triacylglycerols (Beveridge *et al.* 1959). In the Faribault study (National Diet-Heart Study 1968), the addition of about 500 mg cholesterol to an unsaturated fat diet resulted in elevations of 4 and 7 mg/dL of plasma cholesterol versus 13 and 14 mg/dL when added to a saturated fat diet.

In general, crystalline cholesterol was less effective at increasing plasma cholesterol than egg yolk cholesterol (McGill 1979). In addition, the effect of dietary cholesterol on plasma cholesterol was more linearly related between 0 to 634 mg/day of intake, tending to plateau after this level (Beveridge *et al.* 1960) and was most evident in population samples consuming low levels of cholesterol to start with (McGill 1979). Whether the response to plasma cholesterol is curvilinear or linear, reaching a plateau or not, is still a matter of controversy (Keys 1984; Hegsted 1986; Grundy *et al.* 1988).

Dietary Cholesterol and Plasma Lipoproteins

Recent studies have focused on the effect of dietary cholesterol on specific lipoprotein or apolipoprotein fractions. This attention has been prompted by the notion that lipoprotein and apolipoprotein concentrations may be better indicators of cardiovascular risk than plasma lipid levels. Dietary intake of cholesterol (and saturated fat) may induce changes in lipoprotein composition, which may be atherogenic, even in the absence of changes in levels of plasma total cholesterol and/or of lipoprotein cholesterol.

All the absorbed cholesterol enters the circulation in chylomicrons (chylos) which are partially degraded into a cholesterol-ester-enriched remnant for which an atherogenic potential has been postulated (Zilversmit 1973). More recent work indicates that lipolytic surface remnants of triacylglycerol-rich lipoproteins (chylos, VLDL) may be a major atherogenic plasma component (Chung *et al.* 1987). Cholesterol feeding increases the plasma levels of these remnants (Mistry *et al.* 1981; Nestel *et al.* 1982) and their ability to be cleared from plasma depends on which isoform of apo E is present on their surface (Weintraub *et al.* 1987). Furthermore, it appears that post prandial lipemia may be prolonged in individuals at risk for coronary artery disease. This latent dyslipoproteinemia has been recorded by measuring plasma lipids at the eighth hour of fasting (De Gennes *et al.* 1972).

The most consistent effect of cholesterol feeding is an increase in LDL-cholesterol which reflects the changes observed in total cholesterol (Applebaum-Bowden *et al.* 1979; Mistry *et al.* 1981; Schonfeld *et al.* 1982; Packard *et al.* 1983; Applebaum-Bowden *et al.* 1984; Sacks *et al.* 1984) with only a few exceptions (Flaim *et al.* 1981; Nestel *et al.* 1982; MacNamara *et al.* 1987). Plasma apo B is concomitantly increased (Cole *et al.* 1983). In healthy subjects this effect is attributed to an increased LDL production rate and a reduced LDL catabolic rate (Packard *et al.* 1983). The reduction in LDL catabolism is associated with a reduction in LDL receptor activity (Mistry *et al.* 1981; Packard *et al.* 1983; Applebaum-Bowden *et al.* 1984). In subjects who are non-responders to a cholesterol load, LDL production rate is not affected (Ginsberg *et al.* 1981). Miettinen and colleagues have obtained preliminary evidence that plasma LDL-cholesterol response to a dietary cholesterol load is a function of apo E polymorphism (Miettinen T., personal communication). Alteration of LDL composition after cholesterol feeding has also been reported. Beynen and Katan (1985) showed that the core becomes enriched in cholesteryl esters at the expense of triacylglycerols and that the ratio of core to surface components increases by 7%. Cholesterol enrichment of LDL in response to cholesterol feeding has been observed in several other studies (Sacks *et al.* 1984; Schonfeld *et al.* 1982).

Total HDL-cholesterol levels are not always significantly affected by cholesterol feeding because of variability in individual response and influence of other dietary components. (Flaim *et al.* 1981; Ginsberg *et al.* 1981; Packard *et al.* 1983; Sacks *et al.* 1984; McNamara 1987). In several studies demonstrating an HDL increase, it is the HDL2 fraction, not the HDL3, that is raised (Mistry *et al.* 1981; Schonfeld *et al.* 1982; Cole *et al.* 1983; Beynen and Katan 1985). The overall lipoprotein change in "responders" is a more pronounced effect on LDL than on HDL so that the LDL/HDL ratio, the atherogenic index, may be increased (Lin and Connor 1980; Tan *et al.* 1980; Schonfeld *et al.* 1982; Cole *et al.* 1983; Sacks *et al.* 1984) or unchanged (Mistry *et al.* 1981; Nestel *et al.* 1982 after two weeks of feeding; McNamara *et al.* 1987) but rarely lowered (Nestel *et al.* 1982 after four weeks; Beynen and Katan 1985). Functional properties of HDL can be altered by cholesterol feeding (Mahley *et al.* 1978; Cole *et al.* 1983). Mahley *et al.* (1978) showed an increased affinity of the HDL fraction for the fibroblast's LDL-receptor after cholesterol feeding, as measured from the displacement of radiolabelled LDL by cold HDL. This effect is independent of the changes induced in total plasma cholesterol and is not accompanied by a change in HDL cholesterol level. It is attributed to a specific increase in an apo E rich HDL1 fraction, such as occurs in animals fed cholesterol. The long-term biological significance of this effect is still a matter of speculation. The study of Cole *et al.* (1983) concurs with these findings and also shows some enrichment of HDL2 in cholesteryl esters on a high-fat, high-cholesterol diet. It has been hypothesized that the HDL increase with a cholesterol load was an attempt to enhance the return of cholesterol to the liver for excretion.

Adaptive Mechanisms to Excess Dietary Cholesterol

Several mechanisms are available to the body for adjusting to changes in the intake of dietary cholesterol. There is variability between populations and among individuals within a population that could be ascribed to genetically determined differences in adaptive mechanisms. Let us consider these adaptive mechanisms.

There is a decreased efficiency of cholesterol absorption in man at high intake of dietary cholesterol, and hypocholesterolemia may occur in malabsorption (Myant 1981). Individual differences in efficiency of cholesterol absorption may explain some of the variability in plasma cholesterol response to cholesterol feeding (McNamara *et al.* 1987). Recently, Kesaniemi and co-workers (1987) have shown an influence of apo E polymorphism on cholesterol absorption. Subjects bearing the epsilon 4 allele (phenotypes E4/4 and E4/3) absorb dietary cholesterol more efficiently than bearers of the epsilon 2 allele (E3/2, E2/2), whereas the common E3/3 individuals have an intermediate efficiency. This is the first account of a genetic influence on individual variation in cholesterol absorption.

When cholesterol is added to the diet, the increase in net absorption of cholesterol leads to a decrease in its rate of synthesis in the whole body (Nestel and Poyser 1976). There has been controversy (Myant 1981) regarding the extent to which cholesterol synthesis in the human body is suppressible, but considerable evidence now shows that cholesterol synthesis in humans is under feedback control by absorbed cholesterol. Although feeding of cholesterol has no effect on bile acid synthesis, the human liver has considerable capacity for increasing the rate at which absorbed cholesterol is re-excreted into the bile as neutral sterol (Quintao *et al.* 1971). Since biliary cholesterol is incompletely reabsorbed, this mechanism results in an increased rate of fecal excretion of neutral steroids of endogenous origin in response to increased absorption of dietary cholesterol. Person-to-person variability in plasma cholesterol response to dietary cholesterol may be due to differences in this adaptive mechanism.

In response to a dietary cholesterol load, what are the mechanisms used to prevent accumulation of cholesterol, and what proportion of them compensate successfully? This has been examined in 50 male volunteers by McNamara *et al.* (1987). The authors found that 69% compensated for the increase in dietary cholesterol with a decreased cholesterol fractional absorption and/or suppression of endogenous cholesterol synthesis. There was an inverse correlation between the amount of dietary cholesterol absorbed (mg/kg per day) and the intracellular cholesterol synthesis in plasma mononuclear cells. Dietary fat quality had a larger and more consistent effect on plasma cholesterol than dietary cholesterol: the reduction due to the shift in P/S from 0.3 to 1.5 was 6%, and to dietary cholesterol 2%. It was concluded that a reduction in dietary cholesterol would benefit 31% of the population who are "noncompensators", i.e. lacking precise feedback control of endogenous cholesterol synthesis. The same authors were of the opinion that reducing dietary cholesterol from 450 to 300 mg/day in the population at large, to lower plasma cholesterol, was not worthwhile. On the other hand the proportion of "responders" to a cholesterol load varies widely among studies from about 20% to 75% (Connor *et al.* 1964; McGill 1979; Jacobs *et al.* 1983; Katan *et al.* 1986).

In this controversial area with its problems inherent in sampling procedure, population selection, associated factors influencing plasma cholesterol and intraindividual variability, it is difficult to get a precise estimate of "responsiveness" or "sensitivity" to a cholesterol load or to a cholesterol restriction. It is worthwhile noting that in the Lipid Research Clinics Coronary Primary Prevention Trial, 6801 subjects with a cholesterol level over 265 mg/dL (and LDL-cholesterol >190 mg/dL) were instructed in a moderately low cholesterol diet; within the next two visits 2156 of these were excluded because their LDL-cholesterol had decreased below 175 mg/dL (Lipid Research Clinics Program 1983). Thus 31.7% of these hypercholesterolemics may be considered "diet responders". Recently, dietary factors relating to cardiovascular risk factors in early life were studied in the Bogalusa Heart Study (Nicklas *et al.* 1988). Data from this study confirmed the relationship between dietary cholesterol and serum, total and LDL-cholesterol levels in young children. Children with high intakes of dietary cholesterol had higher (14 mg/dL at ages four and seven, upper tertile vs lower tertile) serum cholesterol levels than children with lower intakes of cholesterol. Children on high intake of animal fat were heavier. These results indicate that tracking of dietary components and their relationships with cardiovascular disease risk factors can be detected at an early age (Lauer *et al.* 1988).

Chylomicrons constitute the major carriers of cholesterol into the body. Their catabolism leads to the formation of cholesterol-enriched remnant particles which are taken up by the liver apo E receptor. Brown and Goldstein (1986) have proposed that an excessive entry of dietary cholesterol via this pathway leads to the accumulation of cholesterol in the liver cell because the apo E receptor is not regulated (Kovanen *et al.* 1981; Angelin *et al.* 1983). This excessive entry of cholesterol into the liver cell has several consequences: most importantly it down-regulates the LDL (B,E) receptor resulting in a decreased catabolism of LDL-cholesterol and its accumulation in plasma. Several observations support this concept. In cholesterol feeding experiments the changes in plasma LDL-cholesterol levels are inversely related with the LDL receptor activity (Mistry *et al.* 1981; Applebaum-Bowden *et al.* 1984; Kesaniemi *et al.* 1987; Kesaniemi and Miettinen 1987). More recently it was found by Weintraub *et al.* (1987) that apo E polymorphism had an influence on the clearance rate of plasma chylomicron remnants after a fat load test with retinyl palmitate, but not on chylomicron clearance. The bearer of the epsilon 4 allele (phenotypes E4/3 and E4/4) cleared chylomicron remnants more effectively than subjects with the epsilon 2 allele (phenotypes E3/2, E4/2 and E2/2), while individuals with the E3/3 phenotype had an intermediate response. Thus a gene at the apo E locus may have an influence at two sites of cholesterol homeoregulation. There are, however, questions raised regarding regulation of the apo E receptor in humans as opposed to other species (Hoeg *et al.* 1985), and the nature of this receptor (Beisiegel *et al.* 1988). It should be kept in mind that apo E, independently of apo B, is necessary and sufficient for the binding of large triacylglycerol-rich lipoproteins to the LDL-receptor.

Dietary Cholesterol and Atherosclerosis

Experimental Evidence

Dietary factors have long been considered primary suspects in the causation of atherosclerosis and, for over a century now, attention has been focused on cholesterol (Spain 1960, 1966; Davignon 1977; Myant 1981; Davignon *et al.* 1983). As early as 1847, Vogel, a German anatomist, demonstrated that atherosclerotic arteries invariably contained cholesterol. In 1909, Ignatovsky, a Russian army medical officer, noticed that the meat-eating army officers had many more heart attacks than the "vegetarian peasants", and tested the atherogenic potential of meat in the rabbit. His experiment demonstrated that rabbits fed animal products developed aortic atherosclerosis. In 1913, Anitschkow and Chalatow, in a classical series of feeding experiments, were able to ascribe this effect to cholesterol (Anitschkow 1967). As cholesterol rose in the rabbits' plasma with feeding of crystalline cholesterol and fat, atherosclerotic plaques appeared in their arteries, and lipids gradually disappeared from these plaques after discontinuation of cholesterol feeding.

Since then, experimental atherosclerosis has been induced by feeding cholesterol not only in herbivorous and carnivorous species but also in omnivores and in primates closely related to humans (Armstrong and Megan 1972; Clarkson *et al.* 1981; Wissler and Vesselinovitch 1983). It could be induced with large amounts over a short time but also over a longer period, with a diet not far removed in composition from that of the standard North American diet. It was found that resistant species (rats, dogs) transported most of their cholesterol on HDL, whereas susceptible species (pigs and monkeys) transported it in association with LDL, as is the case in humans.

Epidemiological Evidence

Although long-term cholesterol-feeding experiments cannot be carried out in humans to assess atherogenic potential, there is no evidence that the human species is an exception to the rule. As pointed out by Brown and Goldstein (1986), humans are unique in that they have at birth a low cholesterol level like most animal species, but after a short period of exposure to their natural environment, their cholesterol level increases to as much as four times that of most animals. The highest plasma cholesterol levels are observed in industrialized countries, and about 40% of the individuals are killed by atherosclerotic vascular disease. There is evidence that man is probably among the species most susceptible to atherosclerosis and is sensitive to dietary influences.

In Keys' 7-country study, dietary cholesterol was closely linked to coronary artery disease mortality (Keys 1970, 1980). Similarly, a close correlation between average daily cholesterol intake and death rate from coronary artery disease was observed in males aged 55 to 59 from 24 different countries (Connor and Connor 1972). South African Bantu (Bloomberg *et al.* 1958), among whom death from coronary artery disease is exceedingly rare, have a diet very low in fat (average 17% of total energy), and a mean serum cholesterol level of only 166 mg/dL. Similar findings were reported in Japanese, Yemenite Jews, Chinese and Apache Indians. In contrast, in the U.S. where the coronary artery disease death rate is very high, the average fat intake is 40% of energy and the mean serum cholesterol level is close to 250 mg/dL. Similar situations prevail in Canada, England, Sweden and East Finland. Moreover, there is evidence that people who migrate from a country with a low heart disease death rate to one with a high death rate, and adopt the nutritional and cultural patterns of the latter country, tend to acquire a rise in cholesterol level and an increase in the rate of heart attacks (studies of Yemenite Jews and Japanese) (Kato *et al.* 1973; Marmot *et al.* 1975). One of the most demonstrative studies from this standpoint is that of Ni-Hon-San, where dietary cholesterol, levels of plasma cholesterol, and mortality from heart disease increased progressively in Japanese men living in three cultures: Japan, Hawaii and San Francisco (Kato *et al.* 1973; Robertson *et al.* 1977). Exchange of a high-cholesterol, high-saturated-fat diet for one low in both components, between two countries at the extremes of coronary artery disease risk (North Karelia and Naples), resulted in the expected reciprocal changes in plasma cholesterol and other lipid levels (Enholm *et al.* 1982; Ferro-Luzzi *et al.* 1984).

Four published studies with reliable assessment of cholesterol intakes and adjustment for variation in caloric intake have been reviewed by Grundy *et al.* (1988): the Chicago Western Electric (Shekelle *et al.* 1981), the Zutphen (Kromhout and DeLezenne Coulander 1984), the Ireland-Boston (Kushi *et al.* 1985) and the Honolulu studies (Yano *et al.* 1984). All four found a positive association between cholesterol intake and subsequent rates of coronary artery disease. In some studies this association appeared to be independent of plasma cholesterol concentrations, and in the Chicago Western Electric Study the association between dietary cholesterol and cardiovascular risk was independent of dietary saturated fats. The Western Electric Study provides strong supportive evidence for an impact of *dietary* cholesterol on coronary artery disease that is not only independent of levels at baseline, but also of age, body mass index, systolic blood pressure, cigarette smoking, serum cholesterol, alcohol intake and ethnic origin (Shekelle *et al.* 1981). The implications of such studies for the institution of coronary artery disease prevention programmes have been extensively reviewed by Grundy (1986) and by Stamler (1988). After a thorough review of the evidence by panels of experts in the United States and in 17 European countries, recommendations have been made to reduce the dietary intake of cholesterol to less than 300 mg/day (Consensus Conference 1985; European Atherosclerosis Society 1987). In line with these and other recommendations, major national education programmmes to lower cholesterol have been undertaken (National Cholesterol Education Program Expert Panel 1988) and various strategies established (Lewis *et al.* 1986; Canadian Consensus Conference 1988), in spite of the skepticism of a minority (Oliver 1987; McCormick and Skrabanek 1988).

There is no evidence that such levels of dietary cholesterol (300 mg/day) would be deleterious in infants and children. Human breast milk is richer in cholesterol than most milk formulas and the question may be raised whether this exposure to a cholesterol-enriched milk in infancy has advantages for cholesterol homeostasis in later years. A recent study supports the opposite view (Lewis *et al.* 1988): adolescent baboons, breast-fed as infants and exposed later on to an atherogenic diet, developed more severe atherosclerosis than baboons fed formula with a lower cholesterol content during infancy.

Conclusion

In view of the above, it is concluded that reducing the cholesterol intake of the population towards 300 mg/day or less would be beneficial in the longterm for the reduction of mortality from coronary artery disease in this country. This level of cholesterol consumption is readily achieved without apparent harmful effects in a wide variety of low risk populations. There is evidence that reducing plasma cholesterol by 1% may decrease coronary artery disease risk by at least 2% (it is 4% in the Helsinki Heart trial), or grossly, a 1 mg/dL fall would cause a 1% decline in mortality (Grundy *et al.* 1988). According to controlled clinical trials (Mattson *et al.* 1972; Roberts *et al.* 1981), for an energy intake of 2000 kcal, or 8.4 MJ, a 200 mg/day reduction in dietary cholesterol (500 to 300) should lower plasma cholesterol an average of 24 mg/dL and contribute a 24% reduction in mortality from coronary artery disease (not a negligible figure; it would add to the independent effect of saturated fat reduction). Even the lowest estimates of the effect of dietary cholesterol on plasma cholesterol levels (Keys *et al.* 1965) still predict a 5% to 6% fall in coronary artery disease risk, a change that is not trivial when applied to a whole population. A dietary intake of 300 mg/day of cholesterol or less has become the target for the general population of the United States and 17 European countries as part of a concerted effort to lower coronary artery disease mortality (Consensus Conference 1985; European Atherosclerosis Society 1987).

Cholesterol is a basic structural component of the cell membrane that is indispensible for its survival. Virtually all cells in the body are capable of synthesizing cholesterol. The liver is the prime source of the large amounts of cholesterol that are present in bile, reabsorbed in the intestine, transported in plasma and lymph and made available to the cells. Because of that, the human organism may fulfill its need for cholesterol independently of exogenous sources. No deficiencies or diseases attributable to inadequate dietary intake of cholesterol have been found, and no minimal dietary requirements for cholesterol have been established. On the other hand, there is a wealth of information linking an excess in dietary cholesterol intake and high plasma levels of cholesterol with coronary artery disease and atherosclerotic vascular disease.

Dietary intake of cholesterol is highest in industrialized countries with the highest prevalence of coronary artery disease. The intake of cholesterol is, on average, 400 to 500 mg per day in Canada, where there is an overindulgence in foods rich in saturated fats and cholesterol and a high incidence of coronary artery disease. The intake of cholesterol is much lower in countries with a low incidence of coronary artery disease. The "sick population" concept favors an intervention to lower the mean plasma cholesterol of the population to decrease coronary artery disease mortality (towards 190 mg/dL, 4.9 mmol/L, in Canada according to the Canadian Consensus Conference on Cholesterol). This position is strengthened by the fact that individuals with low plasma cholesterol, moving from a low risk area to one of high risk, acquire higher plasma cholesterol levels and become more susceptible to coronary artery disease as they adopt the dietary habits and lifestyle of the high risk areas. "Spontaneous" induction of atherosclerosis is more prevalent in humans than in any other animal species and it is likely that they rank among species most susceptible to dietary-induced atherosclerosis. A direct relationship has recently been established between plasma LDL-cholesterol levels and the extent of arterial fatty streaks in children and young adults. Furthermore, children with high intakes of dietary cholesterol have higher serum LDL-cholesterol levels than children with lower intakes of cholesterol.

For each 100 mg of cholesterol ingested per 1000 kcal, or 4.2 MJ, there is an average increase in plasma cholesterol of 12 mg/dL. This effect appears to be independent of that of saturated fats. A wide range of variability exists in individual responses to a cholesterol load, and genetically determined adaptive mechanisms may in part prevent cholesterol accumulation in the body. Ingestion of cholesterol may release into circulation triglyceride-rich lipoproteins with atherogenic potential during the post-prandial phase without much change in fasting plasma cholesterol, or alter the lipoprotein profile adversely without necessarily increasing total plasma cholesterol. There is epidemiologic evidence that dietary cholesterol has a "direct" atherogenic effect that is independent of plasma cholesterol concentrations and of dietary saturated fats. Also, experimental evidence shows that cholesterol has a direct damaging effect on the arterial endothelium.

Measures (diet and drugs) aimed at reducing cholesterol in conditions where it is elevated were shown to reduce the incidence of coronary artery disease mortality and induce regression of atherosclerotic lesions both in animals and in humans. From epidemiological observations, autopsy studies, and animal experimentation, it is likely that the reduced incidence of coronary artery disease and the regression of atherosclerosis effected by reducing plasma cholesterol in hypercholesterolemic subjects may be extrapolated to individuals with lower cholesterol levels. Animal experimentation and the natural history of hypercholesterolemia in man indicate that the impact of a rise in plasma cholesterol on atherogenesis is a function of level times duration. One may surmise that even a small increase of plasma cholesterol over time may have deleterious effects on the arterial wall. There is no evidence of a detrimental effect of a low cholesterol diet (i.e. ingestion of <300 mg/day).

Recommendations

In view of the current evidence, it is recommended that the cholesterol intake of the Canadian population be reduced. This should apply to all age groups. In infants and children, caution should be taken to ensure that the dietary changes this recommendation entails do not result in an unbalanced diet, deficient in energy and essential nutrients.

References

Anderson, J.T., Grande, F. and Keys, A. 1976. Independence of the effects of cholesterol and degree of saturation of the fat in the diet on serum cholesterol in man. Am. J. Clin. Nutr. 29:1184-1189.

Angelin, B., Raviola, C.A., Innerarity, T.L. and Mahley, R.W. 1983. Regulation of hepatic lipoprotein receptors in the dog. Rapid regulation of apolipoprotein B,E receptors, but not of apolipoprotein E receptors, by intestinal lipoproteins and bile acids. J. Clin. Invest. 71:816-831.

Anitschkow, N.N. 1967. A history of experimentation on arterial atherosclerosis in animals. *In* Cowdry's arteriosclerosis: a survey of the problem. 2nd ed. Blumenthal, H.T., ed. C.C. Thomas, Springfield, Ill., pp. 21-44.

Applebaum-Bowden, D., Hazzard, W.R., Cain, J., Cheung, M.C., Kushwaha, R.S. and Albers, J.J. 1979. Short-term egg yolk feeding in humans. Increase in apolipoprotein B and low density lipoprotein cholesterol. Atherosclerosis 33:385-396.

Applebaum-Bowden, D., Haffner, S.M., Hartsook, E., Luk, K.H., Albers, J.J. and Hazzard, W.R. 1984. Down-regulation of the low-density lipoprotein receptor by dietary cholesterol. Am. J. Clin. Nutr. 39:360-367.

Armstrong, M.L. 1976. Evidence of regression of atherosclerosis in primates and man. Postgrad. Med. J. 52:456-461.

Armstrong, M.L. and Megan, M.B. 1972. Lipid depletion in atheromatous coronary arteries in rhesus monkeys after regression diets. Circ. Res. 30:675-680.

Arntzenius, A.C., Kromhout, D., Barth, J.D., Reiber, J.H.C., Bruschke, A.V.G., Buis, B., van Gent, C.M., Kempen-Voogd, N., Strikwerda, S. and Van Der Velde, E.A. 1985. Diet, lipoproteins and the progression of coronary atherosclerosis: the Leiden Intervention Trial. N. Engl. J. Med. 312:805-811.

Avogaro, P., Bittolo Bon, G., Cazzolato, G. and Quinci, G.B. 1979. Are apolipoproteins better discriminators than lipids for atherosclerosis? Lancet 1:901-903.

Barbaras, R., Puchois, P., Fruchart, J.C. and Ailhaud, G. 1987. Cholesterol efflux from cultured adipose cells is mediated by LpA_I particles but not by $LpA_I{:}A_{II}$ particles. Biochem. Biophys. Res. Commun. 142:63-69.

Barndt, R., Jr., Blankenhorn, D.H., Crawford, D.W. and Brooks, S.H. 1977. Regression and progression of early femoral atherosclerosis in treated hyperlipoproteinemic patients. Ann. Intern. Med. 86:139-146.

Basta, L.L., Williams, C., Kioschos, J.M. and Spector, A.A. 1976. Regression of atherosclerotic stenosing lesions of the renal arteries and spontaneous cure of systemic hypertension through control of hyperlipidemia. Am. J. Med. 61:420-423.

Beisiegel, U., Weber, W., Havinga, J.R., Ihrke, G., Hui, D.Y., Wernette-Hammond, M.E., Turck, C.W., Innerarity, T.L. and Mahley, R.W. 1988. Apolipoprotein E-binding proteins isolated from dog and human liver. Arteriosclerosis 8:288-297.

Beynen, A.C. and Katan, M.B. 1985. Effect of egg yolk feeding on the concentration and composition of serum lipoproteins in man. Atherosclerosis 54:157-166.

Beveridge, J.M., Connell, W.F., Haust, H.L. and Mayer, G.A. 1959. Dietary cholesterol and plasma cholesterol levels in man. Can. J. Biochem. Physiol. 37:575-582.

Beveridge, J.M.R., Connell, W.F., Mayer, G.A. and Haust, H.L. 1960. The response of man to dietary cholesterol. J. Nutr. 71:61-65.

Blankenhorn, D.H., Nessim, S.A., Johnson, R.L., Sanmarco, M.E., Azen, S.P. and Cashin-Hemphill, L. 1987. Beneficial effects of combined colestipol-niacin therapy on coronary atherosclerosis and coronary venous bypass grafts. J. Am. Med. Assoc. 257:3233-3240.

Bloch, K. 1965. The biological synthesis of cholesterol. Science 150:19-28.

Bloomberg, B.M., Lazarus, F., Mrost, I. and Schneider, R. 1958. Serum lipids in South African Bantu and white subjects. Circulation 17:1021-1028.

Brensike, J.F., Levy, R.I., Kelsey, S.F., Passamani, E.R., Richardson, J.M., Loh, I.K., Stone, N.J., Aldrich, R.F., Battaglini, J.W., Moriarty, D.J., Fisher, M.R., Friedman, L., Friedewald, W., Detre, K.M. and Epstein, S.E. 1984. Effects of therapy with cholestyramine on progression of coronary arteriosclerosis: results of the NHLBI Type II Coronary Intervention Study. Circulation 69:313-324.

Brown, M.S. and Goldstein, J.L. 1986. A receptor mediated pathway for cholesterol homeostasis. Science 232:34-47.

Brunzell, J.D., Sniderman, A.D., Albers, J.J. and Kwiterovich, P.O., Jr. 1984. Apoproteins B and A-I and coronary artery disease in humans. Arteriosclerosis 4:79-83.

Buchwald, H., Moore, R.B., Matts, J.P., Long, J.M., Varco, R.L., Campbell, G.S., Pearce, M.B., Yellin, A.E., Blankenhorn, D.H., Holmes, W.L., Smink, R.D. and Sawin, H.S. 1982. The program on the surgical control of the hyperlipidemias. A status report. Surgery 92:654-662.

Buchwald, H., Moore, R.B., Rucker, R.D., Jr., Amplatz, K., Castaneda, W.R., Francoz, R.A., Pasternak, R.C. and Varco, R.L. 1983. Clinical angiographic regression of atherosclerosis after partial ileal bypass. Atherosclerosis 46:117-128.

Canadian Consensus Conference on the Prevention of Heart and Vascular Disease by Altering Serum Cholesterol and Lipoprotein Risk Factors. 1988. Canadian Consensus Conference on Cholesterol: final report. Can. Med. Assoc. J. 139 (Suppl.):1-8.

Canner, P.L., Berge, K.G., Wenger, N.K., Stamler, J., Friedman, L., Prineas, R.J. and Friedewald, W. 1986. Fifteen year mortality in Coronary Drug Project patients: long-term benefit with niacin. J. Am. Coll. Cardiol. 8:1245-1255.

Carew, T.E., Schwenke, D.C. and Steinberg, D. 1987. Anti-atherogenic effect of probucol unrelated to its hypocholesterolemic effect: evidence that antioxidants in vivo can selectively inhibit low density lipoprotein degradation in macrophage-rich fatty streaks and slow the progression of atherosclerosis in the Watanabe heritable hyperlipidemic rabbit. Proc. Nat. Acad. Sci. USA 84:7725-7729.

Castelli, W.P. 1977. HDL in assessing risk of CHD. Guidelines to Metabolic Therapy 6:1-3.

Chung, B.H., Segrest, J.P., Smith, K. and Griffin, F.M. 1987. Lipolytic surface remnants of triglyceride-rich lipoproteins may be the atherogenic lipoprotein. Circulation, Suppl. 76:IV-296.

Clarkson, T.B., Bond, M.G., Bullock, B.C. and Marzetta, C.A. 1981. A study of atherosclerosis regression in Macaca mulatta. IV. Changes in coronary arteries from animals with atherosclerosis induced for 19 months and then regressed for 24 or 48 months at plasma cholesterol concentrations of 300 or 200 mg/dL. Exp. Mol. Pathol. 34:345-368.

Cole, T.G., Patsch, W., Kuisk, I., Gonen, B. and Schonfeld, G. 1983. Increases in dietary cholesterol and fat raise levels of apoprotein E-containing lipoproteins in the plasma of man. J. Clin. Endocrinol. Metab. 56:1108-1115.

Connor, W.E. 1961. Dietary cholesterol and the pathogenesis of atherosclerosis. Geriatrics 16:407-415.

Connor, W.E. and Connor, S.L. 1972. The key role of nutritional factors in the prevention of coronary heart disease. Prev. Med. 1:49-83.

Connor, W.E. and Lin, D.S. 1982. The effect of shellfish in the diet upon the plasma lipid levels in humans. Metabolism 31:1046-1051.

Connor, W.E., Hodges, R.E. and Bleiler, R.E. 1961. The serum lipids in men receiving high cholesterol and cholesterol-free diets. J. Clin. Invest. 40:894-901.

Connor, W.E., Stone, D.B. and Hodges, R.E. 1964. The interrelated effects of dietary cholesterol and fat upon human serum lipid levels. J. Clin. Invest. 43:1691-1696.

Connor, W.E., Cerqueira, M.T., Connor, R.W., Wallace, R.B., Malinow, M.R. and Casdorph, H.R. 1978. The plasma lipids, lipoproteins and diet of the Tarahumara Indians of Mexico. Am. J. Clin. Nutr. 31:1131-1142.

Consensus Conference. 1985. Lowering blood cholesterol to prevent heart disease. J. Am. Med. Assoc. 253:2080-2086.

Coronary Drug Project Research Group. 1975. Clofibrate and niacin in coronary heart disease. J. Am. Med. Assoc. 231:360-381.

Crouse, J.R., Grundy, S.M. and Ahrens, E.H., Jr. 1972. Cholesterol distribution in the bulk tissues of man: variation with age. J. Clin. Invest. 51:1292-1296.

Davies, J.W., Semenciw, R.M. and Mao, Y. 1988. Cardiovascular disease mortality trends and related risk factors in Canada. Can. J. Cardiol. 4 (suppl. A):16A-20A.

Davignon, J. 1977. Current views on the etiology and pathogenesis of atherosclerosis. *In* Hypertension: physiopathology and treatment. Genest, J., Koiw, E. and Kuchel, O., eds. McGraw-Hill, New York, pp. 961-989.

Davignon, J., Lussier-Cacan, S., Ortin-George, M., Lelièvre, M., Bertagna, C., Gattereau, A. and Fontaine, A. 1977. Plasma lipids and lipoprotein patterns in angiographically graded atherosclerosis of the legs and in coronary heart disease. Can. Med. Assoc. J. 116:1245-1250.

Davignon, J., Leboeuf, N. and Lussier-Cacan, S. 1980. Aspects nutritionnels du traitement des hyperlipidémies et de l'athérosclérose. Union Med. Can. 109:656-665.

Davignon, J., Dufour, R. and Cantin, M. 1983. Atherosclerosis and hypertension. *In* Hypertension: physiopathology and treatment. 2nd ed. Genest, J., Kuchel, O., Hamet, P. and Cantin, M., eds. McGraw-Hill, New York, pp. 810-852.

Davignon, J., Nestruck, A.C., Alaupovic, P. and Bouthillier, D. 1986. Severe hypoalphalipoproteinemia induced by a combination of probucol and clofibrate. Adv. Exp. Med. Biol. 201:111-125.

Davignon, J., Bouthillier, D., Nestruck, A.C. and Sing, C.F. 1987. Apolipoprotein E polymorphism and atherosclerosis: insight from a study in octogenarians. Trans. Am. Clin. Climatol.Assoc. 99:100-110.

Davignon, J., Gregg, R.E. and Sing, C.F. 1988. Apolipoprotein E polymorphism and atherosclerosis. Arteriosclerosis 8:1-21.

De Gennes, J.L., Turpin, G. and Truffert, J. 1972. Dépistage et identification des hyperlipidémies idiopathiques, un nouveau test. Comparaison des concentrations des lipides circulants à la 8e et à la 12e heure de jeûne. Nouv. Presse Méd. 1:1627-1632.

De Palma, R.G., Bellon, E.M., Koletsky, S. and Schneider, D.L. 1979. Atherosclerotic plaque regression in rhesus monkeys induced by bile acid sequestrant. Exp. Mol. Pathol. 31:425-439.

Duffield, R.G.M., Miller, N.E., Brunt, J.N.H., Lewis, B., Jamieson, C.W. and Colchester, A.C.F. 1983. Treatment of hyperlipidaemia retards progression of symptomatic femoral atherosclerosis. A randomized controlled trial. Lancet 2:639-641.

Eisenberg, S. 1987. Lipoprotein abnormalities in hypertriglyceridemia: significance in atherosclerosis. Am. Heart J. 113:555-561.

Enholm, C., Huttunen, J.K., Pietinen, P., Leino, U., Mutanen, M., Kostiainen, E., Pikkarainen, J., Dougherty, R., Iacono, J. and Puska, P. 1982. Effect of diet on serum lipoproteins in a population with a high risk of coronary heart disease. N. Engl. J. Med. 307:850-855.

Erickson, B.A., Coots, R.H., Mattson, F.H. and Kligman, A.M. 1964. The effect of partial hydrogenation of dietary fats, of the ratio of polyunsaturated to saturated fatty acids, and of dietary cholesterol upon plasma lipids in man. J. Clin. Invest. 43:2017-2025.

European Atherosclerosis Society. Study Group. 1987. Strategies for the prevention of coronary heart disease: a policy statement of the European Atherosclerosis Society. Eur. Heart J. 8:77-88.

Ferro-Luzzi, A., Strazzullo, P., Scaccini, C., Siani, A., Sette, S., Mariani, M.A., Mastranzo, P., Dougherty, R.M., Iacono, J.M. and Mancini, M. 1984. Changing the Mediterranean diet: effects on blood lipids. Am. J. Clin. Nutr. 40:1027-1037.

Fielding, C.J. and Fielding, P.E. 1982. Cholesterol transport between cells and body fluids. Role of plasma lipoproteins and the plasma cholesterol esterification system. Med. Clin. North Am. 66:363-373.

Flaim, E., Ferreri, L.F., Thye, F.W., Hill, J.E. and Ritchey, S.J. 1981. Plasma lipid and lipoprotein cholesterol concentrations in adult males consuming normal and high cholesterol diets under controlled conditions. Am. J. Clin. Nutr. 34:1103-1108.

Flynn, M.A., Nolph, G.B., Flynn, T.C., Kahrs, R. and Krause, G. 1979. Effect of dietary egg on human serum cholesterol and triacylglycerols. Am. J. Clin. Nutr. 32:1051-1057.

Frick, M.H., Elo, O., Haapa, K., Heinonen, O.P., Heinsalmi, P., Helo, P., Huttunen, J.K., Kaitaniemi, P., Koskinen, P., Manninen, V., Maenpaa, H., Malkonen, M., Manttari, M., Norola, S., Pasternack, A., Pikkarainen, J., Romo, M., Sjoblom, T. and Nikkila, E.A. 1987. Helsinki Heart Study: primary-prevention trial with gemfibrozil in middle-aged men with dyslipidemia: safety of treatment, changes in risk factors, and incidence of coronary heart disease. N. Engl. J. Med. 317:1237-1245.

Fruchart, J.C., Parra, H., Cachera, C., Clavey, V. and Bertrand, M. 1982. Lipoproteins, apolipoproteins and coronary artery disease. Ric. Clin. Lab. 12:101-106.

Gianturco, S.H., Gotto, A.M., Jr. and Bradley, W.A. 1985. Hypertriglyceridemia: lipoprotein receptors and atherosclerosis. Adv. Exp. Med. 183:47-71.

Ginsberg, H., Le, N.A., Mays, C., Gibson, J. and Brown, W.V. 1981. Lipoprotein metabolism in non-responders to increased dietary cholesterol. Arteriosclerosis 1:463-470.

Goldbourt, U., Holtzman, E. and Neufeld, H.N. 1985. Total and high density lipoprotein cholesterol in the serum and risk of mortality: evidence of a threshold effect. Br. Med. J. 290:1239-1243.

Goldman, L. and Cook, E.F. 1984. The decline in ischemic heart disease mortality rates. An analysis of the comparative effects of medical interventions and changes in lifestyle. Ann. Intern. Med. 101:825-836.

Goldstein, J.L., Ho, Y.K., Basu, S.K. and Brown, M.S. 1979. Binding site on macrophages that mediates uptake and degradation of acetylated low density lipoprotein, producing massive cholesterol deposition. Proc. Nat. Acad. Sci. USA 76:333-337.

Goldstein, J.L., Kita, T. and Brown, M.S. 1983. Defective lipoprotein receptors and atherosclerosis: lessons from an animal counterpart of familial hypercholesterolemia. N. Engl. J. Med. 309:288-296.

Gordon, T. 1970. The Framingham Diet Study: diet and the regulation of serum cholesterol. *In* The Framingham Study: an epidemiological investigation of cardiovascular disease. Section 24. Kannel, W.B. and Gordon, T. eds. United States Government Printing Office, Washington, D.C.

Gregg, R.E., Connor, W.E., Lin, D.S. and Brewer, H.B., Jr. 1986. Abnormal metabolism of shellfish sterols in a patient with sitosterolemia and xanthomatosis. J. Clin. Invest. 77:1864-1872.

Grundy, S.M. 1986. Cholesterol and coronary heart disease - A new era. J. Am. Med. Assoc. 256:2849-2858.

Grundy, S.M., Barrett-Connor, E., Rudel, L.L., Miettinen, T. and Spector, A.A. 1988. Workshop on the impact of dietary cholesterol on plasma lipoproteins and atherogenesis. Arteriosclerosis 8:95-101.

Hegsted, D.M. 1986. Serum-cholesterol response to dietary cholesterol: a re-evaluation. Am. J. Clin. Nutr. 44:299-305.

Hegsted, D.M., McGandy, R.B., Myers, M.L. and Stare, F.J. 1965. Quantitative effects of dietary fat on serum cholesterol in man. Am. J. Clin. Nutr. 17:281-295.

Hesler, C.B., Tall, A.R., Swenson, T.L., Weech, P.K., Marcel, Y.L. and Milne, R.W. 1988. Monoclonal antibodies to the M_r 74 000 cholesteryl ester transfer protein neutralize all of the cholesteryl ester and triglyceride transfer activities in human plasma. J. Biol. Chem. 263:5020-5023.

Hjermann, I., Velvebyre, K., Holme, I. and Leren, P. 1981. Effect of diet and smoking intervention on the incidence of coronary heart disease. Report from the Oslo Study Group of a randomized trial in healthy man. Lancet 2:1303-1310.

Hoeg, J.M., Demosky, S.J., Jr., Gregg, R.E., Schaefer, E.J. and Brewer, H.B., Jr. 1985. Distinct hepatic receptors for low density lipoprotein and apolipoprotein E in humans. Science 227:759-761.

Hopkins, P.N. and Williams, R.R. 1981. A survey of 246 suggested coronary risk factors. Atherosclerosis 40:1-52.

Hopkins, P.N. and Williams, R.R. 1986. Identification and relative weight of cardiovascular risk factors. Cardiol. Clin. 4:3-31.

Huang, Y.S., Eid, K. and Davignon, J. 1981. Cholesteryl sulfate: measurement with beta-sitosteryl sulfate as an internal standard. Can. J. Biochem. 59:602-605.

Jacobs, D.R., Jr., Anderson, J.T., Hannan, P., Keys, A. and Blackburn, H. 1983. Variability in individual serum cholesterol response to change in diet. Arteriosclerosis 3:349-356.

Kakis, G., Feather, T. and Little, J.A. 1983. Plasma high density lipoprotein triglyceride as a risk factor for ischemic vascular disease: a prospective study (abst.). Arteriosclerosis 3:A480.

Kannel, W.B., Castelli, W., Gordon, T. and McNamara, P.M. 1971. Serum cholesterol, lipoproteins, and the risk of coronary heart disease. The Framingham study. Ann. Intern. Med. 74:1-12.

Kannel, W.B., Castelli, W.P. and Gordon, T. 1979. Cholesterol in the prediction of atherosclerotic disease. New perspectives based on the Framingham study. Ann. Intern. Med. 90:85-91.

Kannel, W.B., Neaton, J.D., Wentworth, D., Thomas, H.E., Stamler, J., Hulley, S.B. and Kjelsberg, M.O. 1986. Overall and coronary heart disease mortality rates in relation to major risk factors in 325,348 men screened for the MRFIT. Am. Heart J. 112:825-836.

Katan, M.B., Beynen, A.C., De Vries, J.H.M. and Nobels, A. 1986. Existence of consistent hypo- and hyperresponders to dietary cholesterol in man. Am. J. Epidemiol. 123:221-234.

Kato, H., Tillotson, J., Nichaman, M.Z., Rhoads, G.G. and Hamilton, H.B. 1973. Epidemiologic studies of coronary heart disease and stroke in Japanese men living in Japan, Hawaii and California. Serum lipids and diet. Am. J. Epidemiol. 97:372-385.

Kesaniemi, Y.A. and Miettinen, T.A. 1987. Cholesterol absorption efficiency regulates plasma cholesterol level in the Finnish population. Eur. J. Clin. Invest. 17:391-395.

Kesaniemi, Y.A., Ehnholm, C. and Miettinen, T.A. 1987. Intestinal cholesterol absorption efficiency in man is related to apoprotein E phenotype. J. Clin. Invest. 80:578-581.

Keys, A., ed. 1970. Coronary heart disease in seven countries. Circulation 41: Suppl. I.

Keys, A. 1980. Seven countries: a multivariate analysis of death and coronary heart disease. Harvard Press, Cambridge.

Keys, A. 1984. Serum cholesterol response to dietary cholesterol. Am. J. Clin. Nutr. 40:351-359.

Keys, A., Anderson, J.T. and Grande, F. 1965. Serum cholesterol response to changes in the diet. II. The effect of cholesterol in the diet. Metabolism 14:759-65.

Kita, T., Nagano, Y., Yokode, M., Ishii, K., Kume, N., Ooshima, A., Yoshida, H. and Kawai, C. 1987. Probucol prevents the progression of atherosclerosis in Watanabe heritable hyperlipidemic rabbit, an animal model for familial hypercholesterolemia. Proc. Nat. Acad. Sci. USA 84:5928-5931.

Kokatnur, M.G., Malcom, G.T., Eggen, D.A. and Strong, J.P. 1975. Depletion of aortic free and ester cholesterol by dietary means in rhesus monkeys with fatty streaks. Atherosclerosis 21:195-203.

Koren, E., Puchois, P., Alaupovic, P., Fesmire, J., Kandoussi, A. and Fruchart, J.C. 1987. Quantification of two different types of apolipoprotein A-I containing lipoprotein particles in plasma by enzyme-linked differential-antibody immunosorbent assay. Clin. Chem. 33:38-43.

Kovanen, P.T., Bilheimer, D.W., Goldstein, J.L., Jaramillo, J.J. and Brown, M.S. 1981. Regulatory role for hepatic low density lipoprotein receptors in vivo in the dog. Proc. Nat. Acad. Sci. USA 78:1194-1198.

Kromhout, D. and DeLezenne Coulander, C. 1984. Diet, prevalence and 10-year mortality from coronary heart disease in 871 middle-aged men. The Zutphen Study. Am. J. Epidemiol. 119:733-741.

Kummerow, F.A., Kim, Y., Hull, M.D., Pollard, J., Ilinov, P., Dorossiev, D.L. and Valek, J. 1977. The influence of egg consumption on the serum cholesterol level in human subjects. Am. J. Clin. Nutr. 30:664-673.

Kuo, P.T., Hayase, K., Kostis, J.B. and Moreyra, A.E. 1979. Use of combined diet and colestipol in long-term (7-7 1/2 years) treatment of patients with type II hyperlipoproteinemia. Circulation 59:199-211.

Kushi, L.H., Lew, R.A., Stare, F.J., Ellison, C.R., el Lozy, M., Bourke, G., Daly, L., Graham, I., Hickey, N., Mulcahy, R. and Kevaney, J. 1985. Diet and 20-year mortality from coronary heart disease. The Ireland-Boston Diet-Heart Study. N. Engl. J. Med. 312:811-818.

Langlais, J., Zollinger, M., Plante, L., Chapdelaine, A., Bleau, G. and Roberts, K.D. 1981. Localization of cholesteryl sulfate in human spermatozoa in support of a hypothesis for the mechanism of capacitation. Proc. Nat. Acad. Sci. USA 78:7266-7270.

Lauer, R.M., Lee, J. and Clarke, W.R. 1988. Factors affecting the relationship between childhood and adult cholesterol levels: the Muscatine Study. Pediatrics 82:309-318.

Lee, K.T., Nam, S.C., Florentin, R.A. and Thomas, W.A. 1974. Genesis of atherosclerosis in swine fed high fat-cholesterol diets. Med. Clin. North Am. 58:281-292.

Levy, R.I., Brensike, J.F., Epstein, S.E., Kelsey, S.F., Passamani, E.R., Richardson, J.M., Loh, I.K., Stone, N.J., Aldrich, R.F., Battaglini, J.W., Moriarty, D.J., Fisher, M.L., Friedman, L., Friedewald, W. and Detre, K.M. 1984. The influence of changes in lipid values induced by cholestyramine and diet on progression of coronary artery disease: results of the NHLBI Type II Coronary Intervention Study. Circulation 69:325-337.

Lewis, B., Mann, J.I. and Mancini, M. 1986. Reducing the risks of coronary heart disease in individuals and in the population. Lancet 1:956-959.

Lewis, D.S., Mott, G.E., McMahan, A., Masoro, E.J., Carey, K.D. and McGill, H.C., Jr. 1988. Deferred effects of preweaning diet on atherosclerosis in adolescent baboons. Arteriosclerosis 8:274-280.

Lin, D.S. and Connor, W.E. 1980. The long term effects of dietary cholesterol upon the plasma lipids, lipoproteins, cholesterol absorption, and the sterol balance in man: the demonstration of feedback inhibition of cholesterol biosynthesis and increased bile acid excretion. J. Lipid Res. 21:1042-1052.

Lipid Research Clinics Program. 1983. Pre-entry characteristics of participants in the Lipid Research Clinics' Coronary Primary Prevention Trial. J. Chronic Dis. 36:467-479.

Lipid Research Clinics Program. 1984. The Lipid Research Clinics Coronary Primary Prevention Trial results. J. Am. Med. Assoc. 251:351-374.

Maciejko, J.J., Holmes, D.R., Kottke, B.A., Zinsmeister, A.R., Dinh, D.M. and Mao, S.J.T. 1983. Apolipoprotein A-I as a marker of angiographically assessed coronary-artery disease. N. Engl. J. Med. 309:385-389.

Mahley, R.W. 1979. Dietary fat, cholesterol, and accelerated atherosclerosis. Atheroscler. Rev. 5:1-34.

Mahley, R.W. and Innerarity, T.L. 1983. Lipoprotein receptors and cholesterol homeostasis. Biochim. Biophys. Acta 737:197-222.

Mahley, R.W., Innerarity, T.L., Bersot, T.P., Lipson, A. and Margolis, S. 1978. Alterations in human high-density lipoproteins, with or without increased plasma-cholesterol, induced by diets high in cholesterol. Lancet 2:807-809.

Mahley, R.W., Innerarity, T.L., Rall, S.C., Jr. and Weisgraber, K.H. 1984. Plasma lipoproteins: apolipoprotein structure and function. J. Lipid Res. 25:1277-1294.

Malloy, M.J. and Kane, J.P. 1982. Hypolipidemia. Med. Clin. North Am. 66:469-484.

Marmot, M.G., Syme, S.L., Kagan, A., Kato, H., Cohen, J.B. and Belsky, J. 1975. Epidemiologic studies of coronary heart disease and stroke in Japanese men living in Japan, Hawaii and California: prevalence of coronary and hypertensive heart disease and associated risk factors. Am. J. Epidemiol. 102:514-525.

Mattson, F.H., Erickson, B.A. and Kligman, A.M. 1972. Effect of dietary cholesterol on serum cholesterol in man. Am. J. Clin. Nutr. 25:589-594.

McCormick, J. and Skrabanek, P. 1988. Coronary heart disease is not preventable by population interventions. Lancet 2:839-841.

McGill, H.C., Jr. 1979. The relationship of dietary cholesterol to serum cholesterol concentration and to atherosclerosis in man. Am. J. Clin. Nutr. 32:2664-2702.

McNamara, D.J. 1987. Diet and heart disease: the role of cholesterol and fat. J. Am. Oil Chem. Soc. 64:1565-1574.

McNamara, D.J., Kolb, R., Parker, T.S., Batwin, H., Samuel, P., Brown, C.D. and Ahrens, E.H., Jr. 1987. Heterogeneity of cholesterol homeostasis in man. Response to changes in dietary fat quality and cholesterol quantity. J. Clin. Invest. 79:1729-1739.

Miettinen, M., Turpeinen, O., Karvonen, M.J., Elosuo, R. and Paavilainen, E. 1972. Effect of cholesterol-lowering diet on mortality from coronary heart disease and other causes. A twelve year clinical trial in men and women. Lancet 2:835-838.

Miettinen, T.A., Naukkarinen, V., Huttunen, J.K., Mattila, S. and Kumlin, T. 1982. Fatty-acid composition of serum lipids predicts myocardial infarction. Br. Med. J. 285:993-996.

Miller, G.J. and Miller, N.E. 1975. Plasma high density lipoprotein concentration and development of ischaemic heart disease. Lancet 1:16-19.

Miller, N.E., Hammett, F., Saltissi, S., Rao, S., Van Zeller, H., Coltart, J. and Lewis, B. 1981. Relation of angiographically defined coronary artery disease to plasma lipoprotein subfractions and apolipoproteins. Br. Med. J. 282:1741-1744.

Mistry, P., Miller, N.E., Laker, M., Hazzard, W.R. and Lewis, B. 1981. Individual variation in the effects of dietary cholesterol on plasma lipoproteins and cellular cholesterol homeostasis in man. Studies of low density lipoprotein receptor activity and 3-hydroxy-3-methylglutaryl coenzyme A reductase activity in blood mononuclear cells. J. Clin. Invest. 67:493-502.

Mondeika, T. 1985. Cholesterol content of shellfish. J. Am. Med. Assoc. 254:2970.

Moore, S. 1973. Thromboatherosclerosis in normolipemic rabbits: a result of continued endothelial damage. Lab. Invest. 29:478-487.

Myant, N.B. 1981. The biology of cholesterol and related steroids. Heinemann, London.

Nash, D.T., Gensini, G.G. and Esente, P. 1983. Regression of coronary artery lesions during lipid lowering therapy, demonstrated by scheduled serial arteriography. Int. J. Cardiol. 3:257-260.

National Cholesterol Education Program Expert Panel on Detection, Evaluation and Treatment of High Blood Cholesterol in Adults. 1988. Report. Arch. Intern. Med. 148:36-69.

National Diet-Heart Study Research Group. 1968. Final report. Circulation, Suppl. 37:I-1—I-428.

Nestel, P. and Poyser, A. 1976. Changes in cholesterol synthesis and excretion when cholesterol intake is increased. Metabolism 25:1591-1599.

Nestel, P.J., Whyte, H.M. and Goodman, D.S. 1969. Distribution and turnover of cholesterol in humans. J. Clin. Invest. 48:982-991.

Nestel, P., Tada, N., Billington, T., Huff, M. and Fidge, N. 1982. Changes in very low density lipoproteins with cholesterol loading in man. Metabolism 31:398-405.

Newman, W.P., Freedman, D.S., Voors, A.W., Gard, P.D., Srinivasan, S.R., Cresanta, J.L., Williamson, G.D., Webber, L.S. and Berenson, G.S. 1986. Relation of serum lipoprotein levels and systolic blood pressure to early atherosclerosis. The Bogalusa Heart Study. N. Engl. J. Med. 314:138-144.

Nichols, A.B., Ravenscroft, C., Lamphiear, D.E. and Ostrander, L.D. 1976. Daily nutritional intake and serum lipid levels. The Tecumseh Study. Am. J. Clin. Nutr. 29:1384-1392.

Nicholls, E.S., Jung, J. and Davies, J.W. 1981. Cardiovascular disease mortality in Canada. Can. Med. Assoc. J. 125:981-992.

Nicholls, E., Nair, C., MacWilliam, L., Moen, J. and Mao, Y. 1986. Cardiovascular disease in Canada. Statistics Canada Catalogue No. 82-544. Statistics Canada. Ottawa.

Nicklas, T.A., Farris, R.P., Smoak, C.G., Frank, G.C., Srinivasan, S.R., Webber, L.S. and Berenson, G.S. 1988. Dietary factors relate to cardiovascular risk factors in early life. The Bogalusa Heart Study. Arteriosclerosis 8:193-199.

Nikkila, E.A, Viikinkoski, P., Valle, M. and Frick, M.H. 1984. Prevention of progression of coronary atherosclerosis by treatment of hyperlipidaemia: a seven year prospective angiographic study. Br. Med. J. 289:220-223.

Noma, A., Yokosuka, T. and Kitamura, K. 1983. Plasma lipids and apolipoproteins as discriminators for presence and severity of angiographically defined coronary artery disease. Atherosclerosis 49:1-7.

Norum, R.A., Lakier, J.B., Goldstein, S., Angel, A., Goldberg, R.B., Block, W.D., Noffze, D.K., Dolphin, P.J., Edelglass, J., Bogorad, D.D. and Alaupovic, P. 1982. Familial deficiency of apolipoprotein A-I and C-III and precocious coronary-artery disease. N. Engl. J. Med. 306:1513-1519.

Oliver, M.F. 1987. Dietary fat and coronary heart disease. Br. Heart J. 58:423-428.

Olsson, A.G., Carlson, L.A., Erikson, U., Helmius, G., Hemmingsson, A. and Ruhn, G. 1982. Regression of computer estimated femoral atherosclerosis after pronounced serum lipid lowering in patients with asymptomatic hyperlipidaemia. Lancet 1:1311.

Ost, C.R. and Stenson, S. 1967. Regression of peripheral atherosclerosis during therapy with high doses of nicotinic acid. Scand. J. Clin. Lab. Invest. Suppl. 99:241-245.

Packard, C.J., McKinney, L., Carr, K. and Shepherd, J. 1983. Cholesterol feeding increases low density lipoprotein synthesis. J. Clin. Invest. 72:45-51.

Parthasarathy, S., Fong, L.G., Otero, D. and Steinberg, D. 1987. Recognition of solubilized apoproteins from delipidated, oxidized low density lipoprotein (LDL) by the acetyl-LDL receptor. Proc. Nat. Acad. Sci. U.S.A. 84:537-540.

Peto, R., Yusuf, S. and Collins, R. 1985. Cholesterol-lowering trial results in their epidemiologic context (abst.). Circulation 72:III-451.

Porter, M.W., Yamanaka, W., Carlson, S.D. and Flynn, M.A. 1977. Effect of dietary egg on serum cholesterol and triglyceride of human males. Am. J. Clin. Nutr. 30:490-495.

Pooling Project Research Group. 1978. Relationship of blood pressure, serum cholesterol, smoking habit, relative weight and ECG abnormalities to incidence of major coronary events: final report of the Pooling Project. J. Chronic Dis. 31:201-306.

Puchois, P., Bertrand, M., Lablanche, J.M. and Fruchart, J.C. 1985. Decrease of plasma apo A-I in coronary artery disease is related to lipoprotein particles which contain apo A-I but not apo A-II (abst.). Circulation, Suppl. 72:III-199.

Quintao, E., Grundy, S.M. and Ahrens, E.H., Jr. 1971. Effects of dietary cholesterol on the regulation of total body cholesterol in man. J. Lipid Res. 12:233-247.

Rhoads, G.G., Dahlen, G., Berg, K., Morton, N.E. and Dannenberg, A.L. 1986. Lp(a) lipoprotein as a risk factor for myocardial infarction. J. Am. Med. Assoc. 256:2540-2544.

Rhomberg, H.P. and Braunsteiner, H. 1976. Excessive egg consumption, xanthomatosis, and hypercholesterolaemia. Br. Med. J. 1:1188-1189.

Roberts, K.D., Bandi, L., Calvin, H.I., Drucker, W.D. and Lieberman, S. 1964. Evidence that steroid sulfates serve as biosynthetic intermediates. IV. Conversion of cholesterol sulfate in vivo to urinary C19 and C21 steroidal sulfates. Biochemistry 3:1983-1988.

Roberts, S.L., McMurry, M.P. and Connor, W.E. 1981. Does egg feeding (i.e., dietary cholesterol) affect plasma cholesterol levels in humans? The results of a double-blind study. Am. J. Clin. Nutr. 34:2092-2099.

Robertson, T.L., Kato, H., Rhoads, G.G., Kagan, A., Marmot, M., Syme, S.L., Gordon, T., Worth, R., Belsky, J.L., Dock, D.S., Miyanishi, M. and Kawamoto, S. 1977. Epidemiologic studies of coronary heart disease and stroke in Japanese men living in Japan, Hawaii and California. Incidence of myocardial infarction and death from coronary heart disease. Am. J. Cardiol. 39:239-249.

Robbins, L. and Robichon-Hunt, L. 1986. Nutrients available for consumption from the Canadian food supply, 1963-1983. Food Mark. Comment. 7:34-41.

Ross, R. 1981. Atherosclerosis: a problem of the biology of arterial wall cells and their interactions with blood components. Arteriosclerosis 1:293-311.

Sacks, F.M., Salazar, J., Miller, L., Foster, J.M., Sutherland, M., Samonds, K.W., Albers, J.J. and Kass, E.H. 1984. Ingestion of egg raises plasma low density lipoproteins in free-living subjects. Lancet 1:647-649.

Schaefer, E.J., Heaton, W.H., Wetzel, M.G. and Brewer, H.B., Jr. 1982. Plasma apolipoprotein A-I absence associated with a marked reduction of high density lipoproteins and premature coronary heart disease. Arteriosclerosis 2:16-26.

Schonfeld, G., Patsch, W., Rudel, L.L., Nelson, C., Epstein, M. and Olson, R.E. 1982. Effects of dietary cholesterol and fatty acids on plasma lipoproteins. J. Clin. Invest. 69:1072-1080.

Shekelle, R.B., MacMillan Shryock, A., Oglesby, P., Lepper, M., Stamler, J., Liu, S. and Raynor, W.J. 1981. Diet, serum cholesterol, and death from coronary heart disease. The Western Electric Study. N. Engl. J. Med. 304:65-70.

Simons, L.A. 1984. The lipid hypothesis is proven. Med. J. Aust. 140:316-317.

Sing, C.F. and Davignon, J. 1985. Role of the apolipoprotein E polymorphism in determining normal plasma lipid and lipoprotein variation. Am. J. Hum. Genet. 37:268-285.

Slater, G., Mead, J., Dhopeshwarker, G., Robinson, S. and Alfin-Slater, R.B. 1976. Plasma cholesterol and triacylglycerols in men with added eggs in the diet. Nutr. Rep. Int. 14:249-260.

Sniderman, A.D. 1988. Apolipoprotein B and apolipoprotein AI as predictors of coronary artery disease. Can. J. Cardiol. 4 (suppl. A):24A-30A.

Solberg, L.A. and Strong, J.P. 1983. Risk factors and atherosclerotic lesions. A review of autopsy studies. Arteriosclerosis 3:187-198.

Spain, D.M. 1960. Problems in the study of coronary atherosclerosis in population groups. Ann. N.Y. Acad. Sci. 84:816-834.

Spain, D.M. 1966. Atherosclerosis. Sci. Am. 215:49-59.

Srinivasan, S.R., Patton, D., Radhakrishnamurthy, B., Foster, T.A., Malinow, M.R., McLaughlin, P. and Berenson, G.S. 1980. Lipid changes in atherosclerotic aortas of Macaca fascicularis after various regression regimens. Atherosclerosis 37:591-601.

Stamler, J. 1987. Epidemiology, established major risk factors, and the primary prevention of coronary heart disease. *In* Cardiology. Parmley, W.W. and Chatterjee, K., eds. Lippincott, Philadelphia, pp. 1-41.

Stamler, J. 1988. Risk factor modification trials: implications for the elderly. Eur. Heart J. 9(suppl. D):9-53.

Stamler, J. and Shekelle, R. 1988. Dietary cholesterol and human coronary heart disease: the epidemiological evidence. Arch. Pathol. Lab. Med. 112:1032-40.

Stamler, J., Wentworth, D. and Neaton, J. 1986. Is relationship between serum cholesterol and risk of premature death from coronary heart disease continuous and graded? J. Am. Med. Assoc. 256:2823-2828.

Stehbens, W.E. 1986. An appraisal of cholesterol feeding in experimental atherogenesis. Prog. Cardiovasc. Dis. 29:107-128.

Steiner, A., Howard, E.J. and Akgun, S. 1962. Importance of dietary cholesterol in man. J. Am. Med. Assoc. 181:186-190.

Steinberg, D. 1983. Lipoproteins and atherosclerosis: a look back and a look ahead. Arteriosclerosis 3:283-301.

Stephen, A.M. 1988. Trends in individual fat consumption in the United States from 1920-1984. Circulation, Suppl. 78:II-20.

Strong, J.P. and McGill, H.C. 1969. The pediatric aspects of atheroclerosis. J. Atheroscler. Res. 9:251-265.

Tan, M.H., Dickinson, M.A., Albers, J.J., Havel, R.J., Cheung, M.C. and Vigne, J-L. 1980. The effect of a high cholesterol and saturated fat diet on serum high density lipoprotein-cholesterol, apoprotein A-I, and apoprotein E levels in normolipidemic humans. Am. J. Clin. Nutr. 33:2559-2565.

Thompson, G. 1984. Apoproteins: determinants of lipoprotein metabolism and indices of coronary risk. Br. Heart J. 51:585-588.

Vergani, C. and Bettale, G. 1981. Familial hypo-alphalipoproteinemia. Clin. Chim. Acta 114:45-62.

Walldius, G., Carlson, L.A., Erikson, U., Olsson, A.G., Johansson, J., Molgaard, J., Nilsson, S., Stenport, G., Kaijser, L., Lassvik, C. and Holme, I. 1988. Development of femoral atherosclerosis in hypercholesterolemic patients during treatment with cholestyramine and probucol/placebo: Probucol Quantitative Regression Swedish Trial (PQRST): a status report. Am. J. Cardiol. 62:37B-43B.

Watanabe, Y. 1980. Serial inbreeding of rabbits with hereditary hyperlipidemia (WHHL-rabbit) - Incidence and development of atherosclerosis and xanthoma. Atherosclerosis 36:261-268.

Weintraub, M.S., Eisenberg, S. and Breslow, J.L. 1987. Dietary fat clearance in normal subjects is regulated by genetic variation in apolipoprotein E. J. Clin. Invest. 80:1571-1577.

Wells, V.M. and Bronte-Stewart, B. 1963. Egg yolk and serum-cholesterol levels: importance of dietary cholesterol intake. Br. Med. J. 1:577-81.

Wen, C.-P. and Gershoff, S.N. 1973. Changes in serum cholesterol and coronary heart disease mortality associated with changes in the postwar Japanese diet. Am. J. Clin. Nutr. 26:616-619.

Wissler, R.W. and Vesselinovitch, D. 1983. Combined effects of cholestyramine and probucol on regression of atherosclerosis in rhesus monkey aortas. Appl. Pathol. 1:89-96.

Witztum, J.L., Mahoney, E.M., Branks, M.J., Fisher, M., Elam, R. and Steinberg, D. 1981. Nonenzymatic glucosylation of low density lipoprotein alters its biological activity. Diabetes 31:283-291.

Yano, K., Reed, D.M. and McGee, D.L. 1984. Ten-year incidence of coronary heart disease in the Honolulu Heart Program. Relationship to biologic and lifestyle characteristics. Am. J. Epidemiol. 119:653-666.

Zelis, R., Mason, D.T., Braunwald, E. and Levy, R.I. 1970. Effects of hyperlipoproteinemias and their treatment on the peripheral circulation. J. Clin. Invest. 49:1007-1015.

Zilversmit, D.B. 1973. A proposal linking atherogenesis to the interaction of endothelial lipoprotein lipase with triglyceride-rich lipoproteins. Circ. Res. 33:633-638.

Protein

Dietary requirements for protein are based on needs for both total amino nitrogen (N) and essential amino acids (EAA) to support protein turnover and special functions of amino acids, such as neurotransmitter synthesis. Of the 20 common amino acids, eight are currently considered essential for adults and nine (including histidine) for infants, although evidence suggests that histidine may be essential for the adult as well. Thus, in expressing protein requirements, consideration is given to both total nitrogen needs to maintain balance in adults as well as to the ability of the habitual Canadian diet to meet the requirements for EAA (protein quality). Adjustments are then made for periods of accretion such as growth, pregnancy and lactation.

Despite the complexity of defining protein requirements, the habitual Canadian diet appears adequate to meet protein requirements provided that energy needs are met in almost all individuals. There is currently no evidence to recommend a change from current consumption patterns with respect to protein intake in the healthy Canadian.

Protein Requirements

Current estimates of protein requirements are provided in the 1983 Recommended Nutrient Intakes for Canadians (Canada. Health and Welfare 1983). These requirements were estimated using a combination of factorial and nitrogen-balance approaches, and then corrected for digestibility and protein quality of the habitual Canadian diet. A detailed explanation of both the philosophical and practical aspects of this approach is provided in the former report and will only be briefly summarized here.

The factorial method of estimating protein requirements measures obligatory nitrogen losses (urinary, fecal and dermal losses) during periods of little or no protein intake. This method has the advantage that measurements can be made relatively easily, and hence a substantial volume of data is available. However, it is known that this approach systematically underestimates protein requirements (FAO/WHO 1973; Beaton *et al.* 1979), since efficiency of protein utilization increases as protein intakes fall below protein requirements.

Nitrogen-balance studies, on the other hand, measure the amount of dietary protein necessary to maintain nitrogen-balance (i.e. intake = output) in adults. While this approach provides a more direct measurement of protein requirements, results from earlier studies were clouded for two reasons. First, earlier nitrogen-balance studies tended to provide individuals with energy intakes in excess of their energy requirements. It is now known that there is an interaction between energy intake and the amount of protein necessary to maintain nitrogen-balance within the range of intakes that approximate both energy and protein requirements (Beaton *et al.* 1979; FAO/WHO/UNU 1985). Second, earlier studies tended to use a broad range of protein intakes above and below requirements. Since the efficiency of protein utilization increases as protein intakes fall below requirements, it is known that it is inappropriate to apply linear regression analysis to the data to determine protein requirements (FAO/WHO/UNU 1985).

Due to concerns associated with both methods, a combination approach was taken in estimating protein requirements. That is, data from factorial studies (the larger data base) were adjusted by a factor felt to represent the degree to which this approach underestimated protein requirements. The average requirement for adults determined by this approach was then increased by 30% to allow for individual variability.

In the intervening years since the 1983 publication of the Recommended Nutrient Intakes for Canadians, data bases have evolved to the extent that minor variations to the approach and estimate of protein requirements are warranted. Recently a limited number of nitrogen-balance studies (both short-term and long-term) have been performed on adults in energy balance and on a narrow range of protein intakes around mean protein requirements. Results from these studies (reviewed in FAO/WHO/UNU 1985) suggest that average protein requirements are approximately 0.6 g/kg body weight (BW)/d or 100 mg N/kg BW/d. These data appear to provide the best estimate of adult protein requirements and are the ones currently in use by the FAO/WHO/UNU (1985).

Protein requirements to support periods of accretion are not accurately known, and are best estimated by the factorial model used by the FAO/WHO/UNU committee (1985) in which

mean dietary protein requirement =

$$\left[\text{maintenance need for dietary protein} + \text{protein accretion associated with growth}\right] \frac{100}{\text{utilization efficiency}}$$

In this model, maintenance requirement was estimated as dietary protein (with efficiency of utilization taken into account), derived predominantly from nitrogen-balance studies, whereas growth requirement was estimated from protein accretion data and then adjusted for theoretical efficiency of protein utilization. While the philosophical approach is sound, recently it has been argued that protein requirements for infants using this approach were overestimated.

The concern arose from applying an epidemiological approach to validate protein requirements in infants (Beaton and Chery 1988). That is, predicted protein intakes from human milk were compared with protein requirements. For example, the FAO/WHO/UNU committee (1985) reported average crude protein requirements which were higher than average protein intakes from human milk in infants 1-2 and 2-3 months of age, implying that human milk would not meet an infant's protein needs up to three months of age. Furthermore, the average crude protein requirement for infants 3-4 months of age was estimated at 1.47 g/kg/d, with the safe level of intake (increased by 2 SD; coefficient of variability = 18.3%) being 2.02 g/kg/d. The average protein intake of exclusively breast-fed infants at this age would be approximately 1.49 g/kg/d (i.e. average intake = average requirement). Since there is currently no indication that the protein composition of an individual mother's breast milk varies to meet the needs of her infant, the numbers become inconsistent with the assumption that human milk provides an adequate source of protein even for infants 3-4 months of age.

Using a simulation analysis based on consumption data and the assumptions that breast milk provides adequate protein intake once energy needs are met for an infant 3-4 months of age and that protein and energy requirements are not correlated (i.e. the infant with the lowest energy requirement may have the highest protein requirement), Beaton and Chery (1988) estimated that average protein requirements would be about 1.1 ± 0.1-0.2 g protein/kg/d for this age group.

Upon re-evaluation of the FAO/WHO/UNU report (1985), it can be seen that two factors used in their calculations may account for the difference. First, it was assumed that maintenance requirements for infants of this age were 120 mg N/kg/d. This estimate is derived predominantly from nitrogen-balance data reported by Huang *et al.* (1980). However, in these studies infants' energy requirements were not met, suggesting that protein requirements were overestimated. A study by Torun and colleagues (1981), cited in the FAO/WHO/UNU report, suggests that mean maintenance requirements may be as low as 80 mg N/kg/d. If one takes the mean of these two estimates (100 mg N/kg/d) as the best indicator of requirement for maintenance, the value is identical to the adult maintenance requirement. Concern was raised that this value may not adequately reflect the differences in the proportion of lean body mass in infants versus adults; however, based on available data, this appeared the best estimate of maintenance requirement for all age groups.

Second, in determining protein requirements for growth, the FAO/WHO/UNU committee increased the average accretion values reported by Fomon *et al.* (1982) for different age groups by 50% to cover the needs of infants growing more rapidly, or at different chronological ages. Therefore, the average protein requirement for the most rapidly growing infant was provided; this shifted the requirement curve to the right. Since average requirements have been traditionally increased by 2 SD (assuming a 35% CV for growth in the case of the FAO/WHO/UNU committee) to determine a safe level of intake, it would appear that the FAO/WHO/UNU committee corrected twice for differences in growth rates amongst infants and hence overestimated this portion of the requirement estimate.

For the purpose of this report, the factorial model used by the FAO/WHO/UNU committee was adopted; however, modifications in the approach were made. First, it was assumed that maintenance requirements do not change throughout the lifespan, with a value of 100 mg N/kg/d representing our best estimate of this requirement. Second, nitrogen requirement for growth was based on average accretion values provided by Fomon *et al.* (1982). Similar to the FAO/WHO/UNU committee, it was assumed that efficiency of protein utilization was 70%. The sum of these two values then represents average nitrogen requirement. In order to determine a safe level of intake, a value representing 2 SD above the mean requirement was determined assuming that the CV for maintenance was 12.5% and that the CV for growth was 32%, as suggested by Beaton and Chery (1988). Nitrogen requirement was then converted to crude protein using a factor of 6.25 (crude protein = N × 6.25). This value then represents a safe level of protein intake expressed as an ideal protein (i.e. casein or albumin) and is presented in Table 9. An underlying assumption is that the high coefficient of variability for growth will adjust for the differences in growth rates observed amongst individuals of the same chronological age.

To validate this approach to estimating protein requirements, the safe level of crude protein intake was calculated at monthly intervals for the first 6 months of age (Table 10). Average protein consumption from breast milk (as reported in the FAO/WHO/UNU report 1985) is similar to the predicted safe level of intake for infants 3-4 months of age. However, average intake is above average protein requirement, but falls below the predicted safe level of intake for infants 1-2 and 2-3 months of age. Therefore it would appear that this approach to predicting protein requirements in infants overestimates actual protein requirements provided that the underlying assumption that breast milk is an adequate food (diet) for infants of this age is valid. These data, nevertheless, support the opinion presented by Beaton and Chery (1988) that the FAO/WHO/UNU committee overestimated infant protein requirements.

Adjustment for Protein Quality

To adjust for protein quality, both the EAA composition and digestibility of the habitual Canadian diet must be addressed. The overall approach used is taken from the Recommended Nutrient Intakes for Canadians (Canada. Health and Welfare 1983). The correction factors are based on information on the amino acid composition of the average diet and on the biological utilization of mixed dietary proteins. Derivation of these factors are explained in detail in the preceeding report and will only be briefly explained here.

Table 9
Derivation of the Recommended Intake of Canadian Dietary Protein

Age	Mainte-nance	Growth	Average N Requirement	+2SD	CV%[a]	Recommended Intake of Egg or Milk Protein (g/kg/day)	Quality Adjustment	Safe Level of Dietary Protein (g/kg/day)
	(mg/kg/day)							
Months								
0-2	100	147	247	334	19.7	2.15	1.0	2.15[b]
3-5	100	64	164	212	14.6	1.32	1.1	1.46[b]
6-8	100	48	148	188	13.4	1.17	1.2	1.41
9-11	100	39	139	174	12.7	1.09	1.26	1.37
Years								
1	100	24	124	153	11.8	0.96	1.26	1.21
2-3	100	19	119	147	11.7	0.92	1.26	1.16
4-6	100	13	113	139	11.7	0.87	1.22	1.06
7-9	100	11	111	137	11.7	0.86	1.20	1.03
10-12 M	100	11	111	137	11.7	0.86	1.18	1.01
F	100	12	112	138	11.7	0.86	1.18	1.01
13-15 M	100	12	112	138	11.7	0.86	1.14	0.98
F	100	8	108	133	11.8	0.83	1.14	0.95
16-18 M	100	7	107	132	11.9	0.83	1.12	0.93
F	100	1	101	126	12.4	0.79	1.12	0.88
19+	100	0	100	125	12.5	0.78	1.10	0.86

a. CV for maintenance taken as 12.5%; CV for growth taken as 32%.

$$CV_{total} = \sqrt{\frac{(\text{maintenance} \times CV_{maintenance})^2 + (\text{growth} \times CV_{growth})^2}{\text{maintenance} + \text{growth}}}$$

b. Safe level of protein intake in infants up to four months of age is based on the assumption that human breast milk is providing the sole source of protein. If other protein sources are being consumed, the safe level of intake must be calculated correcting for the essential amino acid profile and digestibility of the protein sources in question.

Table 10.
Crude Protein Requirements for Infants

Age (Months)	Mainte-nance	Growth	Average N[a] Requirement (mg/kg/day)	Avg Protein Requirement (g/kg/day)	CV%[b]	Safe Level of Intake as Milk Protein	Average Intake from Breast Milk (g/kg/day)
1-2	100	160	260	1.63	20.2	2.28[c]	1.93
2-3	100	114	214	1.34	18.0	1.82[c]	1.74
3-4	100	79	179	1.12	15.7	1.47[c]	1.49
4-5	100	63	163	1.02	14.6	1.32	--
5-6	100	59	159	0.99	14.2	1.28	--
6-9	100	53	153	0.96	13.8	1.22	--
9-12	100	43	143	0.89	13.0	1.13	

a. Average N increment based on data provided by Fomon *et al.* (1982) and corrected for 70% efficiency of utilization.

b. CV_{total} calculated as described in Table 9.

c. Safe level of protein intake in infants up to four months of age is based on the assumption that human breast milk is providing the only protein source. If other protein sources are being consumed, the safe level of intake must be calculated correcting for the essential amino acid profile and digestibility of the protein sources in question.

Correction for the EAA composition of the habitual Canadian diet can be made by comparing the apparent EAA composition of mixed proteins disappearing in the Canadian diet with the provisional pattern of EAA in an ideal reference protein suggested by the FAO/WHO/UNU committee (Table 11). It should be noted that expression of EAA requirements in this report as mg/g protein are higher than those in the FAO/WHO/UNU (1985) report. This is due to the fact that the estimates of recommended intake of egg or milk protein reported here are lower than those in the FAO/WHO/UNU report. Values for the EAA composition of the habitual Canadian diet were taken from the 1983 report (Canada. Health and Welfare) which was based on food disappearance data (Ballantyne and McLaughlan 1968). It can be seen that the habitual Canadian diet supplies EAA in excess of that suggested in the provisional pattern for all EAA. The predicted amino acid score of the habitual diet (rather than the score of individual foods) is 100%; hence no correction for protein quality is necessary for adults. To correct for bioavailability of amino acids, it is generally assumed that the digestibility of the mixed diet is approximately 90% in comparison to that of egg or milk. Therefore the theoretical adjustment factor would be (100/90) or 1.1.

In determining the safe level of protein intake for infants and children, corrections for both protein quality and digestibility may be required. In comparing the FAO/WHO/UNU provisional pattern of EAA for children two years of age with the pattern of EAAs in the habitual Canadian diet, it would appear that lysine, threonine and valine may be limiting amino acids. The predicted amino acid score for infants on the habitual diet would be approximately 88%, in comparison with the FAO/WHO/UNU reference protein. Assuming that the correction for digestibility is constant throughout the lifespan, the theoretical correction factor would then be (100/88) × (100/90) or 1.26. This correction factor may be an overestimate for children, since data for the havitual Canadian diet are based on food disappearance figures. The greater milk consumption observed in infants and children would theoretically increase the amino acid score of their habitual diet (eg. cow's milk contains 78 mg lysine/g protein) (FAO/WHO/UNU 1985). However, given the lack of information regarding food consumption patterns for infants and children, the value of 1.26 was used.

Table 11.
Amino Acid Composition of the Average Mixed Protein in Diet of Canadians and Comparison with the Provisional Amino Acid Pattern

	(Canadian) Diet[a]	FAO/WHO/UNU Provisional Pattern[b]				
		Adults		Children (2 yrs)		Infants (3-4 mos.)
	(mg/g)	(mg/kg)	(mg/g)	(mg/kg)	(mg/g)	(mg/kg)
Histidine[c]		[8-12]	[10-15]	[19]	[27]	28
Isoleucine	46.7	10	12.8	31	33.7	70
Leucine	79.1	14	17.9	73	79.3	161
Lysine	61.6	12	15.4	64	70.0	103
Methionine + Cystine	34.1	13	16.7	69	29.3	58
Phenylalanine + Tyrosine	81.8	14	17.9	27	75.0	125
Threonine	38.4	7	9.0	37	40.2	87
Tryptophan	12.3	3.5	4.5	12.5	13.6	17
Valine	57.6	10	12.8	38	41.3	93

a. Based on information presented in previous report (Canada. Health and Welfare 1983). Apparent amino acid composition of the mixed protein disappearing from the Canadian food supply.

b. FAO/WHO/UNU estimates of amino acid requirements (FAO/WHO/UNU 1985), expressed in mg/kg body weight. Converted to mg/g protein by dividing the amino acid requirement/kg by the recommended intake of egg or milk protein/kg. For adults the recommended intake was taken as 0.78 g/kg; for children the recommended intake was taken as 0.92 g/kg.

c. Histidine is also required by the infant and perhaps the adult, but is not thought to be limiting in the mixed proteins in the Canadian diet. Values for histidine requirements taken by extrapolation from the FAO/WHO/UNU estimates of requirement.

Further consideration is given to the correction factor when applying it to all age groups. First, it is assumed that the relative dependence on breast milk as a source of food declines during the first year of life. Therefore during the early months of life, no correction is necessary since milk is the sole source of food. As solid foods are incorporated into the diet, the need for adjustment increases up to a value of 1.26 by one year of age. Second, EAA requirements (expressed as mg/kg body weight) decline from infancy through to adulthood, such that the EAA content of the habitual Canadian diet is adequate to meet the requirements for the adult, and correction is only necessary for protein digestibility. Hence a factor of 1.1 is applied to the adult. It is then assumed that the dependence on EAA composition of the diet declines linearly from one year of age to adulthood, thus providing the various correction factors used during the growth periods (Table 9). Using these correction factors, the safe level of intake of Canadian dietary protein can be calculated (Table 9).

While these values are based on the omnivorous Canadian diet, it is generally felt that no additional corrections for protein quality are necessary for a mixed vegetarian diet provided that some milk, cheese and/or eggs are included (MacMillan and Smith 1975; Canada. Health and Welfare 1980). However, in children consuming strictly vegetarian diets, particularly if they are based principally on cereal or are very restrictive in types of foods, the values presented may be a slight underestimate due to the poorer quality and digestibility of plant proteins. Furthermore, estimates for safe levels of protein intake during the first months of life are based on the assumption that breast milk provides the sole source of foods. These values are not directly transferable to infant formulas; rather the recommended intake of milk protein should be adjusted for the EAA profile, and digestibility of the protein sources used to determine the safe level of intake for individual formulas.

The present dietary recommendations contained within this report will result in a shift of protein-containing foods towards leaner cuts of meats, poultry, fish and higher intakes of whole grain plant products; however, no appreciable effect on protein quality would be anticipated within the range of guidelines presented.

It should be noted that adjustment for protein quality is based upon the FAO/WHO/UNU provisional pattern of EAA in a reference protein. These values are derived primarily from nitrogen-balance studies in which requirements for individual EAAs were assessed. Recently, on the basis of amino acid oxidation and flux measurements using stable isotope methodology, some investigators have suggested that EAA requirements in adults, for certain EAA including lysine, leucine, threonine and valine, may have been underestimated in these earlier studies (Young *et al.* 1985; Young and Bier 1987). Unfortunately, the physiological significance of the more recent stable isotope studies is poorly understood. At present there are insufficient data to alter EAA requirements for adults based on stable isotope studies. However, even if these investigators are correct, it would appear that the amino acid score of the habitual Canadian diet is still sufficient to provide adequate amounts of EAAs and no adjustment in the calculation of safe level of intake is necessary.

Pregnancy and Lactation

Estimates for additional protein requirements to support pregnancy and lactation are based on rates of nitrogen-accretion and nitrogen-retention during pregnancy and nitrogen content of breast milk respectively. These nitrogen values can then be used to convert to daily protein requirements assuming the same factorial model used for infants.

During pregnancy, protein requirements can be broken down into two components: one to support growth of fetal and maternal tissues, and the other to maintain these additional body stores. Due to rapid fetal growth, especially during the last trimester of pregnancy, estimates of protein requirements are based on growth and body composition at the end of each trimester, to ensure adequacy of protein intake to support normal fetal growth throughout gestation.

Requirements for the growth component are based on mean daily increments of protein in fetus and maternal body as reported by Hytten and Leitch (1971). Mean daily increments of stored protein are approximately 6 g/d during the last trimester of pregnancy. To convert this to dietary protein requirements, it is assumed that dietary protein has a 70% efficiency of utilization (correction factor = 1.43). The variability of protein requirement is assumed to be similar to that of birth weight (15%; correction factor = 1.3) and the sensitivity to protein quality to support fetal and maternal tissue growth is assumed to be similar to that of infants (correction factor = 1.26). Therefore, the recommended increase to support growth would be
$6 \times 1.43 \times 1.3 \times 1.26 = 14.1$ g/d.

The second component of requirement would then be the cost of supporting the increased maternal and fetal tissues. Average total protein accretion at 40 weeks of gestation is 925 g (Hytten and Leitch 1971). Assuming that maintenance requirements for these tissues are similar to those observed in the adult, then the value of 100 mg N/kg BW can be used once conversion relative to body protein is made. If it is assumed that the average adult body composition is 10% protein, then requirement would be equivalent to 1 mg N/g protein. Therefore an additional 925 mg nitrogen (or 5.8 g protein) would be necessary for maintenance of the protein accreted. Once again, assuming a coefficient of variability of 15% and a sensitivity to quality similar to that of the infant, the additional maintenance requirement would be
$5.8 \times 1.3 \times 1.26 = 9.5$ g/d. Total requirements for the third trimester of pregnancy would then be
$14.1 + 9.5 = 23.6$ g/d. Using the same approach (Table 12), estimates for protein requirements at the end of the first and second trimester of pregnancy would be 5 g/d and 15 g/d, respectively. These estimates of protein requirement for pregnancy are in addition to prepregnancy protein requirements.

The protein requirements for lactation are based on the average nitrogen content of breast milk. Although not all of the nitrogen is in the form of protein or amino acids, it is considered to be so for the purpose of estimating requirements. The average nitrogen content of mature breast milk is 200 mg/100 mL. Therefore an average daily secretion of 750 mL provides about 9.4 g of protein (FAO/WHO/ UNU 1985). If the efficiency of protein utilization is assumed to be 70%, the coefficient of variation 15% and the sensitivity to protein quality similar to that required for the infant (i.e. during periods of protein accretion), then the additional recommended intake for lactation would be
$9.4 \times 1.43 \times 1.3 \times 1.26 = 22$ g/d.

Table 12
Additional Protein Requirements for Pregnancy

	Growth		Maintenance		
Weeks of Pregnancy	Mean Protein Accretion[a] (g/d)	Dietary Protein Requirement (g/d)	Total Protein Accretion (g)	Dietary Protein Requirement (g/d)	Total (g/d)
13	1.6	3.7	170	1.7	5.4
26	4.9	11.5	350	3.6	15.1
40	6.0	14.1	925	9.5	23.6

a. Values for mean daily protein accretion taken from Hytten and Leitch (1971).

Dietary Protein and Chronic Diseases

Effects of High Intakes

As well as serving as a source of amino acids for the synthesis of tissue proteins, dietary protein and amino acids are sources of energy. Under normal conditions, the human body seems capable of metabolizing much higher intakes of protein than the amounts recommended in this report without apparent detrimental effect. Slight anorexia is observed when animals are shifted to a high protein diet (50-60% of calories), but this anorexic effect is short lasting and presumably related to hepatic induction of amino acid catabolic enzymes (Harper *et al.* 1970). Following this adaptation period, no differences in food consumption or growth rate are observed.

The real upper limit of the safe range of intake would appear to be set by the body's ability to excrete the end products of metabolism, notably urea, which in turn depends upon water consumption and kidney function. There is concern that high protein intakes may result in glomerular capillary hypertension and lead to glomerular sclerosis (Brenner *et al.* 1982). Glomerular capillary hypertension is associated with increased glomerular filtration rate and capillary blood flow and both of these increase in response to high protein intakes (Bosch *et al.* 1983). However, there is currently no epidemiologic data to support the hypothesis that high protein intakes increase the incidence of glomerular sclerosis associated with aging.

Cardiovascular Disease

A number of epidemiological studies have investigated the role of dietary protein as a risk factor in either cardiovascular disease or cancer. Specific interest has been placed on the role that animal versus plant proteins may play. These studies have been complicated by the fact that diets high in animal proteins are often also high in fat. Thus it has been difficult to dissociate the risk of high fat diets in the etiology of chronic diseases from that of animal proteins.

With regard to cardiovascular disease, findings from major cohort studies of coronary heart disease (CHD) have failed to demonstrate an association between total dietary protein intake and risk of CHD (Gordon *et al.* 1981; Keys *et al.* 1986). Present interest in the relationship between dietary protein and CHD relates to the potential cholesterol-lowering effect of plant relative to animal proteins. That is, data from animal experimentation (e.g. Huff and Carroll 1980; Wolfe and Grace 1987) suggest that substitution of plant protein for meat and dairy protein may have a cholesterol-lowering effect. A similar cholesterol-lowering effect of plant (soy) protein is apparent in hypercholesterolemic individuals, with the major decrease being observed in the low-density lipoprotein fraction (Sirtori *et al.* 1979; Descovich *et al.* 1980; Wolfe *et al.* 1981; Verrillo *et al.* 1985). However, the cholesterol-lowering effect of plant proteins in subjects with normal cholesterol levels is variable, with both no effect (van Raaij *et al.* 1979; Terpstra *et al.* 1983) and a decreased serum cholesterol (van Raaij *et al.* 1981; Wolfe *et al.* 1986) being reported.

It has been repeatedly observed that vegetarians have lower blood pressure in comparison to individuals who consume meat and meat products (e.g. Armstrong *et al.* 1977; Ophir *et al.* 1983; Rouse and Beilin 1984). Unfortunately, results from these studies do not allow for a determination of the effects of animal proteins in isolation from other dietary and nondietary factors. Therefore, while there is limited indication that a shift from animal proteins to vegetable proteins may have a positive effect with respect to cardiovascular disease, it would appear that the major impact of this dietary change would relate to the lower fat content of diets high in vegetable proteins, rather than to the actual change in protein sources *per se*. Therefore, at present, it would appear inappropriate to make a specific recommendation on dietary protein sources with regard to cardiovascular disease.

Cancer

Studies on cancer risk and protein intake have concentrated by and large on cancers of the large bowel and breast. Once again, the impact of both total protein and animal versus vegetable proteins has been investigated. In general, results from these studies have failed to identify either total protein intake or animal protein intake as independent risk factors. For example, in two case-control studies, while protein consumption was associated with risk of colon and rectal cancer (Jain *et al.* 1980; Potter and McMichael 1986), this association could not be clearly separated from the effects of dietary fat and/or total calories. Furthermore, results from other case-control (Macquart-Moulin *et al.* 1986; Kune *et al.* 1987) and prospective cohort studies (Stemmermann *et al.* 1984; Garland *et al.* 1985) have failed to observe an association between protein intake and colon cancer risk.

Similar results have been observed with regards to breast cancer risk. An association between protein intake, and particularly animal protein intake, and the risk of breast cancer has been reported (Armstrong and Doll 1975; Gaskill *et al.* 1979; Gray *et al.* 1979); however, the association with dietary fat appears stronger (Armstrong and Doll 1975), suggesting that animal protein intake may be serving as a proxy for fat. Furthermore, several case-control studies have failed to observe an association between protein intake and risk of breast cancer (Miller *et al.* 1978; Hirohata *et al.* 1985). Therefore, as with cardiovascular disease, it would appear at present that there are insufficient data to suggest that either high protein intakes, or intake of animal proteins, are independent risk factors.

Osteoporosis

Concern with regards to the high protein intake of the Canadian population and risk of osteoporosis relates to the observation that high intakes of protein, consumed as a purified isolated nutrient, increases calcium excretion (Margen *et al*. 1974; Kim and Linkswiler 1979; Hegsted and Linkswiler 1981). Results from these studies, however, should not be extended to the normal diet since it appears that high protein intakes increase urinary calcium excretion only if phosphorus intake is held constant. Since phosphorus intake increases in conjunction with protein intake, when protein is consumed in normal foods, the impact of high protein intakes on calcium balance is minimal (Hegsted and Linkswiler 1981; Schuette and Linkswiler 1982). Therefore, there is presently no evidence to suggest that high dietary protein intakes serve as a risk factor in osteoporosis.

Recommendation for Protein Intake

It must be noted that the present report estimates safe levels of protein intake for Canadians. However, it is well known that protein intakes exceed this value in almost all individuals. This is primarily due to the distribution of protein in foods commonly consumed in the Canadian diet. Results from the Nutrition Canada Survey (Canada. Health and Welfare 1975) suggested that mean protein intakes were well above protein requirements for virtually all age groups except for those 65+ years of age. Mean protein intakes for women 65+ years was 0.78 g/kg BW — a value below the present recommendation of 0.86 g/kg BW. Men 65+ years fared slightly better, with a mean intake of 0.93 g/kg BW. Assuming that protein requirements do not change with age during adulthood, these observations would suggest that a proportion of seniors, especially women, are at risk for dietary protein inadequacy. Attention should be given to the elderly Canadian population to ensure adequacy of nutrient intake.

Despite the high levels of protein intake observed in most Canadians, to lower protein consumption, food selection patterns would have to be dramatically altered. There is currently no evidence to suggest that the high level of protein intake observed in the Canadian diet has any deleterious effects for the healthy individual with normal hepatic and renal function. It must be emphasized that the recommendations are to maintain current patterns of protein consumption, and not to lower them to the safe level of intake.

Recommendations for Protein Density of the Diet

There is generally great concern and controversy regarding the appropriateness of expressing protein requirements relative to energy, since these two requirements differ amongst individuals, each having their own independent distributions. That is, the ideal protein/energy (PE) ratio of a diet for an individual with a high protein requirement yet low energy requirement will be higher than that for the individual with high requirements for both protein and energy. Therefore, it is not possible to define the optimal PE ratio of the diet for an individual without knowing his/her requirement for both protein and energy. Interpretation of PE ratios should be made with caution when applying them to the individual. However, for the purpose of expressing the ideal distribution of macronutrient calories in the diet, an attempt at defining PE ratios must be made.

A requirement curve similar to that for other nutrients can theoretically be generated, in which a mean and mean + 2SD of PE ratios can be determined. Thus, a safe PE ratio (mean + 2SD) would ideally cover the protein needs of an individual with a high protein requirement yet low energy requirement provided that his/her energy requirements were met. One such approach to describing the distribution of satisfactory PE ratios is currently in the FAO/WHO/UNU report (1985), based on the statistical and conceptual models of Beaton and Swiss (1974). Reasonable estimates of average requirements for protein and energy, the coefficient of variation of these requirements and the correlation between requirements for protein and energy are needed to predict PE ratios at any given probability (or risk) level. For the purpose of this report, calculations are based on ideal energy intakes rather than on actual energy intakes (i.e. a normative rather than status quo approach) and assume that moderate activity levels are maintained throughout the lifespan. Obviously, as energy intakes shift from the ideal, an effect on ideal PE ratios will be observed. Beaton and Swiss (1974) attempted to obtain estimates of the correlation between energy and protein requirements per unit body weight and concluded that if a correlation existed, it was very low and not likely to exceed 0.2. Using these calculations, a correlation of 0.2 yields values very close to those with a correlation of 0; a correlation of zero has been assumed. A probability (or risk) level of 97.5% has been used, to be consistent with the approach used for nutrient requirements.

The second factor requiring consideration is that both activity levels and chronological age have a major impact on energy requirements throughout the lifespan, while protein requirements do not change beyond adulthood. Therefore it is inappropriate to express one ideal P/E ratio for the adult years; rather the P/E ratio will increase with age, reflecting the decline in energy requirements. The impact of age (i.e. declining energy requirements) on an ideal P/E ratio can be observed (Table 13), with ideal P/E ratios increasing from 10.4% at 19 years of age to 12.2% at age 75 and over in men and from 12.4% to 13.4% over the same age span in women.

In examining Canadian consumption patterns, there is a remarkable consistency in P/E ratios, ranging from 13-15% (Canada. Health and Welfare 1975). This consumption pattern would therefore appear to be appropriate until adulthood. However, this protein density may be low for senior citizens, with a small proportion of female seniors expected to be at risk for protein status. This observation is consistent with the results of the Nutrition Canada survey (Canada. Health and Welfare 1975), suggesting that a portion of senior women are consuming inadequate protein levels.

Table 13
Required Protein/Energy Ratio of the Canadian Diet

Age (Years)		Protein/Energy Ratio[a,b] g protein per 1000 kcal	g protein per 5000 MJ	protein energy per 1000 kcal	protein energy per 5000 MJ
19-24	M	26	31	10.4	12.4
	F	31	37	12.4	14.8
25-49	M	27	32	10.8	13.0
	F	31	37	12.4	14.8
50-74	M	29.5	35	11.8	14.1
	F	33.5	40	13.1	15.7
75+	M	30.5	36	12.2	14.6
	F	33.5	40	13.4	16.0

a. Calculated on the basis of theoretical daily energy requirements according to age, sex and activity (see chapter on energy) assuming maintenance of a moderate activity level.

b. Calculated according to equation provided in FAO/WHO/UNO report (1985; Annex 9) with $\alpha = 0.025$ and assuming the correlation between energy and protein requirements among individuals is zero. Hence

$$R\alpha = \frac{E^2}{E^2 - Z\alpha^2 S_E^2}\left[\frac{P}{E} + \frac{Z\alpha Q}{E}\right]$$

$$\text{and } Q = \sqrt{Sp^2 + \frac{P^2 S_E^2}{E^2} - \frac{Z\alpha^2 S_p^2 S_E^2}{E^2}}$$

Where

$R\alpha$ is the value of the protein energy ratio requirement that would be expected to be exceeded by a certain proportion (α) of individuals

$Z\alpha$ is the standardized normal deviation above which α of the distribution lies (e.g., $Z_{0.025} = 1.96$)

E is the average energy requirement for the specific class of individuals

P is the average protein requirement for the specific class of individuals, expressed as energy equivalents

S_E is the standard deviation of energy requirements

Sp is the standard deviation of protein requirements

Based on these observations, it is recommended that the Canadian diet remain at 13-15% of calories as protein throughout adulthood. However, the protein density of the diet should increase, especially in female seniors, to 15-20% of calories to ensure adequacy of protein intake.

References

Armstrong, B. and Doll, R. 1975. Environmental factors and cancer incidence and mortality in different countries, with specific reference to dietary practices. Int. J. Cancer 15:617-631.

Armstrong, B., Van Merwyk, A.J. and Coates, H. 1977. Blood pressure in Seventh-Day Adventist vegetarians. Am. J. Epidemiol. 105:444-449.

Ballantyne, R.M. and McLaughlan, J.M. 1968. The quality of the "protein" of the Canadian diet. Can. Nutr. Notes 24:79-80.

Beaton, G.H. and Swiss, L.D. 1974. Evaluation of the nutritional quality of food supplies: the prediction of "desirable" or "safe" protein:calorie ratios. Am. J. Clin. Nutr. 27:485-504.

Beaton, G.H. and Chery, A. 1988. Protein requirements of infants: a reexamination of concepts and approaches. Am. J. Clin. Nutr. 48:1403-1412.

Beaton, G.H., Calloway, D.H. and Waterlow, J. 1979. Protein and energy requirements: a joint FAO/WHO memorandum. Bull. WHO 57:65-79.

Bosch, J.P., Saccaggi, A., Lauer, A., Ronco, C., Belledonne, M. and Glabman, S. 1983. Renal functional reserve in humans: effect of protein intake on glomerular filtration rate. Am. J. Med. 75:943-950.

Brenner, B.M., Meyer, T.W. and Hostetter, T.H. 1982. Dietary protein intake and the progressive nature of kidney disease: the role of hemodynamically mediated glomerular injury in the pathogenesis of progressive glomerular sclerosis in aging, renal ablation, and intrinsic renal disease. N. Engl. J. Med. 307:652-659.

Canada. Health and Welfare. Nutrition Canada. Health Protection Branch. Bureau of Nutritional Sciences. 1975. The Ontario survey report. Ottawa.

Canada. Health and Welfare. Health Protection Branch. Nutrition Research Division. 1980. An amino acid profile of a vegetarian diet. Ottawa.

Canada. Health and Welfare. Health Protection Branch. Bureau of Nutritional Sciences. 1983. Recommended nutrient intakes for Canadians. Ottawa.

Descovich, G.C., Gaddi, A., Mannino, G., Cattin, L., Senin, U., Caruzzo, C., Fragiacomo, C., Sirtori, M., Ceredi, C., Benassi, M.S., Colombo, L., Fontana, G., Mannarino, E., Bertelli, E., Noseda, G. and Sirtori, C.R. 1980. Multicentre study of soybean protein diet for outpatient hypercholesterolemic patients. Lancet 2:709-712.

FAO/WHO. 1973. Energy and protein requirements. Report of a Joint FAO/WHO Ad Hoc Expert Committee. W.H.O. Tech. Rep. Ser. 522.

FAO/WHO/UNU. 1985. Energy and protein requirements. Report of a Joint FAO/WHO/UNU Expert Consultation. W.H.O. Tech. Rep. Ser. 724.

Fomon, S.J., Haschke, F., Ziegler, E.E. and Nelson, S.E. 1982. Body composition of reference children from birth to age 10 years. Am. J. Clin. Nutr. 35:1169-1175.

Garland, C., Shekelle, R.B., Barrett-Connor, E., Criqui, M.H., Rossof, A.H. and Paul, O. 1985. Dietary vitamin D and calcium and risk of colorectal cancer: a 19-year prospective study in men. Lancet 1:307-309.

Gaskill, S.P., McGuire, W.L., Osborne, C.K. and Stern, M.P. 1979. Breast cancer mortality and diet in the United States. Cancer Res. 39:3628-3637.

Gordon, T., Kagan, A., Garcia-Palmieri, M., Kannel, W.B., Zukel, W.J., Tillotson, J., Sorlie, P. and Hjortland, M. 1981. Diet and its relation to coronary heart disease and death in three populations. Circulation 63:500-515.

Gray, G.E., Pike, M.C. and Henderson, B.E. 1979. Breast-cancer incidence and mortality rates in different countries in relation to known risk factors and dietary practices. Br. J. Cancer 39:1-7.

Harper, A.E., Benevenga, N.J. and Wohlhueter, R.M. 1970. Effects of ingestion of disproportionate amounts of amino acids. Physiol. Rev. 50:428-558.

Hegsted, M. and Linkswiler, H.M. 1981. Long-term effects of level of protein intake on calcium metabolism in young adult women. J. Nutr. 111:244-251.

Hirohata, T., Shigematsu, T., Nomura, A.M., Nomura, Y., Horie, A. and Hirohata, I. 1985. Occurrence of breast cancer in relation to diet and reproductive history: a case-control study in Fukuoka, Japan. Nat. Cancer Inst. Monogr. 69:187-190.

Huang, P.C., Lin, C.P. and Hsu, J.Y. 1980. Protein requirements of normal infants at the age of about 1 year: maintenance nitrogen requirements and obligatory nitrogen losses. J. Nutr. 110:1727-1735.

Huff, M.W. and Carroll, K.K. 1980. Effects of dietary proteins and amino acid mixtures on plasma cholesterol levels in rabbits. J. Nutr. 110:1676-1685.

Hytten, F.E. and Leitch, I. 1971. The physiology of human pregnancy. 2nd ed. Blackwell Scientific Publications, Oxford.

Jain, M., Cook, G.M., Davis, F.G., Grace, M.G., Howe, G.R. and Miller, A.B. 1980. A case-control study of diet and colo-rectal cancer. Int. J. Cancer 26:757-768.

Keys, A., Menotti, A., Karvonen, M.J., Aravanis, C., Blackburn, H., Buzina, R., Djordjevic, B.S., Dontas, A.S., Fidanza, F., Keys, M.H., Kromhout, D., Nedeljkovic, S., Punsar, S., Seccareccia, F. and Toshima, H. 1986. The diet and 15-year death rate in the Seven Countries Study. Am. J. Epidemiol. 124:903-915.

Kim, Y. and Linkswiler, H.M. 1979. Effect of level of protein intake on calcium metabolism and on parathyroid and renal function in the adult human male. J. Nutr. 109:1399-1404.

Kune, S., Kune, G.A. and Watson, L.F. 1987. Case-control study of dietary etiological factors: the Melbourne Colorectal Cancer Study. Nutr. Cancer 9:21-42.

MacMillan, J.B. and Smith, E.B. 1975. Development of a lacto-ovo vegetarian food guide. J. Can. Diet. Assoc. 36:110-117.

Macquart-Moulin, G., Riboli, E., Cornée, J., Charnay, B., Berthezène, P. and Day, N. 1986. Case-control study on colorectal cancer and diet in Marseilles. Int. J. Cancer 38:183-191.

Margen, S., Chu, J.Y., Kaufmann, N.A. and Calloway, D.H. 1974. Studies in calcium metabolism. I. The calciuretic effect of dietary protein. Am. J. Clin. Nutr. 27:584-589.

Miller, A.B., Kelly, A., Choi, N.W., Matthews, V., Morgan, R.W., Munan, L., Burch, J.D., Feather, J., Howe, G.R. and Jain, M. 1978. A study of diet and breast cancer. Am. J. Epidemiol. 107:499-509.

Ophir, O., Peer, G., Gilad, J., Blum, M. and Aviram, A. 1983. Low blood pressure in vegetarians: the possible role of potassium. Am. J. Clin. Nutr. 37:755-762.

Potter, J.D. and McMichael, A.J. 1986. Diet and cancer of the colon and rectum: a case-control study. J. Nat. Cancer Inst. 76:557-569.

Rouse, I.L. and Beilin, L.J. 1984. Vegetarian diet and blood pressure. J. Hypertens. 2:231-240.

Schuette, S.A. and Linkswiler, H.M. 1982. Effects on Ca and P metabolism in humans by adding meat, meat plus milk, or purified proteins plus Ca and P to a low protein diet. J. Nutr. 112:338-349.

Sirtori, C.R., Gatti, E., Mantero, O., Conti, F., Agradi, E., Tremoli, E., Sirtori, M., Fraterrigo, L., Tavazzi, L. and Kritchevsky, D. 1979. Clinical experience with the soybean protein diet in the treatment of hypercholesterolemia. Am. J. Clin. Nutr. 32:1645-1658.

Stemmermann, G.N., Nomura, A.M.Y. and Heilburn, L.K. 1984. Dietary fat and the risk of colorectal cancer. Cancer Res. 44:4633-4637.

Terpstra, A.H.M., Hermus, R.J.J. and West, C.E. 1983. The role of dietary protein in cholesterol metabolism. World Rev. Nutr. Diet. 42:1-55.

Torun, B., Cabrera-Santiago, M.I. and Viteri, F.E. 1981. Protein requirements of preschool children: milk and soybean protein isolate. *In* Protein-energy requirements of developing countries: evaluation of new data: report of a working group. Torun, B., Young, V.R. and Rand, W.M., eds. United Nations University, Tokyo, pp. 182-190.

van Raaij, J.M.A., Katan, M.B. and Hautvast, J.G.A.J. 1979. Casein, soya protein, serum-cholesterol. Lancet 2:958.

van Raaij, J.M.A., Katan, M.B., Hautvast, J.G.A.J. and Hermus, R.J.J. 1981. Effects of casein versus soy protein diets on serum cholesterol and lipoproteins in young healthy volunteers. Am. J. Clin. Nutr. 34:1261-1271.

Verrillo, A., de Teresa, A., Giarrusso, P.C. and La Rocca, S. 1985. Soybean protein diets in the management of type II hyperlipoproteinaemia. Atherosclerosis 54:321-331.

Wolfe, B.M. and Grace, D.M. 1987. Substitution of mixed amino acids resembling soy protein for mixed amino acids resembling casein in the diet reduces plasma cholesterol in slowly, but not rapidly fed nor fasted baboons. Metabolism 36:223-229.

Wolfe, B.M., Giovannetti, P.M., Cheng, D.C.H., Roberts, D.C.K. and Carroll, K.K. 1981. Hypolipidemic effect of substituting soybean protein isolate for all meat and dairy protein in the diets of hypercholesterolemic men. Nutr. Rep. Int. 24:1187-1198.

Wolfe, B.M., Taves, E.H. and Giovannetti, P.M. 1986. Low protein diet decreases serum cholesterol in healthy human subjects (abst.). Clin. Invest. Med. 9 (Suppl.):A43.

Young, V.R. and Bier, D.M. 1987. A kinetic approach to the determination of human amino acid requirements. Nutr. Rev. 45:289-298.

Young, V.R., Meredith, C., Hoerr, R., Bier, D.M. and Matthews, D.E. 1985. Amino acid kinetics in relation to protein and amino acid requirements: the primary importance of amino acid oxidation. *In* Substrate and energy metabolism in man. Garrow, J.S. and Halliday, D., eds. Libbey, London, pp. 119-134.

Fat-Soluble Vitamins

Carotene and Vitamin A

Chemistry and Biochemistry of Vitamin A

The term vitamin A can be used to describe all substances that possess such nutritional activity, or it can refer specifically to the isoprenoid primary alcohol, retinol. Although it is usual to identify vitamin A with the free alcohol, most of the naturally occurring preformed vitamin is in the form of long-chain retinyl fatty acid esters.

Retinyl esters, accompanied by smaller amounts of the free alcohol and related derivatives, are found only in animal tissues. They are formed during the metabolism of certain carotenoids, known as provitamins, that are present in foods derived from plants and microorganisms. The most abundant provitamin, β-carotene, is structurally equivalent to two molecules of retinol joined tail-to-tail, whereas the resemblance to vitamin A exists in only one half of the molecule of other provitamins.

Hundreds of carotenoids have been identified as natural pigments of foods, but barely fifty have provitamin activity, and only a fifth of these have any nutritional significance. β-Carotene accounts for most of the provitamin activity of North American diets, and in nutrition, other forms need be considered only when individual fruits and vegetables are evaluated in isolation. Until recently, most of the remaining carotenoids were considered to have little importance in human nutrition, other than that they often interfered in the analysis for β-carotene and thus were responsible for serious errors in vitamin A values in tables of food composition.

From time to time, it has been suggested that carotenoids, in addition to sometimes functioning as precursors of vitamin A, might have other biochemical roles in higher animals. This theory is understandably encouraged by observations that carotenoids are often accumulated in visibly high concentrations in certain tissues, although often with marked variations among species. The skin and appendages of birds, for example, are sometimes deeply coloured by carotenoids, and ovaries and eggs of many animals are similarly heavily pigmented. The results of most nutritional investigations have been negative, however, and a vital role for carotenoids, other than that as a precursor of vitamin A, has yet to be demonstrated. Although some observations indicated that carotenoids might affect reproduction in cattle (Lotthammer 1979), the existence of a special role for carotene in reproduction has not been confirmed (Chew and Archer 1983; Marcek *et al.*1985; Wang *et al.*1988). Moreover, many nutritional experiments have involved rearing animals, sometimes for several generations, on carotenoid-free diets. Other than lack of pigmentation, no deleterious effects have been reported.

It has been suggested that carotenes, and perhaps other carotenoids, are antioxidants in tissues and thus quench or deactivate free radicals and excited oxygen (Packer *et al.* 1981; Krinsky and Deneke 1982; Burton and Ingold 1984). Such properties can be used imaginatively to explain how carotenoids might protect animals against carcinogens and related noxious chemicals and even harmful radiations, but evidence that these mechanisms are more than theory is less easily obtained.

Unlike carotene and other carotenoids, retinol has well-established biochemical roles in maintaining epithelial tissues, bone growth, vision and reproduction. Diets that lack vitamin A lead to deficiency disease and, when consumed for long periods, are fatal. The most prominent signs of deficiency differ with age and species: in many animals, metaplasia of epithelial tissues leads to infection and death; in others, such as growing birds, stunting of bone growth compresses the nervous system and causes paralysis.

In humans, the first symptom of deficiency is night blindness, which can be attributed to reduced sensitivity of rod receptors in the retina. In more extreme and protracted deficiency, mucous-secreting epithelia in several locations in the body undergo a keratinizing metaplasia which is associated with dryness and increased susceptibility to infection. The epithelia of the cornea and conjunctiva are especially vulnerable during metaplasia and the consequences of damage to the surface of the eye (xerophthalmia) are far more serious than those resulting from depletion of visual pigment in the retina. Whereas night-blindness is reversible, xerophthalmia can involve irreparable damage. It was once estimated that 25% of the survivors of severe vitamin A deficiency are totally blind, many are partially blind and only 15-25% regain unimpaired sight (WHO/USAID 1976). In some parts of the world, xerophthalmia is a common manifestation of serious deficiency. The overt disease is often associated with high mortality and low resistance to infection.

The role of the aldehyde, retinal, in the formation of visual pigments has been elucidated in detail and the importance of vitamin A in maintaining visual receptor cells is well understood. The other biochemical actions of the vitamin, however, have not been satisfactorily explained.

Although only the initial steps in the metabolism of the vitamin have been traced, much has been learned concerning the digestion, absorption and storage of the vitamin and provitamins, and this information explains most of the biochemical processes important to nutrition. Absorbed retinol is esterified in mucosal cells (Helgerud *et al.* 1983) and passes, mainly in the form of the palmitate, into chylomicrons which, after passage in the circulation, are taken up by hepatocytes (Blomhoff *et al.* 1985a). When more than trace amounts of the vitamin are ingested, a substantial proportion, estimated to reach one-half of the amount consumed, is retained in liver stellate and parenchymal cells (Blomhoff *et al.* 1985b). The liver vitamin A is often viewed as a nutritional "reserve" or "store" because it can protect against deficiency during prolonged periods on a deficient diet.

Vitamin A is released from the liver to the blood on a carrier, retinol binding protein (RBP), and the serum level is maintained relatively constant by homeostatic mechanisms. Values fall only when dietary deprivation is sufficiently prolonged to permit exhaustion of the liver reserves, and at the other extreme, blood levels increase slowly, if at all, when dietary intakes are high. Measurements of serum vitamin A are thus useful for confirming the onset of serious deficiency, but they reveal little concerning the magnitudes of generous dietary intakes or the size of the corresponding liver stores. Although the blood level of vitamin A is of limited use in evaluating nutritional status, especially when frank deficiency is rare or absent, it is easily measured and thus is usually recorded in nutrition surveys. The vitamin A content of the liver is the best index of status, and much effort has been directed at developing methods to estimate it indirectly in living subjects. Most of these techniques have proved to be too expensive or unreliable (Olson 1982), but a "relative dose response test" (Loerch *et al.* 1979) is currently gaining limited acceptance (Flores *et al.* 1984).

The intestinal absorption of carotene benefits when conditions in the lumen encourage emulsification of fats, and suffers, during digestive diseases for example, when they are otherwise. β-Carotene is converted to retinol in the wall of the intestine. Two mechanisms have been proposed, one involving gradual shortening of the molecule (Sharma *etal.*1977), and the second involving central cleavage (Goodman and Huang 1965). Carotenoid levels in blood, unlike those of retinol, are apparently not maintained constant and, in parallel with those in tissues, they vary roughly in proportion to the amounts ingested in the diet.

The efficiency with which dietary β-carotene can be absorbed and converted to retinol is important in the assessment of vitamin A activity of diets, but considerable variation exists, and no accurate representation is possible. Carotene dispersed or dissolved in oil, for example, is utilised more efficiently than that occurring in vegetables. A simple approximation that is now often employed is to assume that the activity of β-carotene is one-sixth of that of an equal weight of retinol, and on this basis, vitamin A activities can be expressed as "retinol equivalents" (RE) each of which corresponds to either one microgram of retinol or six micrograms of carotene (FAO/WHO 1967).

Sources of Vitamin A and the Prevalence of Deficiency in North America

In industrialized countries, vitamin A deficiency is rarely reported. It is generally assumed that the availability of fruits and vegetables, combined with food fortification, has eliminated all risk of deficiency of vitamin A.

Although the public is encouraged to consume recommended amounts of vitamin A, there appears to be neither a clear definition of what constitutes an inadequate diet nor information on how often such diets are likely to be consumed.

Reports of frank deficiency in earlier times seem to have little relevance to present day nutrition. It is true that prior to the discovery of vitamins, night blindness and sometimes xerophthalmia occurred sporadically in Europe and America, but usually only during wars or in groups enduring severe poverty (McLaren 1980). At the beginning of the century, Little (1912) noted night blindness in Newfoundland, at a time when vegetables and game were scarce, and the diet was often no more than bread, tea and molasses. Night blindness was probably still a problem in Newfoundland (Aykroyd 1928; Steven and Wald 1941) until deficiency was eliminated by improvements to the diet, including the use of fortified margarine (Aykroyd *et al.*1949). By the late thirties, serious vitamin A deficiency was considered to be rare in American cities, although night blindness was suspected to be not uncommon.

Many tests of dark adaptation were made before the Second World War, with conflicting results. Although the occurrence of deficiency was probably overestimated, the reports included observations that indicate how mild deficiency might occur even today. Jeghers (1937), for example, found that among university students responding abnormally in tests of dark adaptation, many reported annoying night blindness. The extreme dietary habits of one with especially marked symptoms illustrated how a low intake of vitamin A might be accidentally achieved in the absence of poverty or forced deprivation: for a long period, meals consisted of doughnuts and coffee, meat sandwiches, or meat, bread, potatoes, dessert and a small portion of vegetable. By choice, no milk, fruit, spinach, carrots, liver or cheese was consumed for years.

Jeghers emphasized that deficiency disease occurred because of avoidance of foods containing vitamin A for very long periods of time. Such monotonous habits, which must be uncommon, presumably allow depletion of liver reserves. Most individuals have sufficient vitamin in the liver to protect against deficiency disease for months. This was demonstrated a short time later in an experiment in Sheffield, England (Hume and Krebs 1949) in which volunteers were given deficient diets. The blood levels did not fall for eight months, and only three of the 16 participants displayed markedly abnormal visual sensitivity even after 18 months.

In more recent surveys, such as Nutrition Canada, vitamin A status has been assessed in large numbers of individuals, mainly from measurements of blood levels. The interpretation of such data has been difficult. Some differences in blood levels appear to be related to dietary intakes, such as the relatively low values found in Indians and Eskimos compared to other groups, but the implications concerning health are unclear (Hoffer *et al.* 1981). In the United States, low blood levels of vitamin A have been observed in certain ethnic groups, such as Hispanic children (Looker *et al.* 1988).

The most revealing modern data concerning the general population have been obtained from measurements of liver reserves in individuals who have met sudden, accidental death. A survey in Canada indicated that the mean concentration was 173 µg/g, a value in the same range as those observed in similar surveys in British and American cities (Huque 1982). A significant finding was the wide variation in levels, indicating presumably proportional differences in long-term intake. Although no values below 40 µg/g were observed in accident victims from London, 19% were in this category in Ottawa, 35% in New York City (Underwood *et al.* 1970) and 11-30% in surveys in Missouri, Iowa, Ohio, California and Texas (Raica *etal.* 1972). The significance to health of such relatively low reserves is uncertain but Huque (1982) regards them as "being indicative of low or marginal vitamin A status."

Vitamin A, Carotenoids and Cancer

Research concerning vitamin A in cancer can be classified in two categories. The first concerns the use of vitamin A and related substances (retinoids), sometimes in large doses, in the treatment of cancer (Hill and Grubbs 1982; Pawson *et al.*1982). Usually the purpose of such work has been the development of drugs, an objective not directly relevant to nutrition recommendations.

The second issue which has been investigated in the last decade is the possibility that dietary intakes of vitamin A and carotene are related to the development of cancer in the general population. Evidence that individuals developing cancer have a low vitamin A status has been obtained by measuring blood levels and estimating dietary intakes. Although conclusions based on available data (Peto *et al.* 1981) have attracted much publicity and stimulated long-term research, most studies are compromised by the unavoidable practical difficulties in obtaining conclusive information. While many investigations have yielded evidence of statistically significant associations, evaluation of biochemical and nutritional factors suggests that the implied relationships between nutrition and cancer are suspect, in that they should not have been so easily detectable. Blood retinol levels, for example, are not clearly related to vitamin A status in most of the population. Measurements of serum levels of retinol in cancer patients have provided the least convincing evidence, being confounded by depressed appetites and other secondary changes associated with severe illness. Prospective studies, while more reliable, require surveys of large groups over periods of many years. Some of the reports published so far have concerned samples that were too small, and data have not always been properly adjusted for confounding effects (Palgi 1984).

It is difficult to obtain reliable estimates of dietary vitamin A in any circumstances because of the wide day-to-day variations in intake, and uncertainty concerning the levels of vitamin A in foods. Difficulties are further increased in surveys in which intakes must be recalled from the past, sometimes by surviving relatives. Palgi (1984) has provided more detailed comments on the inconsistencies and limitations in published studies concerning dietary vitamin A and cancer.

The evidence obtained so far is thus inconclusive and lacks specificity. Early studies in this area are reviewed by Peto *et al.*(1981) and Kummet *et al.*(1983). More recent findings indicate that reduced cancer risk is probably not linked to an increased intake of preformed vitamin A (Olson 1986a). On the contrary, intakes of retinol have been positively correlated with colon cancer (Potter and McMichael 1986; Tuyns *et al.* 1987a), oesophageal cancer (Tuyns *et al.* 1987b) and prostate cancer (Graham *et al.* 1983; Heshmat *et al.* 1985; Kolonel *et al.* 1987). Moreover, no beneficial effects in the prevention of oesophageal cancer were observed in an intervention trial with retinol and other micronutrients (Munoz *et al.* 1985).

Although Basu *et al.* (1982) reported low serum vitamin A levels in women with breast cancer, other studies failed to confirm this association (Wald *et al.* 1984; Willett *et al.* 1984) and recent investigations concerning breast cancer suggest either no relationship with dietary carotene or retinol (Marubini *et al.* 1988) or a connection primarily with the consumption of green vegetables (La Vecchia *et al.* 1987; Katsouyanni *et al.* 1988).

On the other hand, an association has been consistently observed between increased consumption of total vitamin A, carotene or green and yellow fruits and vegetables, and decreased risk of cancer in epithelial tissues (Underwood 1986) such as in bladder (Mettlin and Graham 1979; Michalek *et al.* 1987), uterus and cervix (La Vecchia 1984), oral cavity (Marshall *et al.* 1982; Winn *et al.* 1984; Stich *et al.*1986) and especially in lung (Peto *et al.* 1981; Palgi 1984; Underwood 1986; Bond *et al.* 1987; Pastorino *et al.* 1987).

It remains possible, however, that carotene is only an indicator of other substances that are present or missing from protective diets. More decisive proof that carotene has a direct role in cancer prevention requires intervention studies. Several trials of the effectiveness of β-carotene in cancer prevention are underway (Mathews-Roth 1985; Underwood 1986; Bertram *et al.* 1987), but results will not be obtained for several years.

Toxicity

Vitamin A is toxic and teratogenic when consumed in large amounts (Geelen 1979). Excessive intakes, however, have most often occurred because of the use of vitamin supplements or high-potency preparations (Lippe *et al.* 1981; Anon. 1982). Although there are concerns about the potential toxicity of high levels of vitamin A in liver, as in the etiology of diseases in arctic explorers and pibloktoq (hysteria) in Inuit (Landy 1985), reasonable quantities of other foods, even when fortified, contain innocuous amounts of the vitamin.

Supplements of vitamin A should be used cautiously or not at all by pregnant women (Rosa *et al.* 1986; Teratology Society 1987). The recommended amounts of naturally occurring vitamin A in a mixed diet, however, are far from levels associated with teratogenic effects or other symptoms of hypervitaminosis.

Requirements for Vitamin A

The literature concerning requirements for vitamin A was comprehensively reviewed in 1972 (Rodriguez and Irwin 1972) and has been evaluated many times in dietary standards (FAO/WHO 1967) including those from Canada (Canadian Council on Nutrition 1964; Canada. Health and Welfare 1975a, 1983). Although substantial progress has been made since the appearance of these documents in the investigation of the metabolism and function of vitamin A , little has been added to the basic information used to establish national "recommended intakes" and similar standards concerning the prevention of vitamin A deficiency disease. The issue has been complicated, however, by the numerous investigations of the possibility that vitamin A or carotenoids might be involved in the prevention of cancer. One consequence of debate over practical implications of these findings has been the publication of reviews suggesting increases (Anon. 1985; Hegsted 1986) or reductions (Olson 1986b, 1987a,b) to previously accepted values for recommended intakes for vitamin A in the United States.

Information from experiments with humans (Rodriguez and Irwin 1972) suggests that 400 RE is needed by the adult for the prevention of deficiency symptoms, but the figure is acknowledged to be approximate (FAO/WHO 1967). The liver reserves in normal adults are such that it is difficult to induce deficiency, even when the diet contributes little vitamin A. Vitamin A deficiency disease is most likely to occur in infants and children under the age of five years. The recommendations concerning infants have been based on the composition of human milk and have been estimated to be 200-400 RE/day (FAO/WHO 1967).

Recommendations

In 1967, the FAO/WHO group recommended 750 RE/day for adults. This value was apparently based on the demonstration in the Sheffield experiment that an intake of approximately this magnitude was sufficient to prevent impairment of dark adaptation in two individuals (Hume and Krebs 1949). The level was considered to be compatible with the goal of maintaining a liver reserve, but no evidence was provided to indicate the magnitude. A study in the U.S. in 1971 confirmed that 500-600 RE/day was required to prevent deficiency symptoms (Sauberlich *et al.*1974).

As stated in a previous Dietary Standard for Canada (Canada. Health and Welfare 1975a) it would be imprudent for Canadians to limit their intake to the minimum requirement for the prevention of deficiency disease, and thus approach or remain at the brink of serious illness. In some parts of the world, a marginal intake of vitamin A is obtained with difficulty, and a recommendation that prevents deficiency represents a worthwhile and realistic target. In more affluent societies, however, deficiency disease has been virtually eliminated and it is apparent that diets are being consumed which make even isolated deficiencies of vitamin A unlikely in populations of hundreds of millions. There is little evidence of overt vitamin A deficiency in North America, and suggestions to the contrary (Anon. 1985) are usually based on the interpretation of serum vitamin levels rather than the occurrence of definitive symptoms. It is certain that this circumstance reflects the fact that many individuals obtain more vitamin A than they actually require. It is almost as certain that if most individuals obtained a barely adequate amount, a substantial number in the population would show signs of deficiency.

The elimination of vitamin A deficiency is readily explained by the availability of a variety of appropriate foods and prudent application of knowledge of vitamins in the fortification of foods. Resistance to deficiency can be attributed to the accumulation of liver reserves, which can be calculated to be capable of preventing deficiency even during several months of consumption of a diet devoid of vitamin A. It is difficult to estimate how often such reserves have actually prevented deficiency disease in North America. During periods of normal health and dietary practices, probably only a small fraction of the reserves are used to maintain constant levels of vitamin A in the blood. When diseases, dietary restrictions or other stresses are experienced, however, the reserves may be of greater importance. There is some evidence that the utilization and requirements for vitamin A are increased during illness, and it is clearly established that deficiency of vitamin A will aggravate the consequences of disease. It is therefore reasonable to expect a satisfactory diet in Canada to maintain a significant liver store of vitamin A in all individuals, which would guarantee protection against deficiency during periods of dietary deprivation and disease, and in mothers, provide for transfer of the vitamin to infants through the placenta and milk.

It has been established from studies with various species of animals that up to one-half of the preformed vitamin A in the diet can be stored in the liver, and lesser proportions of the vitamin occurring in the form of carotenoids. With respect to practical dietary recommendations for humans, the most useful guide has been obtained from measurements of the average dietary intake of vitamin A in large groups which can be compared with measurements of typical liver stores. In Canada, the Nutrition Canada Survey indicated that the mean intake of vitamin A in adult males was 1550 RE/day (Canada. Health and Welfare 1975b, Table 9-1) and the median value was 1120 RE/day (Canada. Health and Welfare 1977, p 99, Tables 6.1-6.2); values for females were 80% those for males. Surveys of liver stores (Hoppner *et al.* 1968) revealed a mean concentration of 125 μg retinol/g liver in accident victims. It can be concluded that an intake of 1000 RE in adult males and 800 RE in females will provide liver stores in the range of 50-150 μg/g. These values are approximations and attempts to obtain more precise data would be difficult and unlikely to be worthwhile.

Although liver reserves can be closely correlated with dietary intakes in laboratory and farm animals given diets of fixed composition, an equivalent situation does not exist in humans enjoying a free selection of foods. Dietary intakes of vitamin A are erratic in most individuals, and absorption from the intestine is affected by several factors, some transitory, such as cooking practices and the levels of fat and antioxidants in each meal, and others more serious and permanent, such as diseases affecting the digestive system.

Liver reserves of various magnitudes could be considered to be almost equally acceptable, and there is little to be gained in attempting precise or detailed calculations based on data concerning the metabolism and turnover of vitamin A in the liver. Olson (1987b) has attempted to calculate requirements for storage assuming 0.5% loss per day. He deduced that 506 RE are required daily to maintain a liver store of 20 μg/g and on this basis has justified modest and rather precise recommendations. It should be noted that a wide range of recommendations reaching up to 2500 RE/day can be calculated from the formulas by reasonably arguing that liver stores should be, and often are, over 100 μg/g. Such calculations must be applied cautiously in the development of practical recommendations. Recent experiments with animals (Green *et al.* 1987) confirm previous work indicating that depletion of liver reserves is actually a complex process.

The liver reserves of vitamin A in most Canadians are known to provide adequate protection against deficiency. It appears from surveys that such levels are accumulated when dietary intakes are centred near or above those recommended previously. No changes to previous recommendations are considered to be necessary.

It is difficult to justify different recommendations for males and females of various ages, but in the interest of consistency, recommendations can be related to body size. On this basis, 1000 RE/day can be recommended for adult males and 800 RE/day for females. An increased intake of vitamin A is not recommended during pregnancy, but the consumption of foods that are good natural sources of vitamin A is recommended during lactation. There appear to be no grounds for revision of previous recommendations for infants.

Consideration of the possible role of vitamin A and carotenoids in the occurrence of cancer may need to go beyond the conservative and cautious approach normally used in the interpretation of data concerning nutritional requirements. In all recommendations it is necessary to balance the possible benefits with associated risks. In cancer prevention, the importance of even small benefits, the importance of acting early in life, and the long delay before decisive evidence will be obtained, are all factors which could be used to justify positive recommendations based on available inconclusive data. As there is no risk in consuming generous amounts of common foods rich in carotenoids or provitamins, it can be argued that individuals have nothing to lose in making reasonable changes to their dietary habits in what, for other reasons, can be described as a desirable direction. Although it is a remote possibility, they would have much to gain if claims concerning cancer prevention later prove to be justified.

Although increased consumption of foods rich in carotenoids can be safely recommended, it must be acknowledged that there is a high probability that hopes that cancer can be avoided will not be fulfilled. There is certainly insufficient evidence to justify fortifying more foods with preformed vitamin A, or recommending the use of supplements.

A prudent but cautious approach would be limited to endorsing previous Canadian recommendations concerning vitamin A, which should provide a substantial liver reserve of vitamin A, and reinforcing the general advice to consume vegetables and fruits.

References

Anonymous. 1982. The pathophysiological basis of vitamin A toxicity. Nutr. Rev. 40:272-274.

Anonymous. 1985. Vitamin A deficiency — a global disease. Nutr. Rev. 40:240-243.

Aykroyd, W.R. 1928. Vitamin A deficiency in Newfoundland. Ir. J. Med. Sci. 6:161-165.

Aykroyd, W.R., Jolliffe, N., Lowry, O.H., Moore, P.E., Sebrell, W.H., Shank, R.E., Tisdall, F.F., Wilder, R.M. and Zamecnik, P. C. 1949. Medical resurvey of nutrition in Newfoundland 1948. Can. Med. Assoc. J. 60:329-352.

Basu, T.K., Rowlands, L., Jones, L. and Kohn, J. 1982. Vitamin A and retinol-binding protein in patients with myelomatosis and cancer of epithelial origin. Eur. J. Cancer Clin. Oncol. 18: 339-342.

Bertram, J.S., Kolonel, L.N. and Meyskens, F.L., Jr. 1987. Rationale and strategies for chemoprevention of cancer in humans. Cancer Res. 47:3012-3031.

Blomhoff, R., Rasmussen, M., Nilsson, A., Norum, K.R., Berg, T., Blaner, W.S., Kato, M., Mertz, J.R., Goodman, D.S., Eriksson, U. and Peterson, P.A. 1985a. Hepatic retinol metabolism. Distribution of retinoids, enzymes, and binding proteins in isolated rat liver cells. J. Biol. Chem. 260:13560-13565.

Blomhoff, R., Norum, K.R. and Berg, T. 1985b. Hepatic uptake of [^{3}H] retinol bound to the serum retinol binding protein involves both parenchymal and perisinusoidal stellate cells. J. Biol. Chem. 260:13571-13575.

Bond, G.G., Thompson, F.E. and Cook, R.R. 1987. Dietary vitamin A and lung cancer: results of a case-control study among chemical workers. Nutr. Cancer 9:109-121.

Burton, G.W. and Ingold, K.U. 1984. β-Carotene: an unusual type of lipid antioxidant. Science 224:569-573.

Canada. Health and Welfare. Health Protection Branch. Bureau of Nutritional Sciences. 1975a. Dietary standard for Canada. Ottawa.

Canada. Health and Welfare. Nutrition Canada. Health Protection Branch. Bureau of Nutritional Sciences. 1975b. The Ontario survey report. Ottawa.

Canada. Health and Welfare. Nutrition Canada. Health Protection Branch. Bureau of Nutritional Sciences. 1977. Food consumption patterns report. Ottawa.

Canada. Health and Welfare. Health Protection Branch. Bureau of Nutritional Sciences. 1983. Recommended nutrient intakes for Canadians. Ottawa.

Canadian Council on Nutrition. 1964. Dietary standard for Canada. Can. Bull. Nutr. 6:1-76.

Chew, B.P. and Archer, R.G. 1983. Comparative role of vitamin A and β-carotene on reproduction and neonate survival in rats. Theriogenology 20:459-472.

FAO/WHO. 1967. Requirements of vitamin A, thiamine, riboflavine and niacin: report of a joint FAO/WHO Expert Group. W.H.O. Tech. Rep. Ser. 362.

Flores, H., Campos, F., Araujo, C.R.C. and Underwood, B.A. 1984. Assessment of marginal vitamin A deficiency in Brazilian children using the relative dose response procedure. Am. J. Clin. Nutr. 40: 1281-1289.

Geelen, J.A.G. 1979. Hypervitaminosis A induced teratogenesis. CRC Crit. Rev. Toxicol. 6:351-375.

Goodman, D.S. and Huang, H.S. 1965. Biosynthesis of vitamin A with rat intestinal enzymes. Science 149:879-880.

Graham, S., Haughey, B., Marshall, J., Priore, R., Byers, T., Rzepka, T., Mettlin, C. and Pontes, J.E. 1983. Diet in the epidemiology of carcinoma of the prostate gland. J. Nat. Cancer Inst. 70:687-692.

Green, M.H., Green, J.B. and Lewis, K.C. 1987. Variation in retinol utilization rate with vitamin A status in the rat. J. Nutr. 117:694-703.

Hegsted, D.M. 1986. Dietary standards - guidelines for prevention of deficiency or prescription for total health? J. Nutr. 116:478-481.

Helgerud, P., Petersen, L.B. and Norum, K.R. 1983. Retinol esterification by microsomes from the mucosa of human small intestine. J. Clin. Invest. 71:747-753.

Heshmat, M.Y., Kaul, L., Kovi, J., Jackson, M.A., Jackson, A.G., Jones, G.W., Edson, M., Enterlin, J.P., Worrell, R.G. and Perry, S.L. 1985. Nutrition and prostate cancer: a case-control study. Prostate 6:7-17.

Hill, D.L. and Grubbs, C.J. 1982. Retinoids as chemopreventive and anticancer agents in intact animals. Anticancer Res. 2:111-124.

Hoffer, J., Ruedy, J. and Verdier, P. 1981. Nutritional status of Quebec Indians. Am. J. Clin. Nutr. 34:2784-2789.

Hoppner, K., Phillips, W.E.J., Murray, T.K. and Campbell, J.S. 1968. Survey of liver vitamin A stores of Canadians. Can. Med. Assoc. J. 99:983-986.

Hume, E.M. and Krebs, H.A., eds. 1949. Vitamin A requirement of human adults. Report of the Vitamin A Sub-committee of the Accessory Food Factors Committee. M.R.C. Spec. Rep. Ser. No. 264. H.M.S.O., London.

Huque, T. 1982. A survey of human liver reserves of retinol in London. Br. J. Nutr. 47:165-172.

Jeghers, H. 1937. The degree and prevalence of vitamin A deficiency in adults. J. Am. Med. Assoc. 109:756-762.

Katsouyanni, K., Willett, W., Trichopoulos, D., Boyle, P., Trichopoulou, A., Vasilaros, S., Papadiamantis, J. and MacMahon, B. 1988. Risk of breast cancer among Greek women in relation to nutrient intake. Cancer 61:181-185.

Kolonel, L.N., Hankin, J.H. and Yoshizawa, C.N. 1987. Vitamin A and prostate cancer in elderly men: enhancement of risk. Cancer Res. 47:2982-2985.

Krinsky, N.I. and Deneke, S.M. 1982. Interaction of oxygen and oxy-radicals with carotenoids. J. Nat. Cancer Inst. 69:205-210.

Kummet, T., Moon, T.E. and Meyskens, F.L., Jr. 1983. Vitamin A: evidence for its preventive role in human cancer. Nutr. Cancer 5: 96-106.

Landy, D. 1985. Pibloktoq (hysteria) and Inuit nutrition: possible implications of hypervitaminosis A. Soc. Sci. Med. 21: 173-185.

La Vecchia, C., Franceschi, S., Decarli, A., Gentile, A., Fasoli, M., Pampallona, S. and Tognoni, G. 1984. Dietary vitamin A and the risk of invasive cervical cancer. Int. J. Cancer 34:319-322.

La Vecchia, C., Decarli, A., Franceschi, S., Gentile, A., Negri, E. and Parazzini, F. 1987. Dietary factors and the risk of breast cancer. Nutr. Cancer 10:205-214.

Lippe, B., Hensen, L., Mendoza, G., Finerman, M. and Welch, M. 1981. Chronic vitamin A intoxication. A multisystem disease that could reach epidemic proportions. Am. J. Dis. Child. 135:634-636.

Little, J. M. 1912. Beriberi caused by fine white flour. J. Am. Med. Assoc. 58:2029-2030.

Loerch, J.D., Underwood, B.A. and Lewis, K.C. 1979. Response of plasma levels of vitamin A to a dose of vitamin A as an indicator of hepatic vitamin A reserves in rats. J. Nutr. 109:778-786.

Looker, A.C., Johnson, C.L., Woteki, C.E., Yetley, E.A. and Underwood, B.A. 1988. Ethnic and racial differences in serum vitamin A levels of children aged 4-11 years. Am. J. Clin. Nutr. 47:247-252.

Lotthammer, K.H. 1979. Importance of β-carotene for the fertility of dairy cattle. Feedstuffs 51:16,37-38,50.

Marcek, J.M., Appell, L.H., Hoffman, C.C., Moredick, P.T. and Swanson, L.V. 1985. Effect of supplemental β-carotene on incidence and responsiveness of ovarian cysts to hormone treatment. J. Dairy Sci. 68:71-77.

Marshall, J., Graham, S., Mettlin, C., Shedd, D. and Swanson, M. 1982. Diet in the epidemiology of oral cancer. Nutr. Cancer 3: 145-149.

Marubini, E., Decarli, A., Costa, A., Mazzoleni, C., Andreoli, C., Barbieri, A., Capitelli, E., Carlucci, M., Cavallo, F., Monferroni, N., Pastorino, U. and Salvini, S. 1988. The relationship of dietary intake and serum levels of retinol and beta-carotene with breast cancer. Cancer 61:173-180.

Mathews-Roth, M.M. 1985. Carotenoids and cancer prevention — experimental and epidemiological studies. Pure Appl. Chem. 57: 717-722.

McLaren, D.S. 1980. Nutritional ophthalmology. Academic Press, London.

Mettlin, C. and Graham, S. 1979. Dietary risk factors in human bladder cancer. Am. J. Epidemiol. 110:255-263.

Michalek, A.M., Cummings, K.M. and Phelan, J. 1987. Vitamin A and tumor recurrence in bladder cancer. Nutr. Cancer 9:143-146.

Munoz, N., Wahrendorf, J., Bang, L.J., Crespi, M., Thurnham, D.I., Day, N.E., Ji, Z.H., Grassi, A., Yan, L.W., Lin, L.G., Quan, L.Y., Yun, Z.C., Fang, Z.S., Yao, L.J., Correa, P., O'Conor, G.T. and Bosch, X. 1985. No effect of riboflavine, retinol, and zinc on prevalence of precancerous lesions of oesophagus. Randomised double-blind intervention study in high-risk population of China. Lancet 2:111-114.

Olson, J.A. 1982. New approaches to methods for the assessment of nutritional status of the individual. Am. J. Clin. Nutr. 35: 1166-1168.

Olson, J.A. 1986a. Carotenoids, vitamin A and cancer. J. Nutr. 116:1127-1130.

Olson, J.A. 1986b. Letter to the editor. Nutr. Rev. 44:121-123.

Olson, J.A. 1987a. Should vitamin A intakes be two- to fivefold higher than currently recommended? J. Nutr. 117:998-999.

Olson, J.A. 1987b. Recommended dietary intakes (RDI) of vitamin A in humans. Am. J. Clin. Nutr. 45:704-716.

Packer, J.E., Mahood, J.S., Mora-Arellano, V.O., Slater, T.F., Wilson, R.L. and Wolfenden, B.S. 1981. Free radicals and singlet oxygen scavengers: reaction of a peroxy-radical with β-carotene, diphenyl furan and 1,4-diazobicyclo (2,2,2)-octane. Biochem. Biophys. Res. Commun. 98:901-906.

Palgi, A. 1984. Vitamin A and lung cancer: a perspective. Nutr. Cancer 6:105-120.

Pastorino, U., Pisani, P., Berrino, F., Andreoli, C., Barbieri, A., Costa, A., Mazzoleni, C., Gramegna, G. and Marubini, E. 1987. Vitamin A and female lung cancer: a case-control study on plasma and diet. Nutr. Cancer 10:171-179.

Pawson, B.A., Ehmann, C.W., Itri, L.M. and Sherman, M.I. 1982. Retinoids at the threshold: their biological significance and therapeutic potential. J. Med. Chem. 25:1269-1277.

Peto, R., Doll, R., Buckley, J.D. and Sporn, M.B. 1981. Can dietary beta-carotene materially reduce human cancer rates? Nature 290:201-208.

Potter, J.D. and McMichael, A.J. 1986. Diet and cancer of the colon and rectum: a case-control study. J. Nat. Cancer Inst. 76: 557-569.

Raica, N., Jr., Scott, J., Lowry, L. and Sauberlich, H.E. 1972. Vitamin A concentration in human tissues collected from five areas in the United States. Am. J. Clin. Nutr. 25:291-296.

Rodriguez, M.S. and Irwin, M.I. 1972. A conspectus of research on vitamin A requirements in man. J. Nutr. 102:909-968.

Rosa, F.W., Wilk, A.L. and Kelsey, F.O. 1986. Teratogen update: vitamin A congeners. Teratology 33:355-364.

Sauberlich, H.E., Hodges, R.E., Wallace, D.L., Kolder, H., Canham, J.E., Hood, J., Raica, N., Jr. and Lowry, L.K. 1974. Vitamin A metabolism and requirements in the human studied with the use of labeled retinol. Vitam. Horm. 32:251-275.

Sharma, R.V., Mathur, S.N., Dmitrouskii, A.A., Das, R.C. and Ganguly, J. 1977. Studies on metabolism of beta-carotene and apo-beta-carotenoids in rats and chickens. Biochim. Biophys. Acta 486:183-194.

Steven, D. and Wald, G. 1941. Vitamin A deficiency: a field study in Newfoundland and Labrador. J. Nutr. 21:461-476.

Stich, H.F., Hornby, A.P. and Dunn, B.P. 1986. Beta-carotene levels in exfoliated mucosa cells of population groups at low and elevated risk for oral cancer. Int. J. Cancer 37:389-393.

Teratology Society. 1987. Teratology Society position paper: recommendations for vitamin A use during pregnancy. Teratology 35:269-275.

Tuyns, A.J., Haelterman, M. and Kaaks, R. 1987a. Colorectal cancer and the intake of nutrients: oligosaccharides are a risk factor, fats are not. A case-control study in Belgium. Nutr. Cancer 10:181-196.

Tuyns, A.J., Riboli, E., Doornbos, G. and Péquinot, G. 1987b. Diet and esophageal cancer in Calvados (France). Nutr. Cancer 9:81-92.

Underwood, B.A. 1986. The diet-cancer conundrum. Public Health Rev. 14:191-212.

Underwood, B.A., Siegel, H., Weisell, R.C. and Dolinski, M. 1970. Liver stores of vitamin A in a normal population dying suddenly or rapidly from unnatural causes in New York City. Am. J. Clin. Nutr. 23:1037-1042.

Wald, N.J., Boreham, J., Hayward, J.L. and Bulbrook, R.D. 1984. Plasma retinol, beta-carotene and vitamin E levels in relation to the future risk of breast cancer. Br. J. Cancer 49:321-324.

Wang, J.Y., Owen, F.G. and Larson, L.L. 1988. Effect of beta-carotene supplementation on reproductive performance of lactating Holstein cows. J. Dairy Sci. 71:181-186.

WHO/USAID. 1976. Vitamin A deficiency and xerophthalmia. Report of a joint WHO/USAID meeting. W.H.O. Tech. Rep. Series 590.

Willett, W.C., Polk, B.F., Underwood, B.A., Stampfer, M.J., Pressel, S., Rosner, B., Taylor, J.O., Schneider, K. and Hames, C.G. 1984. Relation of serum vitamins A and E and carotenoids to the risk of cancer. N. Engl. J. Med. 310:430-434.

Winn, D.M., Ziegler, R.G., Pickle, L.W., Gridley, G., Blot, W.J. and Hoover, R.N. 1984. Diet in the etiology of oral and pharyngeal cancer among women from the southern United States. Cancer Res. 44:1216-1222.

Vitamin D

Vitamin D consists of two secosteroid parent compounds, vitamin D_2 and vitamin D_3, and certain biologically active metabolites which occur in foods. Vitamin D_2 (ergocalciferol) is synthesized from ergosterol in dead plant tissue exposed to ultraviolet or sunlight irradiation. Vitamin D_3 (cholecalciferol) is similarly synthesized from 7-dehydrocholesterol in the skin. The two vitamins have equal activity, but under most circumstances vitamin D_3 is the main source of biological activity in the body (Fraser 1983).

Vitamin D Deficiency

Vitamin D deficiency causes rickets in children and osteomalacia in adults. A decline in calcium absorption causes hypocalcemia and a consequent increase in parathyroid hormone synthesis, which in turn produces phosphaturia and hypophosphatemia. Affected infants may develop convulsions and tetany. In the absence of sufficient concentrations of calcium and phosphorus in the blood and extracellular fluids to effect normal bone mineralization, skeletal changes occur which include costochondral beading and bowed legs in children and rarefied, weakened bones in adults.

Overt rickets in Canada is limited almost entirely to unsupplemented infants consuming unfortified milk. These infants are usually either breastfed or fed vegetarian or so-called natural diets from which fortified milk has been excluded. There are no data on the prevalence of osteomalacia in Canada or the United States, but this condition is reportedly common among the elderly in Britain (Parfitt *et al.* 1982). The major predisposing factors in the UK are limited sunlight exposure and little food fortification. These factors pose less risk of osteomalacia in Canada.

Metabolism

The absorption of vitamin D is similar to that of other lipids, i.e. after emulsification with the aid of bile salts it is absorbed from the intestine and transported to the liver via the lymphatic system. Vitamins D_2 and D_3 in their parent forms have virtually no biological activity. They undergo two transformations which result in their conversion to metabolically active forms (DeLuca 1988). The first is 25-hydroxylation by a hepatic mixed function oxidase system to form 25-OHD (calcidiol), the main transport form of the vitamin in the blood. This metabolite is further hydroxylated by a renal mitochondrial mixed function oxidase system to produce 1,25-$(OH)_2D$ (calcitriol), the metabolically active form of the vitamin. The synthesis of 1,25-$(OH)_2D$ is stimulated by hypocalcemia, hypophosphatemia and parathyroid hormone, and is inhibited by hypercalcemia and by 1,25-$(OH)_2D$ itself. Extrarenal synthesis of 1,25-$(OH)_2D$ has been reported in bone and intestinal cells grown in culture and in various other tissues, but the physiological significance of these findings is still unclear. The kidney also forms other metabolites of vitamin D, notably 24,25-$(OH)_2D$, which is on a catabolic pathway but also exhibits biological activity.

Vitamin D and its metabolites circulate in blood plasma bound to a specific carrier, the vitamin D binding protein (DBP). The main circulating form of the vitamin is 25-OHD, which normally consists predominantly of 25-OHD_3. This metabolite occurs at concentrations of 12-45 ng/mL in plasma (Chesney 1981), where it has a half-life of 3-4 weeks. The parent vitamin binds weakly to the DBP, turns over rapidly and, except at high intakes, occurs in plasma at low concentrations (<5 ng/mL). It is stored mainly in adipose tissue, where it has a half-life of >3 months (Lawson *et al.* 1986).

In adults, 1,25-$(OH)_2D$ normally occurs at concentrations of 30-50 pg/mL of blood plasma and has a half-life of 3-4 hours. Its synthesis is not as tightly regulated in children as in adults and its circulating concentrations are higher (90-140 pg/mL in young children and 30-90 pg/mL in adolescents) (Stern *et al.* 1981). Plasma 25-OHD and 1,25-$(OH)_2D$ concentrations decline with age (Lips *et al.* 1987; Eastell *et al.* 1988).

Physiological Role

The role of the vitamin D endocrine system is to maintain serum calcium and phosphorus at concentrations which will support bone mineralization, neuromuscular function and various other cellular processes which are dependent on these elements (Henry and Norman 1984). These effects are mediated by 1,25-$(OH)_2D$ via a specific intracellular receptor. Because vitamin D functions in a manner similar to that of steroid hormones and can be synthesized in the body, it has the properties of a hormone as well as a vitamin. 1,25-$(OH)_2D$ derepresses a gene in the nucleus of cells of the intestinal epithelium to increase the synthesis of a calcium binding protein necessary for the active absorption of calcium. It also has an obscure role in the absorption of phosphorus. In conjunction with parathyroid hormone, it increases the resorption of bone cells and the tubular reabsorption of calcium and phosphate by the kidney. Receptors for 1,25-$(OH)_2D$ have been found in many tissues, indicating that it has a pervasive role in the metabolism of calcium and possibly of phosphate, and thereby in many metabolic processes.

Assessment of Vitamin D Status

The circulating concentration of 25-OHD is the best biochemical indicator of vitamin D status. However, the normal range of concentrations varies with age and physiological status, and the critical levels have not been clearly defined for all circumstances. Levels below 10 ng/mL are generally considered to reflect low vitamin D status, although 5 ng/mL appears to be sufficient to prevent symptoms of rickets and osteomalacia. Serum concentrations of 25-OHD rise with intake, whereas 1,25-$(OH)_2D$ levels are homeostatically controlled by feedback regulation of the renal 1-hydroxylase enzyme.

There is a seasonal variation in 25-OHD levels in blood plasma as well as in human and bovine milk. Serum 25-OHD levels also vary among national populations according to differences in climatic conditions and food fortification practices. Serum 25-OHD levels reported for young adults in Britain and Denmark (mean values 9 and 12 ng/mL, respectively) (Lester *et al.* 1980) are lower than those recorded in Canada and the United States (approximately 25 ng/mL) (Chesney 1981). In Britain, biochemical and clinical evidence of vitamin D deficiency has been reported among Asian immigrants, who have a lower dietary intake and capacity for endogenous synthesis of the vitamin than the general population.

Even in countries with liberal sunlight, low 25-OHD levels (<10 ng/mL) have been observed in some older adults. Such levels are generally attributable to an indoor existence and a low intake of fortified foods. A cohort of 96 non-institutionalized postmenopausal Canadian women surveyed in 1982 had a mean serum 25-OHD level of 16.5 ng/mL (Gibson *et al.* 1986). Eleven percent had levels below 10 ng/mL but none were below 5 ng/mL. A sample of 59 male and 54 female East Indian Punjabi immigrants to Canada (mean age 35 years) had average serum 25-OHD levels of 14.2 and 12.3 ng/mL, respectively (Gibson *et al.* 1987). The mean 25-OHD level of low-income elderly subjects living alone in Montreal was found to be 35.9 nmol/L (14.5 ng/mL) in men and 39.7 nmol/L (16.0 ng/mL) in women (Delvin *et al.* 1988). These values are lower than those reported for Caucasian adults of comparable age (Chesney 1981). Twelve percent of the males and 22% of the females had levels <9 ng/mL but none had a level associated with clinically overt vitamin D deficiency.

Vitamin D Intake

Although the vitamin D requirement can be met entirely from solar radiation, the diet must provide enough vitamin D to meet the requirements of individuals who receive little or no direct sunlight. It has been estimated that at least 12.5 µg (500 IU) of dietary vitamin D/day are necessary to maintain serum 25-OHD within the normal range for adults in the absence of sunlight (Fraser 1983). Because solar radiation is normally the predominant source of vitamin D activity, intakes below 5 µg/day have little influence on vitamin D status except when reserves are low (Fraser 1983).

Fortified dairy products are the most important dietary sources of vitamin D in Canada: margarine, fish, liver, eggs and meat are also significant sources. Present intakes of vitamin D appear to be sufficient to maintain adequate status in children and most adults. Healthy older women in the Guelph area were found to consume an average of 4.3 µg/day (Gibson *et al.* 1986). Milk and milk products were the main dietary sources of vitamin D. By comparison, vitamin D intake by a group of women in Britain, where dairy products are unfortified, averaged 2.4 µg/day and the main sources were eggs and fatty fish (Lawson *et al.* 1979).

The vitamin D intake of a sample of young adult Punjabi immigrants to Canada averaged 3.4 µg/day, of which 84% was derived from fortified milk and milk products (Gibson *et al.* 1987). They had lower serum 25-OHD levels than generally observed in young Canadians, a finding which may be attributable to limited exposure to sunlight afforded by their clothing habits and possibly to a high fibre diet, which has inconsistently been reported to inhibit the reabsorption of vitamin D compounds from the intestine.

Vitamin D occurs in human and bovine milk mainly in the form of its hydroxylated derivatives, which are secreted into the milk attached to the plasma DBP (Hollis *et al.* 1981; Kunz *et al.* 1984). 25-OHD is the main source of biological activity. Upon standing, the vitamin D compounds dissociate from the DBP in the whey and migrate to the fat portion of milk. Estimates of the vitamin D potency of milk vary with supplementation and with the values assigned to the biological activity of vitamin D metabolites, particularly 25-OHD. Estimates range from 0.6 to >2 µg vitamin D_3 equivalents (25 to 80 IU) per litre (Hollis *et al.* 1981; Kunz *et al.* 1984). These values indicate that, although unfortified milk is a significant source of vitamin D activity for infants, it does not contain enough activity to assure the prevention of rickets.

Toxicity

The margin of safety for vitamin D, taken orally, is unusually narrow. Excessive intake arising from concurrent consumption of fortified foods and supplements has been implicated in infantile hypercalcemia (American Academy of Pediatrics 1967). Hypercalcemia has been observed in elderly adults consuming 50 µg/day (Parfitt *et al.* 1982), whereas a supplement of 25 µg/day was found to increase calcium absorption without hypercalcemia (Orwoll *et al.* 1988). The intake of vitamin D from all sources by infants and by pregnant and lactating women should not greatly exceed the recommended amounts. Prolonged exposure to sunlight does not appear to pose a danger of toxicity.

Recommendations

Experience has shown that 10 μg (400 IU)/day will prevent rickets, promote growth and maintain calcium and phosphorus homeostasis, even in infants deprived of sunlight, without risk of toxicity (American Academy of Pediatrics 1963). This amount is recommended for children up to two years of age as a safe and effective prophylactic. An additional intake of 10 μg/day has been recommended for infants living in the far north during winter (Canadian Pediatric Society 1988). The recommended intakes are 5 μg/day for children two to six years of age and during the prepubertal growth spurts.

Nutrition Canada data (Canada. Health and Welfare 1975) indicated that a significant fraction of adults received less than 2.5 μg (100 IU) vitamin D/day from fortified sources, yet exhibited no biochemical or clinical evidence of deficiency. This observation indicates that most adults in Canada receive sufficient exposure to sunlight to prevent a deficiency at this level of intake.

The occurrence of suboptimal levels of serum 25-OHD and 1,25-$(OHD)_2D$ in some older adults, a lower efficiency of calcium and of vitamin D absorption and a reduced exposure to sunlight, indicate that the dietary requirement for vitamin D in the elderly is greater than that of young adults (Lukert *et al.* 1987; Eastell *et al.* 1988). Consequently, the recommended intake of adults 50 years and older is increased from 2.5 μg/day to 5 μg/day. In the case of individuals with little or no exposure to sunlight, this recommendation may require the use of a supplement for compliance.

References

American Academy of Pediatrics. Committee on Nutrition. 1963. The prophylactic requirement and the toxicity of vitamin D. Pediatrics 31:512-525.

American Academy of Pediatrics. Committee on Nutrition. 1967. The relationship between infantile hypercalcemia and vitamin D: public health implications in North America. Pediatrics 40:1050-1061.

Canada. Health and Welfare. Nutrition Canada. Health Protection Branch. Bureau of Nutritional Sciences. 1975. Provincial survey reports. Ottawa.

Canadian Paediatric Society. Indian and Inuit Health Committee. 1988. Vitamin D supplementation for northern native communities. Can. Med. Assoc. J. 138:229-230.

Chesney, R.W. 1981. Current clinical applications of vitamin D metabolite research. Clin. Orthop. 161:285-314.

DeLuca, H.F. 1988. The vitamin D story: a collaborative effort of basic science and clinical medicine. FASEB J. 2:224-236.

Delvin, E.E., Imbach, A. and Copti, M. 1988. Vitamin D nutritional status and related biochemical indices in an autonomous elderly population. Am. J. Clin. Nutr. 48:373-378.

Eastell, R., Heath, H., Kumar, R. and Riggs, B.L. 1988. Hormonal factors: PTH, vitamin D, and calcitonin. *In* Osteoporosis: etiology, diagnosis, and management. Riggs, B.L. and Melton, L.J., eds. Raven Press, New York, pp. 373-388.

Fraser, D.R. 1983. The physiological economy of vitamin D. Lancet 1:969-972.

Gibson, R.S., Draper, H.H., McGirr, L.G., Nizan, P. and Martinez, O.B. 1986. The vitamin D status of a cohort of postmenopausal non-institutionalized Canadian women. Nutr. Res. 6:1179-1187.

Gibson, R.S., Bindra, G.S., Nizan, P. and Draper, H.H. 1987. The vitamin D status of East Indian Punjabi immigrants to Canada. Br. J. Nutr. 58:23-29.

Henry, H.L. and Norman, A.W. 1984. Vitamin D: metabolism and biological actions. Annu. Rev. Nutr. 4:493-520.

Hollis, B.W., Roos, B.A., Draper, H.H. and Lambert, P.W. 1981. Vitamin D and its metabolites in human and bovine milk. J. Nutr. 111:1240-1248.

Kunz, C., Niesen, M., von Lilienfeld-Toal, H. and Burmeister, W. 1984. Vitamin D, 25-hydroxy-vitamin D and 1,25-dihydroxy-vitamin D in cow's milk, infant formulas and breast milk during different stages of lactation. Int. J. Vitam. Nutr. Res. 54:141-148.

Lawson, D.E.M., Paul, A.A., Black, A.E., Cole, T.J., Mandal, A.R. and Davie, M. 1979. Relative contributions of diet and sunlight to vitamin D state in the elderly. Br. Med. J. 2:303-305.

Lawson, D.E.M., Douglas, J., Lean, M. and Sedrani, S. 1986. Estimation of vitamin D_3 and 25-hydroxyvitamin D_3 in muscle and adipose tissue of rats and man. Clin. Chim. Acta 157:175-182.

Lester, E., Skinner, R.K., Foo, A.Y., Lund, B. and Sorensen, O.H. 1980. Serum 25-hydroxyvitamin D levels and vitamin D intake in healthy young adults in Britain and Denmark. Scand. J. Clin. Lab. Invest. 40:145-150.

Lips, P., van Ginkel, F.C., Jongen, M.J.M., Rubertus, F., van der Vijgh, W.F.J. and Netelenbos, J.C. 1987. Determinants of vitamin D status in patients with hip fracture and in elderly control subjects. Am. J. Clin. Nutr. 46:1005-1010.

Lukert, B.P., Carey, M., McCarty, B., Tiemann, S., Goodnight, L., Helm, M., Hassanein, R., Stevenson, C., Stoskopf, M. and Doolan, L. 1987. Influence of nutritional factors on calcium-regulating hormones and bone loss. Calcif. Tissue Int. 40:119-125.

Orwoll, E.S., Weigel, R.M., Oviatt, S.K., McClung, M.R. and Deftos, L.J. 1988. Calcium and cholecalciferol: effects of small supplements in normal men. Am. J. Clin. Nutr. 48:127-130.

Parfitt, A.M., Chir, B., Gallagher, J.C., Heaney, R.P., Johnston, C.C., Neer, R. and Whedon, G.D. 1982. Vitamin D and bone health in the elderly. Am. J. Clin. Nutr. 36:1014-1031.

Stern, P.H., Taylor, A.B., Bell, N.H. and Epstein, S. 1981. Demonstration that circulating 1α,25-dihydroxyvitamin D is loosely regulated in normal children. J. Clin. Invest. 68:1374-1377.

Vitamin E

Natural Occurrence

Vitamin E consists of two families of four naturally occurring compounds each, the tocopherols and the tocotrienols (Pennock et al. 1964). In the tocopherols the lipophilic sidechain is saturated, and in the tocotrienols it is unsaturated. The members of each family are designated α, β, γ or δ or according to the number and position of methyl groups attached to the chroman nucleus.

d-α-Tocopherol, which occurs naturally as the stereoisomer RRR-α-tocopherol, is the vitamer of main nutritional importance because of its widespread distribution and high biological activity. However, there is about three times as much γ-tocopherol in the diet, and despite its much lower biological activity, γ-tocopherol makes a significant contribution to total vitamin E activity. α-Tocotrienol and β-tocotrienol occur in significant amounts in cereal grains such as wheat, oats and barley, but they have a lower biopotency than their saturated homologues and have little nutritional significance. It has been estimated that about 80% of the total vitamin E activity in the U.S. diet is attributable to α-tocopherol and most of the remainder to γ–tocopherol (Bieri and Evarts 1973). The various natural forms of vitamin E which occur in foods can be separated and measured using high performance liquid chromatography (Thompson and Hatina 1979).

Biological Activity

Biological activity is expressed in international units or in d-α-tocopherol equivalents. The international unit is based on the activity of 1 mg of synthetic all-rac-α-tocopheryl acetate, which is isomeric at carbons 2, 4′ and 8′. The activities (IU/mg) assigned to other forms of γ-tocopherol are: d-α-tocopheryl acetate 1.36; d-α-tocopherol 1.49. In terms of d-α-tocopherol equivalents, β-tocopherol, d-α-tocotrienol and γ-tocopherol have biopotencies of approximately 0.5, 0.3 and 0.1, respectively. Differences in biological activity are due primarily to differences in turnover rates in the plasma and tissues. Vitamin E supplements may contain d-α-tocopherol, all-rac-α-tocopherol or their acetate esters. Their potency is indicated either in international units or d-α–tocopherol equivalents.

Requirement

The vitamin E requirement is determined primarily by the concentration and composition of polyunsaturated fatty acids (PUFA) in the tissues, and therefore is related to the PUFA content of the diet. This relationship stems from the role of vitamin E as a lipid antioxidant. In this role, vitamin E serves as a donor of hydrogen needed to quench hydroperoxy radicals, and possibly other lipoxy radicals, formed in the oxidation of PUFA by molecular oxygen. This action prevents the occurrence of lipid free radical chain reactions which cause oxidative decomposition of PUFA present in the phospholipids of cell membranes, and thereby the pervasive tissue damage seen in vitamin E deficiency. It has been postulated that the α-tocopheroxy radical formed in this process is reduced to α-tocopherol, enabling the vitamin to be reutilized, but at least in part it is further oxidized to α-tocopheryl quinone and a dimer which are biologically inactive. The four tocopherols appear to have a similar general order of *in situ* antioxidant activity, indicating that the marked differences in their potency when administered in the diet are related to differences in biological half-life.

Attempts to define the vitamin E requirements in terms of fixed ratio to dietary PUFA have been unsuccessful because the optimum ratio is affected by the degree of unsaturation of the fatty acids consumed, and appears not to be a linear function of PUFA intake. Since the synthesis of PUFA and of vitamin E in plants is genetically linked, the risk of a deficiency arising from the increased vitamin E requirement associated with a high intake of PUFA from cereal oils (the main source of both nutrients in the diet) is counteracted by the high vitamin E content of these oils.

Assessment

Vitamin E status is assessed according to the plasma or serum level of the vitamin, which in adults falls within a normal range of 0.5-1.5 mg/dL. High performance liquid chromatography enables vitamin E to be determined in small aliquots of plasma. A sample of 451 healthy male and female Canadian adults consuming a mixed diet was found to have a mean serum concentration of 1.02 mg/dL, of which 13% consisted of γ-tocopherol and virtually all of the remainder of α-tocopherol (Behrens and Madère 1986). Earlier surveys on adults living in Ottawa and Vancouver also yielded values within the normal range (Desai 1968; Hoppner *et al.* 1970). Serum values for Inuit (Canada. Health and Welfare 1975a) and Indians (Canada. Health and Welfare 1975b) sampled in the Nutrition Canada survey, and for three samples of Indian adults residing in western Canada (Desai and Lee 1974), were lower than those for the general adult population. These values were also associated with lower lipid levels and may reflect a difference in the level of transport lipoproteins.

Although the plasma concentration of vitamin E is sometimes expressed on the basis of the concentration of cholesterol, triglycerides or total lipids because their concentrations in adults are significantly correlated, the vitamin E requirement is not related to the level of other plasma lipids and this expression may misrepresent vitamin E status in subjects with dyslipidemias. Erythrocytes from blood containing less than 0.5 mg/dL plasma hemolyze in the presence of a mild oxidizing agent. Such levels in adults are considered undesirable, and survey data indicate that in healthy Canadian adults they are rare (Desai 1968; Behrens and Madère 1986). Plasma vitamin E tends to rise with adult age in association with cholesterol and other lipids. Over 90% of the α-tocopherol is carried by the low density lipoproteins (Behrens *et al.* 1982), more being transported by high density lipoproteins in females than in males.

Plasma vitamin E levels (0.2-0.4 mg/dL) in term infants are substantially lower than those in adults. They rise rapidly during consumption of colostrum (10 mg/dL) and breast milk (3 mg/L), but only slowly, if at all, during consumption of unmodified cow's milk (0.1-1 mg/L) (Jansson *et al.* 1981). Commercial formulas based on cow's milk therefore are supplemented with vitamin E.

Premature infants tend to have lower plasma levels of vitamin E than term infants, and cases of hemolytic anemia have been reported. Some prematures have an impaired capacity for fat digestion arising from limited production of bile or lipolytic enzymes, which results in poor absorption of vitamin E and other fat soluble vitamins. Such infants may also lack adequate serum transport lipoproteins and become frankly vitamin E deficient (Farrell 1979). They are more responsive to water-miscible forms of vitamin E than to oil emulsions administered orally, but may require parenteral administration.

Plasma vitamin E levels rise progressively in growing children but remain below those of adults until at least 12 years of age (Farrell *et al.* 1978). About one-third of children have a concentration below the 0.5 mg/dL level necessary for a negative result in the standard erythrocyte hemolysis test. This illustrates the fact that the hemolysis test is an arbitrary procedure of uncertain clinical significance.

Vitamin E in Clinical Disease

Several clinical conditions involving a defect in the absorption or metabolism of vitamin E are marked by signs of frank deficiency in early childhood. Chronic cholestasis, biliary atresia and certain other hepatobiliary diseases associated with defective bile production or secretion result in vitamin E malabsorption with severe neuropathology and myopathy similar to that seen in vitamin A deficient animals. Abetalipoproteinemia, a condition caused by a rare congenital failure to synthesize apoprotein B, which is necessary for vitamin E absorption, is marked by progressive neurological lesions. The pancreatic exocrine insufficiency of cystic fibrosis is also associated with neurological disease caused by malabsorption of vitamin E. These conditions, which in some cases can be prevented or reversed by giving large doses of vitamin E, reflect the important role of this vitamin in neurological function.

Evidence that lipid free radicals may be involved in carcinogenesis, and that some products of lipid peroxidation are mutagenic in cells grown in culture, have prompted some investigators to propose that intakes of vitamin E in excess of the levels recommended above be consumed as a possible preventative of cancer. In support of this proposal, it has been found that the synthetic food antioxidants butylated hydroxyanisole (BHA) and butylated hydroxytoluene (BHT) have a protective effect against chemical carcinogenesis in experimental animals. However, the protection furnished by BHA and BHT appears to be due to stimulation of the hepatic mixed function oxidase system by these compounds, resulting in accelerated detoxification and elimination of chemical carcinogens, rather than to their antioxidant properties (Draper and Bird 1984). It is noteworthy that vitamin E, which has no stimulatory effect on this detoxification system, provides no protection against chemically induced carcinogenesis. Moreover, BHA and BHT are inactive as biological antioxidants.

Prospective studies on a possible inverse association between plasma vitamin E level and cancer incidence in subsequent years have yielded inconsistent results. Vitamin E prophylaxis for cancer prevention would require the use of supplements, since intakes substantially above the present recommendations would not be readily obtainable from even good quality diets. Use of vitamin E supplements for cancer prevention therefore constitutes a pharmacological, rather than a nutritional intervention. Such an intervention is not justified by current evidence of vitamin E deficiency in the general population or the efficacy of vitamin E supplements in cancer prevention.

Toxicity

Except at intakes of one gram or more per day, which may cause intestinal disturbances, vitamin E appears to be non-toxic. Fractional absorption declines rapidly with increases in intake, thereby preventing the accumulation of toxic concentrations of vitamin E in the tissues.

Recommendations

No new evidence has come forth to justify revision of the recommendations in the 1983 edition of Recommended Nutrient Intakes for Canadians. The rapid rise in plasma vitamin E in nursing term neonates indicates that the 2-2.5 mg of α-tocopherol per day provided by 750 mL of breast milk is adequate. An additional intake of 0.5-1 mg/day is recommended to allow for the increased requirement generated by use of formulas containing added PUFA and iron.

The recommendations for children beyond infancy reflect their increasing intake of PUFA, and those for adults allow for the sex difference in PUFA intake. Although some individuals may require more vitamin E than is recommended because of an exceptionally high PUFA intake, such intakes normally are associated with intakes of vitamin E which exceed the recommendation.

A lack of epidemiological evidence of vitamin E deficiency among growing children and adults indicates that the mixed diet generally consumed in Canada and the United States is adequate in this vitamin. Such diets have been calculated to provide adults with 7 to 9 mg of d-α-tocopherol per day (Bieri and Evarts 1973; Thompson *et al.* 1973). Allowance for other vitamers raises the intake to 8 to 11 mg d-α-tocopherol equivalents per day. These amounts are commensurate with the recommended intakes of 6 to 10 mg/day.

References

Behrens, W.A., Thompson, J.N. and Madère, R. 1982. Distribution of α-tocopherol in human plasma lipoproteins. Am. J. Clin. Nutr. 35:691-696.

Behrens, W.A. and Madère, R. 1986. Alpha- and gamma tocopherol concentrations in human serum. J. Am. Coll. Nutr. 5:91-96.

Bieri, J.G. and Evarts, R.P. 1973. Tocopherols and fatty acids in American diets. J. Am. Diet. Assoc. 62:147-151.

Canada. Health and Welfare. Nutrition Canada. Health Protection Branch. Bureau of Nutritional Sciences. 1975a. The Eskimo survey report. Ottawa.

Canada. Health and Welfare. Nutrition Canada. Health Protection Branch. Bureau of Nutritional Sciences. 1975b. The Indian survey report. Ottawa.

Desai, I.D. 1968. Plasma tocopherol levels in normal adults. Can. J. Physiol. Pharmacol. 46:819-822.

Desai, I.D. and Lee, M. 1974. Plasma vitamin E and cholesterol relationship in Western Canadian Indians. Am. J. Clin. Nutr. 27:334-338.

Draper, H.H. and Bird, R.P. 1984. Antioxidants and cancer. J. Agric. Food Chem. 32:433-435.

Farrell, P.M. 1979. Vitamin E deficiency in premature infants. J. Pediatr. 95:869-872.

Farrell, P.M., Levine, S.L., Murphy, M.D. and Adams, A.J. 1978. Plasma tocopherol levels and tocopherol-lipid relationships in a normal population of children as compared to healthy adults. Am. J. Clin. Nutr. 31:1720-1726.

Hoppner, K., Phillips, W.E.J., Murray, T.K. and Campbell, J.S. 1970. Data on serum tocopherol levels in a selected group of Canadians. Can. J. Physiol. Pharmacol. 48:321-323.

Jansson, L., Akesson, B. and Holmberg, L. 1981. Vitamin E and fatty acid composition of human milk. Am. J. Clin. Nutr. 34:8-13.

Pennock, J.F., Hemming, F.W. and Kerr, J.D. 1964. A reassessment of tocopherol chemistry. Biochem. Biophys. Res. Commun. 17:542-548.

Thompson, J.N., Beare-Rogers, J.L., Erddy, P. and Smith, D.C. 1973. Appraisal of human vitamin E requirement based on examination of individual meals and a composite Canadian diet. Am. J. Clin. Nutr. 26:1349-1354.

Thompson, J.N. and Hatina, G. 1979. Determination of tocopherols and tocotrienols in foods and tissues by high performance liquid chromatography. J. Liq. Chromatogr. 2:327-344.

Vitamin K

Vitamin K is a generic term applied to a family of compounds derived from 2-methyl-1,4-naphthoquinone. The form of the vitamin that occurs in plants has a phytyl side chain at the 3-position of the naphthoquinone ring and is called vitamin K_1 or phylloquinone. A second form of the vitamin, synthesized by bacteria, consists of a group of substances with an unsaturated multiprenyl side chain at the 3-position that, collectively, are called vitamin K_2 or menaquinones. They are designated menaquinone-n or MK-n, where n represents the number of isoprene groups in the side chain (Savage and Lindenbaum 1983; Suttie 1985).

The parent compound of the vitamin K series, 2-methyl-1,4-naphthoquinone, has in the past been referred to as vitamin K_3 or menaquinone, but is now designated menadione. This compound is not found as a natural product, but is widely used as a feed supplement for animals, in which it is converted by hepatic alkylating enzymes to menaquinone-4 (MK-4). It is not used in human nutrition because of its toxicity for neonates. Menaquinones with up to 13 isoprene units in the side chain have been identified in bacteria and most of these forms have been found in the tissues of ruminants. MK-6 through MK-12, along with some biohydrogenated forms, occur in human liver; however, the main forms present are phylloquinone and MK-7 (Duello and Matschiner 1972; Shearer *et al.* 1988).

Vitamin K was first identified as a factor in blood coagulation. It is necessary for the formation of the active forms of coagulation protein factors II (prothrombin), VII, IX and X. Reduced vitamin K participates in the post-translational synthesis of γ-carboxylated glutamic acid residues (Gla) in these clotting proteins, enabling them to bind calcium. In the absence of vitamin K, inactive decarboxy-intermediates accumulate (Savage and Lindenbaum 1983; Olson 1984). Since the discovery of Gla in these proteins, this amino acid has been found in other vitamin K-dependent proteins. Two additional anticoagulant proteins, protein C and protein S, as well as a number of non-clotting proteins containing Gla, have been found in bone, skin, kidney, atherosclerotic plaque, lung, spleen, placenta and reproductive organs (Suttie 1985). The physiological significance and biochemical functions of these non-clotting proteins have yet to be determined.

In spite of the fact that accurate data for the vitamin K content of food are limited, it is generally agreed that the richest sources of vitamin K_1 are green leafy vegetables such as kale, broccoli, spinach, turnip greens and brussel sprouts (>100 µg/100 g). Intermediate amounts of vitamin K_1 can be found in meat and dairy products (50-100 µg/100 g) while cereals and fruits provide lesser amounts (<10 µg/100 g) (Olson 1988).

Vitamin K_1 is absorbed predominantly in the upper part of the small intestine by a process which requires the presence of bile salts and pancreatic juices. Vitamin K_1 is absorbed unchanged from the gut to the extent of 40-70% and enters the chylomicron circulation (Shearer *et al.* 1974; Barkhan and Shearer 1977). The contribution of menaquinones synthesized by bacteria in the intestine to vitamin K nutrition in humans has yet to be clearly established (Shearer *et al.* 1974). The difficulty encountered in experimentally producing a dietary vitamin K deficiency in humans with normal intestinal function suggests that some absorption of intestinal menaquinones occurs. However, the plasma level of menaquinones is normally lower than that of phylloquinone (Shearer *et al.* 1982).

In the absence of lipid malabsorption, chronic gastrointestinal disorders or chronic treatment with antibiotics, individuals consuming a mixed diet are unlikely to develop clincal signs of vitamin K deficiency. In an early study by Frick *et al.* (1967) involving a group of debilitated vitamin K depleted adult patients, phylloquinone (0.1 µg/kg/day) could not maintain normal prothrombin levels, but 1.5 µg/kg/day was sufficient to prevent any decrease in the synthesis of clotting factors. O'Reilly (1971) observed normal prothrombin times in four subjects ingesting approximately 25 µg of phylloquinone/day for 28 days, as did Olson *et al.* (1984) in six subjects fed a diet containing 10 µg/day for 3-8 weeks.

Vitamin K deficiency is usually diagnosed on the basis of a prolonged prothrombin time that can be corrected by vitamin K supplementation. Recently it has been found that the circulating level of abnormal prothrombin (with a reduced number of gamma-carboxyglutamic acid residues) provides a more sensitive test for vitamin K deficiency (Blanchard *et al.* 1981). In a recent study involving college-age students, Suttie *et al.* (1988) reported that daily ingestion of approximately 0.7 µg phylloquinone/kg/day was sufficient to maintain routine one-stage prothrombin times over 21 days, but was insufficient to prevent a decrease in the plasma level of phylloquinone from 0.85 to 0.47 ng/mL and a decrease of 10% in the ratio of carboxylated prothrombin.

Because of the widespread distribution of the vitamin in plants and animal tissues, clinical vitamin K deficiency in healthy persons is rare. However, a hemorrhagic disease of the newborn, especially in breast-fed prematures, has long been known (Savage and Lindenbaum 1983; Suttie 1985). There is little vitamin K storage in the neonate and its synthesis by the intestinal microflora is limited. In addition, breast milk is low in vitamin K (approximately 2 µg/L) (Haroon *et al.* 1982). For the prevention of hemorrhagic disease of the newborn, the Canadian Pediatric Society recommends that all healthy term infants be given a single dose of 2.0 mg of vitamin K_1 orally, or 1.0 mg intramuscularly, within six hours after birth, and that all preterm, low-birthweight and sick newborns be given 1.0 mg intramuscularly. Olson (1987) has proposed that the dietary intake of infants (0-1 year) should be 10-25 µg/day. Following reports of vitamin K toxicity (hemolytic anemia and kernicterus) in premature infants given supplements of water soluble menadione, phylloquinone is considered the preferred form of the vitamin for clinical use (Lane and Hathaway 1985).

Information on vitamin K status in the elderly is scanty. Hypoprothrombinemia was observed in 75% of elderly hospitalized patients, and the majority were responsive to vitamin K treatment (Hazell and Baloch 1970). However, until further studies employing new assay methods, such as the determination of abnormal vitamin K dependent proteins, have been carried out, no statement can be made about vitamin K requirements in the elderly (Munro *et al.* 1987).

References

Barkhan, P. and Shearer, M.J. 1977. Metabolism of vitamin K_1 (phylloquinone) in man. Proc. R. Soc. Med. 70:93-96.

Blanchard, R.A., Furie, B.C., Jorgensen, M., Kruger, S.F. and Furie, B. 1981. Acquired vitamin K-dependent carboxylation deficiency in liver disease. N. Engl. J. Med. 305:242-248.

Canadian Paediatric Society. 1988. The use of vitamin K in the perinatal period. Can. Med. Assoc. J. 139:127-130.

Duello, T.J. and Matschiner, J.T. 1972. Characterization of vitamin K from human liver. J. Nutr. 102:331-335.

Frick, P.G., Riedler, G. and Brögli, H. 1967. Dose response and minimal daily requirement for vitamin K in man. J. Appl. Physiol. 23:387-389.

Haroon, Y., Shearer, M.J., Rahim, S., Gunn, W.C., McEnery, G. and Barkhan, P. 1982. The content of phylloquinone (vitamin K_1) in human milk, cow's milk and infant formula foods determined by high-performance liquid chromatography. J. Nutr. 112:1105-1117.

Hazell, K. and Baloch, K.H. 1970. Vitamin K deficiency in the elderly. Gerontol. Clin. 12:10-17.

Lane, P.A. and Hathaway, W.E. 1985. Vitamin K in infancy. J. Pediatr. 106:351-359.

Munro, H.N., Suter, P.M. and Russell, R.M. 1987. Nutritional requirements of the elderly. Annu. Rev. Nutr. 7:23-49.

Olson, J.A. 1987. Recommended dietary intakes (RDI) of vitamin K in humans. Am. J. Clin. Nutr. 45:687-692.

Olson, R.E. 1984. The function and metabolism of vitamin K. Annu. Rev. Nutr. 4:281-337.

Olson, R.E. 1988. Vitamin K. *In* Modern nutrition in health and disease. 7th ed. Shils, M.E. and Young, V.R., eds. Lea & Febiger, Philadelphia, pp. 328-339.

Olson, R.E., Meyer, R.G., Chao, J. and Lewis, J.H. 1984. The vitamin K requirement of man (abst.). Circulation 70:II-97.

O'Reilly, R.A. 1971. Vitamin K in hereditary resistance to oral anticoagulant drugs. Am. J. Physiol. 221:1327-1330.

Savage, D. and Lindenbaum, J. 1983. Clinical and experimental human vitamin K deficiency. *In* Nutrition in hematology. Lindenbaum J., ed. Churchill Livingstone, New York, pp. 271-320.

Shearer, M.J., McBurney, A. and Barkhan, P. 1974. Studies on the absorption and metabolism of phylloquinone (vitamin K_1) in man. Vitam. Horm. 32:513-542.

Shearer, M.J., Rahim, S., Barkhan, P. and Stimmler, L. 1982. Plasma vitamin K_1 in mothers and their newborn babies. Lancet 2:460-463.

Shearer, M.J., McCarthy, P.T., Crampton, O.E. and Mattock, M.B. 1988. The assessment of human vitamin K status from tissue measurements. *In* Current advances in vitamin K research. Proceedings of the 17th Steenbock Symposium held June 21st-25th, 1987. Suttie, J.W., ed. Elsevier, New York, pp. 437-452.

Suttie, J.W. 1985. Vitamin K. *In* The fat-soluble vitamins: their biochemistry and applications. Diplock, A.T., ed. Heinemann, London, pp. 225-311.

Suttie, J.W., Mummah-Schendel, B.S., Shah, D.V., Lyle, B.J. and Greger, J.L. 1988. Vitamin K deficiency from dietary vitamin K restriction in humans. Am. J. Clin. Nutr. 47:475-480.

Water-Soluble Vitamins

Vitamin C

Humans and other primates, guinea pigs, some flying mammals, birds and fish require a dietary source of vitamin C (ascorbic acid) because they lack the last enzyme, L-gulono-γ-lactone oxidase, required in its synthesis. Vitamin C deficiency produces scurvy, a disease characterized by degeneration of collagenous tissue and capillary hemorrhaging.

Distribution and Intake

Vitamin C is commonly associated with citrus fruits, but numerous foods are good sources of this vitamin, including other fruits, tomatoes, potatoes and leafy vegetables. Animal tissues are poorer sources, but they contain enough of the vitamin to prevent scurvy when eaten in the fresh state. Vitamin C is subject to oxidation during prolonged heating of foods and to leaching from foods cooked by boiling.

Calculations made from family food purchases indicate that the average amount of vitamin C available from the Canadian diet in 1986 was 127 mg per capita per day (Canada. Agriculture Canada 1986). Fresh fruit, processed fruit and fresh vegetables each contributed about one-quarter of the available intake. Allowances for food wastage and cooking losses led to an estimated intake of 114 mg per day. These losses are somewhat compensated by the fact that food composition tables seldom list dehydroascorbic acid, which is equal to ascorbic acid in biological activity and is prevalent in the diet. Overall, the data indicate that diets based on Canada's Food Guide contain adequate amounts of vitamin C to meet the recommended intakes of all Canadians. The calculated vitamin C content of foods purchased by families in 1972 was equivalent to 99 mg per capita per day, indicating that there has been a substantial recent increase in the amount of this vitamin in the food supply.

Metabolism

Vitamin C is 90-95% absorbed at normal intakes. It is transported in the blood plasma in the free form and is readily taken up by the blood cells and body tissues. The main urinary metabolite at intakes below 100 mg per day is oxalic acid (Jaffe 1984). Other metabolites include dehydroascorbic acid, diketogulonic acid, ascorbic acid-2-sulfate, methyl ascorbate and 2-ketoascorbitol, plus four-carbon and five-carbon sugars. The renal threshold begins to be exceeded at 60 mg per day (Kallner *et al.* 1979), and further increases in intake result in rapid increments in the proportion of the vitamin excreted unchanged.

Function

Although many biological processes can be influenced by ascorbic acid at various levels of intake, its exact biochemical function has not been clearly established. There is strong evidence for a role as a cofactor for several monoxygenases and dioxygenases, including the prolyl and lysyl hydroxylases involved in the biosynthesis of collagen (Englard and Seifter 1986). Other reportedly ascorbic acid-dependent hydroxylases include those involved in the hydroxylation of dopamine to form norepinephrine, the amidation of peptide hormones, and possibly those involved in the biosynthesis of homogentisate, carnitine, elastin and nucleosides (Englard and Seifter 1986). The activity of vitamin C in these metalloenzymes appears to be due to its reducing power, which may be necessary to restore their metal components, or the metal ions necessary for their catalytic activity, to the reduced state. The reducing activity of vitamin C also accounts for its stimulatory effect on the absorption of dietary non-heme iron, and probably for a large number of other reported effects, including the prevention of nitrosamine formation, enhancement of drug and xenobiotic catabolism, maintenance of the immune response, synthesis of anti-inflammatory steroids in the adrenal gland, and promotion of wound healing. These effects indicate that vitamin C has a general role in metabolism as a water soluble antioxidant, analogous to that of vitamin E as a lipid soluble antioxidant. However, some such effects have been seen only at pharmacological concentrations.

Efficacy in Disease Prevention

The ingestion of megadoses of vitamin C constitutes a drug use of the vitamin, and therefore is not considered in estimating its requirement as a nutrient or in formulating a recommended intake. Many health claims have been made for intakes above the nutritional range (i.e. 250-10 000 mg per day), including the prevention and/or treatment of colds, infections, cancer, stress-related illnesses, hypercholesterolemia, psychiatric conditions, atherosclerosis and various other diseases. Few of these claims have been tested in controlled studies. In the case of those subjected to such studies (cancer and the common cold) the results have been negative or equivocal. Some investigators, but not others, have observed a diminution of cold symptoms in subjects given pharmacological amounts of vitamin C. The evidence for prevention of colds and other infections is predominantly negative (Briggs 1984). A correlation between vitamin C intake and cancer incidence has been observed in some epidemiological surveys, but the vitamin may be only a marker for diets high in fruits and vegetables and low in fat and calories, which are associated with a lower frequency of some cancers. Vitamin C has been demonstrated to be ineffective in the treatment of colorectal cancer (Moertel *et al.* 1985) and there is no satisfactory evidence for its efficacy in other malignant diseases (Hodges 1982). Ascorbic acid reduces the formation of nitrosamines from nitrites in foods, but is ineffective in reducing the oral carcinogenicity of nitrosamines in animals (Jaffe 1984).

Toxicity

Several adverse effects of pharmacological intakes of vitamin C have been reported, including a risk of renal calculi arising from increased oxalic acid production, destruction of vitamin B_{12} in the tissues, and subsequent "rebound scurvy", but there is little evidence that these effects occur under most circumstances (Miller and Hayes 1982). Intakes above 100 mg per day have no appreciable influence on oxalate formation. Large doses ($\geq$ 1 g per day) cause abdominal distress and diarrhea in some subjects, but have no apparent long-term effects. Nevertheless, chronic ingestion of any vitamin in amounts markedly in excess of those present in normal diets may entail a toxicological risk, and in the case of vitamin C, is unjustified by evidence of efficacy.

Recommendations

Historically, the recommended intake of vitamin C has been marked by unusual variability, arising from the relative importance attached to various criteria used to assess the requirement: the prevention of scurvy, maintenance of specified pool sizes, maximum production of metabolites, maximum reducing activity. There is general agreement that the amount of vitamin C required to prevent scurvy is not more than 10 mg/day (Bartley *et al.* 1953; Hodges *et al.* 1969). The recommended intake initially was set at 30 mg/day on the basis of a sharp decrease in fractional retention of the vitamin observed at higher levels of intake (Canadian Council on Nutrition 1964). This amount was reliably available from the mixed diet consumed by the general population, and there was no evidence of scurvy even among inhabitants of the high Arctic who consumed the native diet.

Studies on the metabolism of radioactive vitamin C led to estimates of pool sizes at various levels of intake, their relationship to the occurrence of deficiency symptoms and to the generation of metabolites. Symptoms of scurvy in adults fed a deficient diet were shown to appear when the pool size fell below 300 mg (Hodges *et al.* 1969; Sauberlich 1981). When subjects habituated to a vitamin C intake of 78 mg/day were switched to a diet free of the vitamin, psychological disturbances, including depression and hysteria, developed when the pool size fell below 600 mg (Kinsman and Hood 1971). The appearance of symptoms at this pool size, rather than at 300 mg, has not been observed in adults subjected to gradual reductions in intake, and may indicate that there is a limit to the rate of equilibration of metabolic pools in the tissues. Behavioural abnormalities also have been observed in individuals habituated to large doses of vitamin C after resumption of a normal intake (so-called rebound scurvy). This phenomenon may be due to induced synthesis of enzymes involved in vitamin C catabolism at high intakes.

A higher estimate of desirable pool size was derived from findings on the metabolism of ^{14}C-ascorbic acid in adults maintained under steady state conditions of vitamin C intake (Kallner *et al.* 1979). A pool size of 1500 mg appeared to reflect the maximum amount of the vitamin that could be metabolized in the tissues: additional amounts were excreted unchanged. On the assumption that maximum production of metabolites reflected maximum biological activity, it was proposed that this pool size was necessary for the vitamin to exert its full physiological effect. The estimated turnover rate of vitamin C in the tissues at this pool size was 60 mg per day. Allowance for incomplete absorption led to an estimated requirement of 70-75 mg per day, and further allowance for variability among individuals led to a proposed recommended intake of 100 mg per day (Kallner *et al.* 1979). In response to these findings, in 1983 the recommended intake of vitamin C was raised from 30 mg to 60 mg per day (Canada. Health and Welfare 1983).

However, subsequent evidence on the biochemical function of vitamin C has indicated that it is ascorbic acid itself, acting as a water soluble reducing agent, rather than its metabolites, that is responsible for its biological activity (Englard and Seifter 1986). None of its metabolites are active in ascorbic acid dependent hydroxylase enzyme systems. A pool size of 1500 mg appears to represent the maximum amount of the vitamin which can be catabolized in the tissues before the renal threshold is exceeded.

Adults

No health benefits have been associated with a pool size >600 mg. However, to allow for individual variability in turnover rate and excretion, a possible effect of environmental conditions on the requirement, and to provide a store of vitamin C sufficient to meet the requirements for at least a month, a pool size of 900 mg is deemed desirable (Baker *et al.* 1971).

Calculated on the basis of this pool size, a turnover rate of 2.7% per day (Baker *et al.* 1971; Kallner *et al.* 1977) and an absorption efficiency of 90% (Baker *et al.* 1969; Kallner *et al.* 1977), the estimated average vitamin C requirement of adult males is 27 mg per day. A 40% margin of safety is provided on the basis of a 20% coefficient of variability observed among the subjects of kinetic studies (Baker *et al.* 1971; Kallner *et al.* 1979). The resulting figure, 38 mg per day, is rounded to a recommended intake of 40 mg per day.

An intake of 40 mg sustains a serum level of 0.6 mg per dL in adult males (Kallner *et al.* 1979). This is three times the serum level at which symptoms of scurvy appear and is substantially higher than the level seen in animals which synthesize vitamin C (0.33-0.40 mg per dL) (Sheahan 1947). Forty mg per day is five times the average amount of ascorbic acid required to prevent scurvy, and is higher than the recommendations of WHO, FAO and most other countries (Truswell *et al.* 1983).

Kinetic studies have not been conducted on women. However, there is good evidence that pool size is proportional to body size, and on the basis of reference weights of 70 kg for men and 55 kg for women, the calculated recommendation for women is 31 mg per day, which is rounded to 30 mg per day.

Individuals with a normal intake of vitamin C who smoke 20 or more cigarettes per day exhibit lower serum and leukocyte levels and a markedly reduced half-life of the vitamin in the blood (Pelletier 1975; Kallner *et al.* 1981). The intake of vitamin C required to maintain a pool size of 900 mg may be increased by as much as 50% in heavy smokers, for whom the recommended intakes are therefore 60 mg and 45 mg per day for men and women, respectively.

Pregnancy

The plasma level of vitamin C declines during pregnancy because of active transport across the placenta and expansion of the pool size. Fetal and infant plasma levels are about 50% higher than the maternal level. The optimal pool size and the kinetics of vitamin C metabolism in the fetus are unknown. If the same relationship between pool size and body weight exists in the fetus as in adults, and the same estimates of fractional turnover rate, efficiency of absorption and overall variance are applied, the calculated increment in the maternal requirement during the third trimester of pregnancy is only 2.3 mg per day (Olson and Hodges 1987). Because this calculation may underestimate pool size and turnover rate in the fetuses, an additional intake of 10 mg per day is recommended during the second and third trimesters of pregnancy.

Lactation

The ascorbic acid content of breast milk increases with maternal intake up to approximately 90 mg per day (Byerley and Kirksey 1985). Most values for the vitamin C content of human milk fall within a range of 3-5 mg/dL, corresponding to an intake by infants of 23-38 mg per day in 750 mL of milk. Clinical experience indicates that this intake is adequate for all infants. The amount of vitamin C required to prevent scurvy in infants has been estimated at 7-12 mg per day (Olson and Hodges 1987). On the basis of these observations, the recommended intake for infants is 20 mg per day. Allowance for a maternal absorption efficiency of 90% results in an increment in the recommended intake during lactation of 25 mg per day.

Growth

On the assumption that the vitamin C requirement is related to body size, the recommended intakes of growing children are increased accordingly until they attain the values recommended for adult males and females (Table 20).

References

Baker, E.M., Hodges, R.E., Hood, J., Sauberlich, H.E. and March, S.C. 1969. Metabolism of ascorbic-1-^{14}C acid in experimental human scurvy. Am. J. Clin. Nutr. 22:549-558.

Baker, E.M., Hodges, R.E., Hood, J., Sauberlich, H.E., March, S.C. and Canham, J.E. 1971. Metabolism of ^{14}C and ^{3}H-labelled L-ascorbic acid in human scurvy. Am. J. Clin. Nutr. 24:444-454.

Bartley, W., Krebs, H.A. and O'Brien, J.R.P. 1953. Vitamin C requirement of human adults. Medical Research Council. Spec. Rep. Ser. No. 280. London.

Briggs, M. 1984. Vitamin C and infectious disease: a review of the literature and the results of a randomized, double-blind, prospective study over 8 years. *In* Recent vitamin research. Briggs, M.H., ed. CRC Press, Boca Raton, Fla., pp. 39-82.

Byerley, L.O. and Kirksey, A. 1985. Effect of different levels of vitamin C intake on the vitamin C concentration in human milk and the vitamin C intakes of breast-fed infants. Am. J. Clin. Nutr. 41:665-671.

Canada. Agriculture Canada. 1986. Nutrient assessment program. Family food expenditure survey component. Ottawa. (Computer data base)

Canada. Health and Welfare. Health Protection Branch. Bureau of Nutritional Sciences. 1983. Recommended nutrient intakes for Canadians. Ottawa.

Canadian Council on Nutrition. 1964. Dietary standard for Canada. Can. Bull. Nutr. 6:1-76.

Englard, S. and Seifter, S. 1986. The biochemical functions of ascorbic acid. Ann. Rev. Nutr. 6:365-406.

Hodges, R.E. 1982. Vitamin C and cancer. Nutr. Rev. 40:289-292.

Hodges, R.E., Baker, E.M., Hood, J., Sauberlich, H.E. and March, S.C. 1969. Experimental scurvy in man. Am. J. Clin. Nutr. 22:535-548.

Jaffe, G.M. 1984. Vitamin C. *In* Handbook of vitamins: nutritional, biochemical, and clinical aspects. Machlin, L.J., ed. Marcel Dekker, New York, pp. 199-244.

Kallner, A., Hartmann, D. and Hornig, D. 1977. On the absorption of ascorbic acid in man. Int. J. Vitam. Nutr. Res. 47:383-388.

Kallner, A., Hartmann, D. and Hornig, D. 1979. Steady-state turnover and body pool of ascorbic acid in man. Am. J. Clin. Nutr. 32:530-539.

Kallner, A.B., Hartmann, D. and Hornig, D.H. 1981. On the requirements of ascorbic acid in man: steady-state turnover and body pool in smokers. Am. J. Clin. Nutr. 34:1347-1355.

Kinsman, R.A. and Hood, J. 1971. Some behavioral effects of ascorbic acid deficiency. Am. J. Clin. Nutr. 24:455-464.

Miller, D.R. and Hayes, K.C. 1982. Vitamin excess and toxicity. III. A. Vitamin C. *In* Nutritional toxicology. Vol. I. Hathcock, J.N., ed. Academic Press, New York, pp. 101-107.

Moertel, C.G., Fleming, T.R., Creagan, E.T., Rubin, J., O'Connell, M.J. and Ames, M.M. 1985. High-dose vitamin C versus placebo in the treatment of patients with advanced cancer who have had no prior chemotherapy. N. Engl. J. Med. 312:137-141.

Olson, J.A. and Hodges, R.E. 1987. Recommended dietary intakes (RDI) of vitamin C in humans. Am. J. Clin. Nutr. 45:693-703.

Pelletier, O. 1975. Vitamin C and cigarette smokers. Ann. N.Y. Acad. Sci. 258:156-168.

Sauberlich, H.E. 1981. Ascorbic acid (vitamin C). *In* Clinics in laboratory medicine. Vol. I. Laube, R.F., ed. W.B. Saunders, Philadelphia, pp. 673-683.

Sheahan, M.M. 1947. The ascorbic acid content of the blood serum of farm animals. J. Comp. Path. Ther. 57:28-35.

Truswell, A.S., Irwin, T., Beaton, G.H., Suzue, R., Haenel, H., Hejda, S., Hou, X.C., Leveille, G., Morava, E., Pedersen, J. and Stephen, J.M.L. 1983. Recommended dietary intakes around the world. A report by Committee 1/5 of the International Union of Nutritional Sciences (1982). Nutr. Abst. Rev. 53:1075-1119.

Thiamin

Thiamin pyrophosphate is a coenzyme in two types of reactions involving carbohydrate metabolism. One of these is the oxidative decarboxylation of α-keto acids such as pyruvic and α-ketoglutaric, a reaction important in the production of energy. The second type of reaction is the formation and degradation of ketols by transketolase which catalyses the interconversion of sugars containing three to seven carbon atoms. The requirement for thiamin is thus related to energy expenditure, and may to some extent be reduced by dietary fat (Reinhold *et al.* 1944; Holt and Snyderman 1955). Most studies on thiamin requirements have been done with subjects on diets similar to those commonly consumed in Canada, in which variation in the ratio of fat to carbohydrate is small in comparison with a ratio that might affect the requirement for thiamin. In general, the intake of thiamin need not be adjusted for the relative amounts of dietary carbohydrate and fat.

Beriberi is the classical pathological condition associated with a deficiency of thiamin (Neal and Sauberlich 1980; Sandstead 1980). In western countries, deficiency is most often associated with alcoholism. During starvation or semi-starvation, tissue stores of thiamin are rapidly depleted (Consolazio *et al.* 1971).

Recommendations

Adults

The requirement for thiamin was found to be proportional to the intake of energy when the dietary energy varied according to the intake of carbohydrate (Sauberlich *et al.* 1979). Thiamin is required for the utilization of energy, even when no food is eaten. Sauberlich *et al.* (1979) found the average requirement for thiamin for adult men to be 0.30 mg/1000 kcal (0.36 mg/5000kJ) on the basis of urinary excretion of the vitamin and transketolase activity in erythrocytes. Others have suggested that the average requirement is approximately 0.33 mg/1000 kcal (0.39 mg/5000kJ) (Ziporin *et al.* 1965; Bamji 1970). On the basis of their findings, Daum *et al.* (1949) proposed 0.63 mg/day or 0.25-0.30 mg/1000 kcal (0.30-0.36 mg/5000 kJ) as the average range of requirement for healthy young women. Elsom *et al.* (1942) also found intakes of 0.60-0.70 mg/day (0.35 mg/1000 kcal or 0.42 mg/5000 kJ) to be adequate for women. Intakes of 0.18-0.22 mg/1000 kcal (0.22-0.26 mg/5000 kJ) by adults have been reported to result in clinical signs indicative of deficiency (Williams *et al.* 1942, 1943; Foltz *et al.* 1944).

Abnormal thiamin status as judged by erythrocyte transketolase activity was found in a cross-section of individuals in a semi-urban medical practice in Great Britain (Anderson *et al.* 1986). A 7-day dietary record indicated that subjects with abnormal biochemical thiamin status had significantly lower mean thiamin intakes (0.89 and 1.08 mg/day for women and men, respectively; 0.52 and 0.47 mg/1000 kcal) than those with higher transketolase activity (1.21 and 1.52 mg/day thiamin for women and men, respectively; 0.64 and 0.58 mg/1000 kcal). The proposal of Anderson *et al.* (1986) that the "absolute" daily thiamin requirement be 1.03 mg for women and 1.22 mg for men was weakened by the overlap in values which occurred in mean daily thiamin intake and the biochemical measure of normal and abnormal thiamin status, especially among the male subjects. Furthermore, a severe cut-off point for abnormal values of erythrocyte transketolase activity was selected.

On the basis of available information, the average requirement for thiamin to prevent signs of depletion is taken to be 0.30 mg/1000 kcal (0.36 mg/5000 kJ), which, on the assumption that the coefficient of variation is 15%, supports a recommended intake of 0.40 mg/1000 kcal (0.48 mg/5000 kJ) (representing a mean + 2 SD). The requirement of older adults may be higher than that of young adults (Oldham 1962) but there are insufficient data upon which to base a different recommendation. There is also no clear evidence that there is a corresponding decrease in the requirement for thiamin when the intake of energy falls to levels of 1800-2000 kcal/day (7600-8400 kJ/day) and below. It is known that a decrease in the intake of food, as in weight reduction programs, does not correspondingly affect the need for thiamin because of its relation to energy expenditure.

The recommended thiamin intake is the same as in the 1983 Canadian standard (Canada. Health and Welfare 1983), namely, 0.40 mg/1000 kcal (0.48 mg/5000 kJ). This value is in keeping with intakes recommended by the majority of countries around the world (Truswell *et al.* 1983).

It is further recommended that the mean daily intake for adults not fall below 0.8 mg per day, even if energy intake falls below 2000 kcal (8400 kJ) per day.

Infants

Because information on the thiamin needs of infants is so limited and there is no indication that they are different from those of older age groups, an intake of 0.40 mg/1000 kcal (0.48 mg/5000 kJ) is recommended. It is recognized that this may be higher than the level secreted in breast milk by well-nourished mothers but likewise there is no evidence that the levels in breast milk are not adequate. The recommended amount should be applied in the formulation of substitutes for breast milk and in the complementary feeding of older infants.

Children and Adolescents

There have been very few studies on the thiamin requirements of children and adolescents. The results of studies with children from pre-school age to 13 years have suggested that intakes of 0.70-1.40 mg/day (Stearns *et al.* 1958) and of 0.45-0.50 mg/1000 kcal (0.54-0.60 mg/5000 kJ) (Bensen *et al.* 1941; Oldham *et al.* 1944) are adequate. On the other hand, average intakes of 0.30 mg/1000 kcal (0.36 mg/5000 kJ) for adolescent girls (Hart and Reynolds 1957) and of 0.28 mg/1000 kcal (0.36 mg/5000 kJ) for adolescent boys (Dick *et al.* 1958) have been considered marginal or inadequate, although an intake of 0.38 mg/1000 kcal (0.45 mg/5000 kJ) was considered adequate for boys (Dick *et al.* 1958). Boyden and Erikson (1966), however, found that an average intake of 0.32 mg/1000 kcal (0.38 mg/5000 kJ) was adequate for pre-adolescent children. Based on these limited data, the recommended amount for adults, 0.40 mg/1000 kcal (0.48 mg/5000 kJ), seems appropriate for children and adolescents.

Pregnancy and Lactation

Studies on the thiamin status of pregnant women have indicated that the requirement is increased during pregnancy (Lockhart *et al.* 1943; Heller *et al.* 1974). Oldham *et al.* (1950), however, did not find evidence for an increased need during pregnancy, and Heller *et al.* (1974) found no correlation between thiamin status and the course and outcome of pregnancy. Consequently, no special recommendation is necessary for pregnancy and lactation except for that associated with the extra energy that is required. The recommendation therefore remains at 0.40 mg/1000 kcal (0.48 mg/5000 kJ).

References

Anderson, S.H., Vickery, C.A. and Nicol, A.D. 1986. Adult thiamine requirements and the continuing need to fortify processed cereals. Lancet 2:85-89.

Bamji, M.S. 1970. Transketolase activity and urinary excretion of thiamin in the assessment of thiamin-nutrition status of Indians. Am. J. Clin. Nutr. 23:52-58.

Bensen, R.A., Witzberger, C.M. and Slobody, L.B. 1941. The urinary excretion of thiamin in normal children. J. Pediatr. 18:617-620.

Boyden, R.E. and Erikson, S.E. 1966. Metabolic patterns in preadolescent children. Thiamine utilization in relation to nitrogen intake. Am. J. Clin. Nutr. 19:398-406.

Canada. Health and Welfare. Health Protection Branch. Bureau of Nutritional Sciences. 1983. Recommended nutrient intakes for Canadians. Ottawa.

Consolazio, C.F., Johnson, H.L., Krzywicki, H.J., Daws, T.A. and Barnhart, R.A. 1971. Thiamin, riboflavin, and pyridoxine excretion during acute starvation and calorie restriction. Am. J. Clin. Nutr. 24:1060-1067.

Daum, K., Tuttle, W.W. and Wilson, M. 1949. Influence of various levels of thiamine intake on physiologic response. VII. Thiamine requirements and their implications. J. Am. Diet. Assoc. 25:398-404.

Dick, E.C., Chen, S.D., Bert, M. and Smith, J.M. 1958. Thiamine requirement of eight adolescent boys as estimated from urinary thiamine excretion. J. Nutr. 66:173-188.

Elsom, K.O., Reinhold, J.G., Nicholson, J.T.L. and Chornock, C. 1942. Studies of the B vitamins in the human subject. V. The normal requirement for thiamine; some factors influencing its utilization and excretion. Am. J. Med. Sci. 203:569-577.

Foltz, E.E., Barborka, C.J. and Ivy, A.C. 1944. The level of vitamin B-complex in the diet at which detectable symptoms of deficiency occur in man. Gastroenterology 2:323-344.

Hart, M. and Reynolds, M.S. 1957. Thiamine requirement of adolescent girls. J. Home Econ. 49:35-37.

Heller, S., Salkeld, R.M. and Korner, W.F. 1974. Vitamin B_1 status in pregnancy. Am. J. Clin. Nutr. 27:1221-1224.

Holt, L.E., Jr. and Snyderman, S.E. 1955. The influence of dietary fat on thiamine loss from the body. J. Nutr. 56:495-500.

Lockhart, H.S., Kirkwood, S. and Harris, R.S. 1943. The effect of pregnancy and puerperium on the thiamine status of women. Am. J. Obstet. Gynecol. 46:358-365.

Neal, R.A. and Sauberlich, H.E. 1980. Thiamin. *In* Modern nutrition in health and disease. 6th ed. Goodhart, R.S. and Shils, M.E., eds. Lea & Febiger, Philadelphia, pp. 191-197.

Oldham, H.G. 1962. Thiamine requirements of women. Ann. N.Y. Acad. Sci. 98:542-549.

Oldham, H., Johnston, F., Kleiger, S. and Hedderich-Arismendi, H. 1944. A study of the riboflavin and thiamine requirements of children of preschool age. J. Nutr. 27:435-446.

Oldham, H., Sheft, B.B. and Porter, T. 1950. Thiamine and riboflavin intakes and excretions during pregnancy. J. Nutr. 41:231-245.

Reinhold, J.G., Nicholson, J.T.L. and Elsom, K.O. 1944. The utilization of thiamine in the human subject: the effect of high intake of carbohydrate or of fat. J. Nutr. 28:51-62.

Sandstead, H.H. 1980. Beriberi. *In* Modern nutrition in health and disease. 6th ed. Goodhart, R.S. and Shils, M.E., eds. Lea & Febiger, Philadelphia, pp. 686-688.

Sauberlich, H.E., Herman, Y.F., Stevens, C.O. and Herman, R.H. 1979. Thiamin requirement of the adult human. Am. J. Clin. Nutr. 32:2237-2248.

Stearns, G., Adamson, L., McKinley, J.B., Linner, T. and Jeans, P.C. 1958. Excretion of thiamine and riboflavin by children. Am. J. Dis. Child. 95:185-201.

Truswell, A.S., Irwin, T., Beaton, G.H., Suzue, R., Haenel, H., Hejda, S., Hou, X.-C., Leveille, G., Morava, E., Pedersen, J. and Stephen, J.M.L. 1983. Recommended dietary intakes around the world. Report by Committee 1/5 of the International Union of Nutritional Sciences.(1982) Part 2. Nutr. Abstr. Rev. 53:1075-1119.

Williams, R.D., Mason, H.L., Smith, B.F. and Wilder, R.M. 1942. Induced thiamine (vitamin B_1) deficiency and the thiamine requirement of man. Arch. Intern. Med. 69:721-738.

Williams, R.D., Mason, H.L. and Wilder, R.M. 1943. The minimum daily requirement of thiamine of man. J. Nutr. 25:71-97.

Ziporin, Z.Z., Nunes, W.T., Powell, R.C., Waring, P.P. and Sauberlich, H.E. 1965. Thiamine requirement in the adult human as measured by urinary excretion of thiamine metabolites. J. Nutr. 85:297-304.

Riboflavin

Riboflavin is a constituent of the coenzymes flavin adenine dinucleotide and riboflavin-5′-phosphate (McCormick 1988). The flavoproteins function as enzymes in tissue respiration and in the direct oxidation of substrates by oxygen.

Recommendations

A deficiency of riboflavin in man is characterized by a variety of symptoms, including soreness of the tongue and lips and seborrheic dermatitis (McCormick 1988).

Recommended dietary intakes of riboflavin have been related to the intakes of energy (Bro-Rasmussen 1958a,b) and of protein (Horwitt 1966; McCormick 1988) and to metabolic size (U.S. N.R.C. 1968). For practical reasons, recommended intakes frequently are expressed in relation to energy utilized. Belko *et al.* (1983) found no relationship between the amount of riboflavin required to maintain a high level of erythrocyte glutathione reductase activity and the energy intake or the lean body mass of young women, but the degree of saturation of this enzyme may be dependent on several different mechanisms (Suzuki *et al.* 1985).

Urinary riboflavin excretion and erythrocyte glutathione reductase activity have been the two most frequently used methods for assessing riboflavin status and for estimating riboflavin requirement (Bates 1987). A number of factors have been shown to affect urinary riboflavin excretion (Bates 1987) and, in turn, the estimates of riboflavin requirement by this method. Similarly, use of erythrocyte glutathione reductase activity to estimate riboflavin requirement has been criticized because riboflavin intake may have an effect not only on coenzyme status but on tissue apoenzyme concentration as well (Horwitt 1984, 1986). Even in normal subjects glutathione reductase was not found to be saturated (Horwitt 1984).

Adults

Clinical signs of riboflavin deficiency have been recorded for adults on diets providing 0.5 mg or less of riboflavin daily (Horwitt *et al.* 1949), whereas no signs of deficiency have been recorded when daily intake was 0.75 mg or greater (Williams *et al.* 1943; Keys *et al.* 1944; Friedemann *et al.* 1949; Horwitt *et al.* 1950). Regression analysis, reported by Oldham *et al.* (1950), based on urinary excretion of riboflavin, suggested that the mean riboflavin requirement for the adult varied between 0.9 mg (Davis *et al.* 1946) and 1.4 mg (Brewer *et al.* 1946) daily. In general, urinary riboflavin excretion was found to increase sharply in both men and women at daily riboflavin intakes above 1.1-1.2 mg (Williams *et al.* 1943; Davis *et al.* 1946; Horwitt *et al.* 1950), a level which equated to an intake of approximately 0.55 mg/1000 kcal (0.66 mg/5000 kJ). By contrast, Belko *et al.* (1984, 1985) suggested, on the basis of their results on erythrocyte glutathione reductase in women on weight-reducing regimens, that the riboflavin requirement was 1.16 mg/1000 kcal (1.39 mg/5000kJ). Under conditions of assumed inadequacy, however, riboflavin continued to be excreted in the urine. Moreover, the suggested level of intake was appreciably greater than the mean intake associated with a marked increase in urinary excretion of riboflavin. It is also much higher than the 1.4-1.8 mg per day or 0.8 mg/1000 kcal (0.96 mg/5000 kJ) intake quoted by Bates (1987). The observations by Belko *et al.* (1983, 1984, 1985) are also difficult to rationalize in light of the study by Bamji (1969), who found that urinary riboflavin excretion increased sharply and the erythrocyte glutathione reductase activity was in the normal range at riboflavin intakes of 0.5 mg/1000 kcal (0.6 mg/5000 kJ) for women on diets providing 2000 kcal (8400 kJ) per day.

It is suggested that 0.5 mg/1000 kcal (0.6 mg/5000 kJ) is adequate to meet the riboflavin needs of adults.

Infants, Children and Adolescents

There is very little information on the riboflavin requirements of infants and children. Snyderman *et al.* (1949), in a study with three children ranging in age from 14 to 32 months, suggested that a daily intake of 0.4 to 0.5 mg of riboflavin resulted in urinary riboflavin excretion above minimum values. However, a plot of urinary excretion increased sharply at intakes of 0.9 mg or greater. Furthermore, two of the three infants were especially small for their age. Oldham *et al.* (1944), in a study with two 5-year-old boys, found that urinary riboflavin excretion increased sharply at daily riboflavin intakes above 0.700-0.725 mg (0.53 mg/1000 kcal or 0.63 mg/5000 kJ). The recommended intake for infants and children would appear to be the same as for adults.

Pregnancy and Lactation

Findings by Oldham *et al.* (1950) suggested that an intake of at least 0.9 mg of riboflavin daily is required during pregnancy. Brzezinski *et al.* (1952) reported some signs of clinical deficiency among pregnant women on intakes of 0.7-1.3 mg/day, and evidence of an increased requirement as pregnancy progresses. Heller *et al.* (1974) also found evidence for an increased requirement for riboflavin during pregnancy, but found no correlation between signs of deficiency and the outcome of pregnancy. More recently, Bates *et al.* (1981) found that a mean riboflavin intake of 1.5 mg/day was inadequate for pregnant and lactating Gambian women, as reflected by the erythrocyte glutathione reductase assay. When a riboflavin supplement of 2 mg per day was provided to give a total intake of 2.5 mg per day in Gambian women, enzyme saturation was within the normative range for 90% of the women (Bates *et al.* 1982), but the criteria of enzyme saturation is controversial. The increase in energy requirement during pregnancy is associated with an increase of about 0.2 mg of riboflavin per day.

The riboflavin content of breast milk varies appreciably. Mean values generally fall between 25 and 40 µg/100 mL (Roderuck *et al.* 1946; Gunther 1952; Jenness 1979; McCormick 1988). An important factor in this variation is the amount of riboflavin in the food consumed. The riboflavin content of breast milk is affected within a matter of hours by riboflavin intake (Roderuck *et al.* 1946; Gunther 1952).

The additional requirement for riboflavin would be, by calculation, 0.22 mg per day, associated with the increased energy requirement of 450 kcal or 1.9 MJ. In view of the lack of experimental data, the recommended increment for pregnancy and lactation remains at 0.3 and 0.4 mg per day respectively.

References

Bamji, M.S. 1969. Glutathione reductase activity in red blood cells and riboflavin nutritional status in humans. Clin. Chim. Acta 26:263-269.

Bates, C.J. 1987. Human riboflavin requirements and metabolic consequences of deficiency in man and animals. World Rev. Nutr. Diet. 50:215-265.

Bates, C.J., Prentice, A.M., Paul, A.A., Sutcliffe, B.A., Watkinson, M. and Whitehead, R.G. 1981. Riboflavin status in Gambian pregnant and lactating women and its implications for recommended dietary allowances. Am. J. Clin. Nutr. 34:928-935.

Bates, C.J., Phil, D., Prentice, A.M., Watkinson, M., Morrell, P., Sutcliffe, B.A., Foord, F.A. and Whitehead, R.G. 1982. Riboflavin requirements of lactating Gambian women: a controlled supplementation trial. Am. J. Clin. Nutr. 35:701-709.

Belko, A.Z., Obarzanek, E., Kalkwarf, H.J., Rotter, M.A., Bogusz, S., Miller, D., Haas, J.D. and Roe, D.A. 1983. Effects of exercise on riboflavin requirements of young women. Am. J. Clin. Nutr. 37:509-517.

Belko, A.Z., Obarzanek, E., Roach, R., Rotter, M., Urban, G., Weinberg, S. and Roe, D.A. 1984. Effects of aerobic exercise and weight loss on riboflavin requirements of moderately obese, marginally deficient young women. Am. J. Clin. Nutr. 40:553-561.

Belko, A.Z., Meredith, M.P., Kalkwarf, H.J., Obarzanek, E., Weinberg, S., Roach, R., McKeon, G. and Roe, D.A. 1985. Effects of exercise on riboflavin requirements: biological validation in weight reducing women. Am. J. Clin. Nutr. 41:270-277.

Brewer, W., Porter, T., Ingalls, R. and Ohlson, M.A. 1946. The urinary excretion of riboflavin by college women. J. Nutr. 32:583-596.

Bro-Rasmussen, F. 1958a. The riboflavin requirement of animals and man and associated metabolic relations. Part I. Technique of estimating requirement and modifying circumstances. Nutr. Abstr. Rev. 28:1-23.

Bro-Rasmussen, F. 1958b. The riboflavin requirement of animals and man and associated metabolic relations. Part II. Relation of requirement to the metabolism of protein and energy. Nutr. Abstr. Rev. 28:369-386.

Brzezinski, A., Bromberg, Y.M. and Braun, K. 1952. Riboflavin excretion during pregnancy and early lactation. J. Lab. Clin. Med. 39:84-90.

Davis, M.V., Oldham, H.G. and Roberts, L.J. 1946. Riboflavin excretions of young women on diets containing varying levels of the B vitamins. J. Nutr. 32:143-161.

Friedemann, T.E., Ivy, A.C., Jung, F.T., Sheft, B.B. and Miller, V. 1949. Work at high altitude. IV. Utilization of thiamin and riboflavin at low and high dietary intake: effect of work and rest. Q. Bull. Northwestern Univ. Med. Sch. 23:177-197.

Gunther, M. 1952. Composition of human milk and factors affecting it. Br. J. Nutr. 6:215-220.

Heller, S., Salkeld, R.M. and Korner, W.F. 1974. Riboflavin status in pregnancy. Am. J. Clin. Nutr. 27:1225-1230.

Horwitt, M.K. 1966. Nutritional requirements of man with special reference to riboflavin. Am. J. Clin. Nutr. 18:458-466.

Horwitt, M.K. 1984. Comments on methods for estimating riboflavin requirements. Am. J. Clin. Nutr. 39:159-161.

Horwitt, M.K. 1986. Interpretations of requirements for thiamin, riboflavin, niacin-tryptophan, and vitamin E plus comments on balance studies and vitamin B-6. Am. J. Clin. Nutr. 44:973-985.

Horwitt, M.K., Hills, O.W., Harvey, C.C., Liebert, E. and Steinberg, D.L. 1949. Effects of dietary depletion of riboflavin. J. Nutr. 39:357-373.

Horwitt, M.K., Harvey, C.C., Hills, O.W. and Liebert, E. 1950. Correlation of urinary excretion of riboflavin with dietary intake and symptoms of ariboflavinosis. J. Nutr. 41:247-264.

Jenness, R. 1979. The composition of human milk. Semin. Perinat. 3:225-239.

Keys, A., Henschel, A.F., Mickelsen, O., Brozek, J.M. and Crawford, J.H. 1944. Physiological and biochemical functions in normal young men on a diet restricted in riboflavin. J. Nutr. 27:165-178.

McCormick, D.B. 1988. Riboflavin. *In* Modern nutrition in health and disease. 7th ed. Shils, M.E. and Young, V.R., eds. Lea & Febiger, Philadelphia, pp. 362-369.

Oldham, H., Johnston, F., Kleiger, S. and Hedderich-Arismendi, H. 1944. A study of the riboflavin and thiamine requirements of children of preschool age. J. Nutr. 27:435-446.

Oldham, H., Sheft, B.B. and Porter, T. 1950. Thiamine and riboflavin intakes and excretions during pregnancy. J. Nutr. 41:231-245.

Roderuck, C., Coryell, M.N., Williams, H.H. and Macy I.G. 1946. Metabolism of women during the reproductive cycle. IX. The utilization of riboflavin during lactation. J. Nutr. 32:267-283.

Suzuki, T., Agar, N.S. and Suzuki, M. 1985. Red blood cell metabolism in experimental animals: pentose phosphate pathway, antioxidant enzymes and glutathione. Exp. Anim. 34:353-366.

Snyderman, S.E., Ketron, K.C., Burch, H.B., Lowry, O.H., Bessey, O.A., Guy, L.P. and Holt, L.E. Jr. 1949. The minimum riboflavin requirement of the infant. J. Nutr. 39:219-232.

U.S. National Research Council. Food and Nutrition Board. 1968. Recommended dietary allowances. 7th ed. Publication 1694. National Academy of Sciences, Washington.

Williams, R.D., Mason, H.L., Cusick, P.L. and Wilder, R.M. 1943. Observations on induced riboflavin deficiency and the riboflavin requirement of man. J. Nutr. 25:361-377.

Niacin

Niacin is the generic term for nicotinic acid and its derivatives of equivalent biological activity (Darby *et al.* 1975; Sauberlich 1987). Nicotinamide, the active form, functions in two coenzymes, nicotinamide adenine dinucleotide (NAD) and its phosphate (NADP) which remove hydrogen from substrates during glycolysis and respiration.

A deficiency of niacin can cause pellagra, which is characterized by dermatitis, inflammation of the mucous membranes and dementia (Sandstead 1980).

An assessment of niacin requirements is complicated by the poor biological availability of preformed niacin from some foods, particularly cereals, and the oxidation of some tryptophan to niacin (Horwitt *et al.* 1956; Bender and Bender 1986). Niacin equivalents (NE) take into account that about 3% of ingested tryptophan is converted, and 60 mg provides 1 mg of niacin. (Horwitt *et al.* 1956, 1981; Goldsmith *et al.* 1961; Vivian 1964). Thus, 1 NE equals 1 mg of niacin or 60 mg of tryptophan. Data from the Nutrition Canada survey (1977) indicated that the average Canadian diet provided approximately 13 NE/1000 kcal (16 NE/5000 kJ). The effective intake would be slightly lower if the biological availability of preformed niacin were taken into account.

Recommendations

Adults

The recommended intake is based on the average amount of niacin that is required to produce a clear increase in urinary excretion of niacin metabolites (Horwitt *et al.* 1956). If this value (viz., 5.5 NE/1000 kcal or 6.6 NE/5000 kJ) is adjusted by a factor of 30% in order to account for individual variation, the recommended intake is 7.2 NE/1000 kcal (8.6 NE/5000 kJ). Although niacin requirements are commonly expressed in terms of energy intakes, little direct evidence exists to demonstrate that the niacin requirement parallels energy expenditures. On the other hand, it can be argued that recommended intakes are somewhat inflated because the minimum intakes required to prevent signs of pellagra, 4.4 NE/1000 kcal (5.3 NE/5000 kJ) (Horwitt 1958) or to produce a noticeable increase in urinary excretion of niacin metabolites (5.5 mg/1000 kcal or 6.6 mg/5000 kJ) were established with diets containing appreciable amounts of cereals. However, the slight over-estimation of niacin requirement is countered by the fact that the usually accepted conversion factor for tryptophan (60:1) may over-estimate the contribution tryptophan makes to the niacin status of the adult human (Vivian 1964). Niacin is utilized even during fasting. There is no information on level of requirements for niacin at low intakes of energy by adults, but for safety it is recommended that the intake should not be lower than that based on 2000 kcal/day (8400 kJ/day), i.e., 14.4 NE/day, by people 19 years of age and older.

The recommended intakes for niacin by Bender and Bender (1986) and average recommended intakes cited in the International Union of Nutritional Sciences (IUNS) report (Truswell *et al.* 1983), support the level of 7.2 NE/1000 kcal (8.6 NE/5000 kJ) in the Recommended Nutrient Intakes for Canadians (1983). This level is slightly higher than the mean value reported in the IUNS report (Truswell *et al.* 1983) for 32 out of 41 countries in which recommendations fell between 6.6 and 6.8 NE/1000 kcal (7.9-8.1 NE/5000 kJ). The recommendation for Canadian adults therefore remains at 7.2 NE/1000 kcal (8.6 NE/5000 kJ).

Infants, Children and Adolescents

There are no data on the niacin requirements of infants, children and adolescents. Breast milk provides 6.2-7.6 NE/1000 kcal (7.4-9.1 NE/5000 kJ) (Macy 1949; Walker 1954; Jenness 1979). The recommended intake is the same as that for adults, and likewise for children and adolescents; namely 7.2 NE/1000 kcal (8.6 NE/5000 kJ). Human milk contains about 180-230 µg of preformed niacin and 19-21 mg of tryptophan per 100 mL (Macy 1949; Walker 1954; Jenness 1979).

Pregnancy and Lactation

There is no indication of an increased requirement for niacin during pregnancy, other than that which accompanies the increased energy intake, 2 NE/day.

The extra intake of energy that is recommended during lactation, 450 kcal/day (1900 kJ/day), would increase the requirement by about 3 NE/day. The recommended intake of niacin during lactation is the same as that for non-lactating women, 7.2 NE/1000 kcal (8.6 NE/5000 kJ).

References

Bender, D.A. and Bender, A.E. 1986. Niacin and tryptophan metabolism: the biochemical basis of niacin requirements and recommendations. Nutr. Abstr. Rev. 56:695-719.

Canada. Health and Welfare. Nutrition Canada. Health Protection Branch. Bureau of Nutritional Sciences. 1977. Food consumption patterns report. Ottawa.

Canada. Health and Welfare. Health Protection Branch. Bureau of Nutritional Sciences. 1983. Recommended nutrient intakes for Canadians. Ottawa.

Darby, W.J., McNutt, K.W. and Todhunter, E.N. 1975. Niacin. Nutr. Rev. 33:289-297.

Goldsmith, G.A., Miller, O.N. and Unglaub, W.G. 1961. Efficiency of tryptophan as a niacin precursor in man. J. Nutr. 73:173-176.

Horwitt, M.K. 1958. Niacin-tryptophan requirements of man. J. Am. Diet. Assoc. 34:914-919.

Horwitt, M.K., Harvey, C.C., Rothwell, W.S., Cutler, J.L. and Haffron, D. 1956. Tryptophan-niacin relationships in man. J. Nutr. 60 (Suppl.1):1-43.

Horwitt, M.K., Harper, A.E. and Henderson, L.M. 1981. Niacin-tryptophan relationships for evaluating niacin equivalents. Am. J. Clin. Nutr. 34:423-427.

Jenness, R. 1979. The composition of human milk. Semin. Perinatol. 3:225-239.

Macy, I.G. 1949. Composition of human colostrum and milk. Am. J. Dis. Child. 78:589-603.

Sandstead, H.H. 1980. Pellagra. *In* Modern nutrition in health and disease. 6th ed. Goodhart, R.S. and Shils, M.E., eds. Lea & Febiger, Philadelphia, pp. 688-690.

Sauberlich, H.E. 1987. Nutritional aspects of pyridine nucleotides. *In* Pyridine nucleotide coenzymes: chemical, biochemical and medical aspects. Vol. 2B. Dolphin, D., Poulson, R. and Avramovic, O., eds. John Wiley, New York, pp. 600-626.

Truswell, A.S., Irwin, T., Beaton, G.H., Suzue, R., Haenel, H., Hejda, S., Hou, X.-C., Leveille, G., Morava, E., Pedersen, J. and Stephen, J.M.L. 1983. Recommended dietary intakes around the world. Report by Committee 1/5 of the International Union of Nutritional Sciences (1982). Part 2. Nutr. Abstr. Rev. 53:1075-1119.

Vivian, V.M. 1964. Relationship between tryptophan-niacin metabolism and changes in nitrogen balance. J. Nutr. 82:395-400.

Walker, A.R.P. 1954. Low niacin concentration in the breast milk of Bantu mothers on a high-maize diet. Nature (London) 173:405-406.

Vitamin B_6

Vitamin B_6 is a collective term for three metabolically interrelated pyridines, namely, pyridoxal, pyridoxamine and pyridoxine (McCoy and Colombini 1972). In the forms of pyridoxal phosphate and pyridoxamine phosphate, vitamin B_6 acts as a cofactor for enzymes which catalyze many reactions involving amino acids, including transamination, decarboxylation, dehydration, desulfhydration and racemization. It is essential for the synthesis of amino acids from the products of carbohydrate metabolism, their oxidation to produce energy, and their utilization for the synthesis of proteins and other nitrogenous compounds. In addition, vitamin B_6 is involved in the metabolism of single carbon units and in the biosynthesis of sphingolipids, neurotransmitters and heme. Pyridoxal phosphate is also covalently bound to glycogen phosphorylase, which may function as a storage form of the vitamin (Black *et al.* 1978).

Vitamin B_6 is widely distributed in small amounts throughout nature. Pyridoxal phosphate and pyridoxamine phosphate are the predominant forms of vitamin B_6 in animal products, while pyridoxine occurs mainly in plant foods (Rabinowitz and Snell 1948). Although vitamin B_6 in animal foods is highly bioavailable, thermal processing may reduce their content by 25% to 30% (Gregory and Kirk 1981). Vitamin B_6 from plant-derived foods is less bioavailable owing to the presence of pyridoxine glucosides that are absorbed but poorly metabolized (Kabir *et al.* 1983).

The B_6 vitamers and their phosphorylated derivatives are absorbed across the intestinal mucosa by nonsaturable, passive diffusion (Buss *et al.* 1980). At the cellular level, uptake of pyridoxal, pyridoxamine and pyridoxine also occurs by passive diffusion, the vitamers being trapped within the cell by pyridoxal kinase dependent phosphorylation (Buss *et al.* 1980; Mehanso *et al.* 1980). Pyridoxine phosphate is oxidized to pyridoxal phosphate, which can be transaminated to pyridoxamine phosphate. Pyridoxic acid, the major excretory product, is formed from pyridoxal by the action of aldehyde oxidase (Schwartz and Kjelgaard 1951) or an NAD-dependent aldehyde dehydrogenase (Stanulovic *et al.* 1976).

Methods to assess vitamin B_6 status in humans include measurement of pyridoxal phosphate dependent enzymes in erythrocytes in the presence and absence of added pyridoxal phosphate, estimation of B_6 vitamers in blood, plasma and urine, and measurement of metabolite excretion levels in response to overloading doses of methionine and tryptophan (Sauberlich *et al.* 1974). It has been proposed that urinary pyridoxic acid indicates recent vitamin B_6 intake, while plasma pyridoxal phosphate is reflective of body stores (Lui *et al.* 1985). Since pyridoxal is the ultimate transport form of vitamin B_6 (Ink and Henderson 1984), the ratio of pyridoxal to pyridoxal phosphate may be a useful measure to assess vitamin B_6 status.

Dietary vitamin B_6 deficiency is rare. Experimental vitamin B_6 deficiency has been produced in humans by feeding a deficient diet in association with a pyridoxine antagonist such as 4-deoxypyridoxine. Deficiency symptoms include seborrhea-like lesions about the eyes, nose and mouth, cheilosis, glossitis and stomatitis (which are morphologically indistinguishable from the oral lesions of niacin and riboflavin deficiency), weight loss, apathy, somnolence and increased irritability, impaired antibody response to antigenic stimuli, and hypochromic microcytic anemia (Sauberlich and Canham 1980). Convulsive seizures and nervous irritability have been observed in infants fed a commercial liquid formula in which the vitamin B_6 content was reduced by inappropriate heat sterilization (Coursin 1954). Deficiency symptoms clear rapidly after administration of pyridoxine.

Estrogens

Excretion of xanthurenic acid in response to a tryptophan load test is abnormal in oral contraceptive users (Leklem *et al.* 1975). This is related to a specific effect of estrogen on enzymes in the tryptophan-kynurenine pathway and is not indicative of vitamin B_6 deficiency. The effect of estrogen on other indices of vitamin B_6 status is equivocal. With anovulatory steroid use, plasma pyridoxal phosphate is reduced (Miller 1985; Leklem 1986), but urinary pyridoxic acid excretion is normal (Leklem 1986). Stimulation of erythrocyte transaminase activity by pyridoxal phosphate is variable (Leklem 1986), and the response to depletion-repletion is similar to that of nonusers (Donald and Bossé 1979). Whether the decrease in pyridoxal phosphate is balanced by an increase in pyridoxal, as occurs in pregnancy (Barnard *et al.* 1987), is not known. Based on these observations, it has been concluded that the requirement for vitamin B_6 in oral contraceptive users is similar to that of nonusers. However, pregnant and lactating women who used anovulatory steroids for longer than 30 months prior to conception had lower levels of vitamin B_6 in their serum at five months gestation, in cord serum at term, and in breast milk at 14 days postpartum (Roepke and Kirksey 1979). This suggests that body reserves of vitamin B_6 in long term users may be reduced.

Estrogen is often used in the management of postmenopausal osteoporosis. Whether estrogen interacts adversely with the normal age-related changes in vitamin B_6 metabolism remains to be determined.

Toxicity

Prolonged excessive intake of vitamin B_6 causes a severe sensory neuropathy. Subjects self-medicating with 500 mg to 6 g/day for two to 40 months developed a syndrome characterized by progressive sensory ataxia and profound distal limb impairment of position and vibration sense (Schaumburg *et al.* 1983; Berger and Schaumburg 1984). Symptoms gradually regressed when supplementation was discontinued. Impaired memorization skill has been noted during ingestion of 100 mg/day (Molimard *et al.* 1980).

Recommendations

Adults

The requirement for vitamin B_6 is related to dietary protein intake. The results of several studies suggest that a ratio of 0.015 mg/g dietary protein will normalize excretion of tryptophan metabolites in almost all young adult subjects (Baker *et al.* 1964; Miller and Linkswiler 1967; Canham *et al.* 1969). This amount includes an allowance for individual variability. Accordingly, this ratio is accepted as the basis for the intake of vitamin B_6 recommended for normal adults. When intake is expressed as milligrams per day, it varies with protein intake. For example, at the level of the recommended intake of protein, 57 and 41 g/day for adult men and women, respectively, the recommended amounts of vitamin B_6 are 0.9 and 0.6 mg/day; at the level of the average intake of protein reported in the Nutrition Canada Survey (Canada. Health and Welfare 1977) by young adult men and women, 120 and 70 g/day, respectively, the recommended amounts of vitamin B_6 are 1.8 and 1.1 mg/day. Although amino acids consumed in excess of the requirement are catabolized, high protein diets increase the efficiency of vitamin B_6 utilization, i.e. more pyridoxal is retained in the body rather than being converted to pyridoxic acid (Miller *et al.* 1985). Therefore a ratio of 0.015 mg/g dietary protein should satisfy the vitamin B_6 requirement over a wide range of dietary protein intakes. A large proportion of protein in the Canadian diet is derived from animal sources which are also rich in vitamin B_6.

Physical exercise is associated with increased gluconeogenesis and glycogenolysis, both processes requiring vitamin B_6 as a cofactor for transaminase enzymes and as a component of glycogen phosphorylase. Exercise in trained, healthy young men and women causes a transient increase in plasma pyridoxal phosphate and urinary pyridoxic acid excretion (Leklem 1985; Dreon and Butterfield 1986; Manore *et al.* 1987). However, the response to a loading dose of tryptophan or methionine indicates that vitamin B_6 status is not compromised, despite the increased rate of catabolism (Leklem 1985). It is proposed that the stimulus of physical activity promotes storage of vitamin B_6, possibly in the form of glycogen phosphorylase, during periods of rest. This store of pyridoxal can then be mobilized to meet the needs imposed by periods of exercise. Thus a diet providing sufficient energy and 0.015 mg/g dietary protein should be adequate.

Elderly

Indices of vitamin B_6 status decrease with age. It is estimated that the plasma pyridoxal phosphate level declines by approximately 0.90 ng/mL per decade (Rose *et al.* 1976). This appears to be a specific effect of aging on vitamin B_6 metabolism, and not the result of poor dietary intake (Rose *et al.* 1976; Lee and Leklem 1985). While the plasma concentration in the elderly will respond to supplementation (Jacobs *et al.* 1968; Lee and Leklem 1985), there is no evidence at this time to suggest that aging increases the vitamin B_6 requirement. The recommended intake therefore is 0.015 mg/g dietary protein, the same as for young adults.

Infants

The concentration of vitamin B_6 in breast milk ranges from 0.008 to 0.16 mg/L during the first few days of lactation and 0.08 to 0.18 mg/L in mature milk (West and Kirksey 1976; Roepke and Kirksey 1979; Styslinger and Kirksey 1985; Bamji *et al.* 1987). No signs of deficiency have been observed in infants receiving milk containing from 0.007 to 0.013 mg/g dietary protein (West and Kirksey 1976; Styslinger and Kirksey 1985; Bamji *et al.* 1987). The vitamin B_6 requirement of all breast-fed infants should be met by consumption of 750 mL of breast milk produced by a mother ingesting an adequate diet. In some cases, vitamin B_6 intake by breast-fed infants may be less than 0.015 mg/g dietary protein. However, it should be noted that vitamin B_6 in breast milk is present predominantly as pyridoxal, a form which may be more readily absorbed (Kirksey and Udipi 1985). In addition, the high level of nitrogen retention in infants (approximately 70%) and the low level of amino acid catabolism may reduce the amount of pyridoxal necessary to support nitrogen metabolism. The vitamin B_6 content of commercial formula is 0.016 mg/g dietary protein. Whole blood total vitamin B_6 levels in formula-fed infants are twice those of breast-fed infants (McCoy *et al.* 1985).

Children and Adolescents

A satisfactory evaluation of the requirements of children and adolescents for vitamin B_6 is not possible based on available data (McCoy 1978; Ritchey *et al.* 1978). Reports on intakes suggest that 0.015 mg/g dietary protein is appropriate for this group as well (Ritchey and Freely 1966; Lewis and Nunn 1977; Kirksey *et al.* 1978).

Pregnancy

The diet in pregnancy must provide sufficient vitamin B_6 to support both fetal and maternal amino acid metabolism, as well as supply a small quantity for deposition in fetal tissues. In pregnancy, plasma pyridoxal phosphate levels are 50% less than nonpregnant values (Schuster *et al.* 1984; Barnard *et al.* 1987). During the last 10 weeks of gestation, pyridoxal phosphate levels drop precipitously, reflecting sequestration by fetal tissues during this period of rapid growth (Schuster *et al.* 1984). Plasma pyridoxal phosphate can be maintained at the nonpregnant level by supplementation (Schuster *et al.* 1984); however, the amount of pyridoxine required is large. This suggests that maternal tissues are resistant to the effects of supplemental vitamin B_6, and that lower plasma pyridoxal phosphate is a normal response to pregnancy. In addition, measurement of both pyridoxal and pyridoxal phosphate at 22 weeks gestation indicates that total vitamin B_6 is unchanged; there is a shift in vitamers such that pyridoxal, not pyridoxal phosphate, is the predominant form in maternal plasma (Barnard *et al.* 1987). Since pyridoxal is the chief transport form, this may represent a physiological adjustment which enhances availability of vitamin B_6 to both maternal and fetal tissues. Based on these observations, a diet providing a 0.015 mg/g dietary protein should be adequate during pregnancy.

Lactation

There is no indication that lactation alters vitamin B_6 metabolism. The amount of the vitamin required to support the formation of milk protein is not known. In general, while the vitamin B_6 content of breast milk reflects dietary intake, there appears to be some inefficiency in the transfer process, as a 10-fold increase in maternal intake produces only a 4-fold increase in breast milk concentration (Styslinger and Kirksey 1985). The recommended intake for non-lactating women provides vitamin B_6 at a somewhat greater level than is secreted in milk (West and Kirksey 1976; Roepke and Kirksey 1979; Styslinger and Kirksey 1985; Bamji *et al.* 1987). On the assumption that protein metabolism is not altered, a diet providing 0.015 mg/g dietary protein should be adequate to support lactation. As with pregnancy, if the intake of dietary protein is increased, intake of vitamin B_6 should be increased proportionately.

References

Baker, E.M., Canham, J.E., Nunes, W.T., Sauberlich, H.E. and McDowell, M.E. 1964. Vitamin B_6 requirement for adult men. Am. J. Clin. Nutr. 15:59-66.

Bamji, M.S., Premakumari, K. and Jacob, C.M. 1987. Pyridoxine status and requirement of breast-fed infants: relationship with maternal status and milk pyridoxine levels. Nutr. Rep. Int. 35:171-177.

Barnard, H.C., deKock, J.J., Vermaak, W.J.H. and Potgieter, G.M. 1987. A new perspective in the assessment of vitamin B_6 nutritional status during pregnancy in humans. J. Nutr. 117:1303-1306.

Berger, A. and Schaumburg, H.H. 1984. More on neuropathy from pyridoxine abuse. N. Engl. J. Med. 311:986-987.

Black, A.L., Guirard, B.M. and Snell, E.E. 1978. The behavior of muscle phosphorylase as a reservoir for vitamin B_6 in the rat. J. Nutr. 108:670-677.

Buss, D.D., Hamm, M.W., Mehansho, H. and Henderson, L.M. 1980. Transport and metabolism of pyridoxine in the perfused small intestine and the hind limb of the rat. J. Nutr. 110:1655-1663.

Canada. Health and Welfare. Nutrition Canada. Health Protection Branch. Bureau of Nutritional Sciences. 1977. Food consumption patterns report. Ottawa.

Canham, J.E., Baker, E.M., Harding, R.S., Sauberlich, H.E. and Plough, I.C. 1969. Dietary protein — its relationship to vitamin B_6 requirements and function. Ann. N.Y. Acad. Sci. 166:16-29.

Coursin, B.B. 1954. Convulsive seizures in infants with pyridoxine deficient diet. J. Am. Med. Assoc. 154:406-408.

Donald, E.A. and Bossé, T.R. 1979. The vitamin B_6 requirement in oral contraceptive users. II. Assessment by tryptophan metabolites, vitamin B_6, and pyridoxic acid levels in urine. Am. J. Clin. Nutr. 32:1024-1032.

Dreon, D.M. and Butterfield, G.E. 1986. Vitamin B_6 utilization in active and inactive young men. Am. J. Clin. Nutr. 43:816-824.

Gregory, J.F., III and Kirk, J.R. 1981. The bioavailability of vitamin B_6 in foods. Nutr. Rev. 39:1-8.

Ink, S.L. and Henderson, L.M. 1984. Effect of binding to hemoglobin and albumin on pyridoxal transport and metabolism. J. Biol. Chem. 259:5833-5837.

Jacobs, A., Cavill, I.A.J. and Hughes, J.N.P. 1968. Erythrocyte transaminase activity. Effect of age, sex, and vitamin B_6 supplementation. Am. J. Clin. Nutr. 21:502-507.

Kabir, H., Leklem, J. and Miller, L.T. 1983. Measurements of glycosylated vitamin B_6 in foods. J. Food Sci. 48:1422-1425.

Kirksey, A., Keaton, K., Abernathy, R.P. and Greger, J.L. 1978. Vitamin B_6 nutritional status of a group of female adolescents. Am. J. Clin. Nutr. 31:946-954.

Kirksey, A. and Udipi, S.A. 1985. Vitamin B_6 in human pregnancy and lactation. *In* Current topics in nutrition and disease. Vol. 13. Vitamin B-6: its role in health and disease. Reynolds, R.D. and Leklem, J.E., eds. A.R. Liss, New York, pp. 57-77.

Lee, C. and Leklem, J.E. 1985. Differences in vitamin B_6 status indicator responses between young and middle-aged women fed constant diets with two levels of vitamin B_6. Am. J. Clin. Nutr. 42:226-234.

Leklem, J.E. 1985. Physical activity and vitamin B_6 metabolism in men and women: interrelationship with fuel needs. *In* Current topics in nutrition and disease. Vol. 13. Vitamin B-6: its role in health and disease. Reynolds, R.D. and Leklem, J.E., eds. A.R. Liss, New York, pp. 57-77.

Leklem, J.E. 1986. Vitamin B_6 requirement and oral contraceptive use — a concern? J. Nutr. 116:475-477.

Leklem, J.E., Brown, R.R., Rose, D.P., Linkswiler, H. and Arend, R.A. 1975. Metabolism of tryptophan and niacin in oral contraceptive users receiving controlled intakes of vitamin B_6. Am. J. Clin. Nutr. 28:146-156.

Lewis, J.S. and Nunn, K.P. 1977. Vitamin B_6 intakes and 24-hour 4-pyridoxic acid excretions of children. Am. J. Clin. Nutr. 30:2023-2027.

Lui, A., Lumeng, L., Aronoff, G.R. and Li, T.K. 1985. Relationship between body store of vitamin B_6 and plasma pyridoxal-P clearance: metabolic balance studies in humans. J. Lab. Clin. Med. 106:491-497.

Manore, M.M., Leklem, J.E. and Walter, M.C. 1987. Vitamin B_6 metabolism as affected by exercise in trained and untrained women fed diets differing in carbohydrate and vitamin B_6 content. Am. J. Clin. Nutr. 46:995-1004.

McCoy, E.E. 1978. Vitamin B_6 requirements of infants and children. *In* Human vitamin B_6 requirements: proceedings of a workshop. Food and Nutrition Board, National Academy of Sciences, Washington, pp. 257-271.

McCoy, E.E. and Colombini, C. 1972. Interconversions of vitamin B_6 in mammalian tissue. J. Agric. Food Chem. 20:494-498.

McCoy, E., Strynadka, K. and Brunet, K. 1985. Vitamin B_6 intake and whole blood levels of breast and formula fed infants: serial whole blood vitamin B_6 levels in premature infants. *In* Current topics in nutrition and disease. Vol. 13. Vitamin B-6: its role in health and disease. Reynolds, R.D. and Leklem, J.E., eds. A.R. Liss, New York, pp. 79-88.

Mehansho, H., Buss, D.D., Hamm, M.W. and Henderson, L.M. 1980. Transport and metabolism of pyridoxine in rat liver. Biochim. Biophys. Acta 631:112-123.

Miller, L.T. 1985. Oral contraceptives and vitamin B_6 metabolism. *In* Current topics in nutrition and disease. Vol. 13. Vitamin B-6: its role in health and disease. Reynolds, R.D. and Leklem, J.E., eds. A.R. Liss, New York, pp. 243-255.

Miller, L.T. and Linkswiler, H. 1967. Effect of protein intake on the development of abnormal tryptophan metabolism by men during vitamin B_6 depletion. J. Nutr. 93:53-59.

Miller, L.T., Leklem, J.E. and Shultz, T.D. 1985. The effect of dietary protein on the metabolism of vitamin B_6 in humans. J. Nutr. 115:1663-1672.

Molimard, R., Marillaud, A., Paille, A., Le Devehat, C., Lemoine, A. and Dougney, M. 1980. Impairment of memorization by high doses of pyridoxine in man. Biomedicine 32:88-92.

Rabinowitz, J.C. and Snell, E.E. 1948. The vitamin B_6 group. XIV. Distribution of pyridoxal, pyridoxamine and pyridoxine in some natural products. J. Biol. Chem. 176:1157-1167.

Ritchey, S.J. and Freely, R.M. 1966. The excretion patterns of vitamin B_6 and B_{12} in preadolescent girls. J. Nutr. 89:411-413.

Ritchey, S.J., Johnson, F.S. and Korslund, M.K. 1978. Vitamin B_6 requirements in the preadolescent and adolescent. *In* Human vitamin B_6 requirements: proceedings of a workshop. Food and Nutrition Board, National Academy of Sciences, Washington, pp. 272-278.

Roepke, J.L.B. and Kirksey, A. 1979. Vitamin B_6 nutriture during pregnancy and lactation. I. Vitamin B_6 intake, levels of the vitamin in biological fluids and condition of the infant at birth. Am. J. Clin. Nutr. 32:2249-2256.

Roepke, J.L.B. and Kirksey, A. 1979. Vitamin B_6 nutriture during pregnancy and lactation. II. The effect of long-term use of oral contraceptives. Am. J. Clin. Nutr. 32:2257-2264.

Rose, C.S., Gyorgy, P., Butler, M., Andres, R., Norris, A.H., Shock, N.W., Tobin, J., Brin, M. and Spiegel, H. 1976. Age differences in vitamin B_6 status of 617 men. Am. J. Clin. Nutr. 29:847-853.

Sauberlich, H.E. and Canham, J.E. 1980. Vitamin B_6. *In* Modern nutrition in health and disease. 6th ed. Goodhart, R.S. and Shils, M.E., eds. Lea & Febiger, Philadelphia, pp. 216-228.

Sauberlich, H.E., Skala, J.H. and Dowdy, R.P. 1974. Laboratory tests for the assessment of nutritional status. CRC Press, Cleveland.

Schaumburg, H., Kaplan, J., Windebank, A., Vick, N., Rasmus, S., Pleasure, D. and Brown, M.J. 1983. Sensory neuropathy from pyridoxine abuse: a new megavitamin syndrome. N. Engl. J. Med. 309:445-448.

Schuster, K., Bailey, L.B. and Mahan, C.S. 1984. Effect of maternal pyridoxine HCl supplementation on the vitamin B_6 status of mother and infant and on pregnancy outcome. J. Nutr. 114:977-998.

Schwartz, R. and Kjelgaard, N.O. 1951. The enzymic oxidation of pyridoxal by liver aldehyde oxidase. Biochem. J. 48:333-337.

Stanulovic, M., Jeremic, V., Leskovac, V. and Chaykin, S. 1976. New pathway of conversion of pyridoxal to 4-pyridoxic acid. Enzyme 21:357-369.

Styslinger, L. and Kirksey, A. 1985. Effects of different levels of vitamin B_6 supplementation on vitamin B_6 concentrations in human milk and vitamin B_6 intakes of breastfed infants. Am. J. Clin. Nutr. 41:21-31.

West, K.D. and Kirksey, A. 1976. Influence of vitamin B_6 intake on content of the vitamin in human milk. Am. J. Clin. Nutr. 29:961-969.

Folate

Forms and Function

Folacin and folate are generic descriptors for a group of coenzymes and their precursors that have a chemical structure similar to and exhibit the biological activity and nutritional properties of folic acid: N-[4-[(2-amino-1,4-dihydro-4-oxo-6-pteridinyl)methyl]amino-benzoyl]-L-glutamic acid, also known as pteroylglutamic acid (PGA; PteGlu). PGA is the completely oxidized form of the molecule and is probably not found as such in nature. It is used both therapeutically and as a reference compound because of its stability. The naturally occurring derivatives, dihydrofolates (H_2) and tetrahydrofolates (H_4) are reduced forms and have additional glutamic acid residues bound in peptide linkage to the gamma-carboxyl group of the glutamate of the parent molecule.

The folate that is absorbed from food and which circulates in body fluids is 5-methyltetrahydrofolate (Chanarin and Perry 1969). Recent evidence suggests the presence of a membrane-associated transport protein that facilitates its entry into the cell (Antony *et al.* 1985). In the cell, additional glutamic acid residues are added in a chain of up to 11 units. These forms are called folate polyglutamates ($PteGlu_n$). Most folates in mammalian tissues, with the exception of plasma, are present as conjugated folylpolyglutamate derivatives. In this form folate is retained in the cell and serves as the active coenzyme in the transfer of single carbon units for purine, pyrimidine, and methionine synthesis. Cells that have lost the ability to make polyglutamates can not grow unless the end products of folate metabolism, such as purines, are supplied (Baugh and Krumdieck 1971; Chanarin et al 1985; Shane and Stokstad 1985; Scrimgeour 1986).

Requirements for the vitamin can be met by the different forms, providing the essential subunit remains intact; if broken, nutritional activity is lost. Deficiency of folate leads to impaired cell division and to alterations in protein synthesis, the effects of which are most pronounced in rapidly growing tissues. Apparently, the dU suppression test, a sensitive indicator of folate-deficient DNA synthesis, becomes clearly abnormal when intracellular folate levels fall below 0.2 ng/10^6 cell (Colman and Herbert 1980; Steinberg *et al.* 1983; Herbert 1985, 1986).

Naturally occurring folates exhibit a variable degree of instability towards endogenous deconjugation by pteroylpolyglutamyl hydrolases which remove glutamate residues but leave an active compound. Heat, oxidation, extreme pH and ultraviolet light can cleave the folate molecule, rendering it inactive. Hence folates are likely to be lost during storage and cooking. Reducing agents, such as ascorbate, preserve folate (O'Broin *et al.* 1975).

All foods of plant and animal origin contain folates: liver, leafy vegetables, fruit, pulses and yeast are especially good sources.

Folate content is expressed in terms of PGA equivalents. Quantitatively, the vitamin is commonly measured by its ability to support the growth of folate-dependent organisms in an otherwise complete chemically defined culture and assay medium. *Lactobacillus casei* is generally accepted as the standard assay organism because it responds to the greatest number of folate derivatives, including those with up to three L-glutamic residues. Prior to assay, foods and tissues must be pre-treated with pteroylpolyglutamyl hydrolase in order to convert polyglutamate folate to the folate monoglutamate form that is available to the organism. The term "total" folate has been used to express folate content after hydrolase pre-treatment. The term "free" folate has been used to designate the forms measurable by *Lactobacillus casei* without hydrolase treatment. Since the amount of "free" folate depends on the activity of endogenous hydrolases and inhibitors, unless stringent precautions have been taken in collecting and handling the sample, the proportion in the diet is so variable that it is not a useful measurement (Rodriguez 1978).

Absorption

Approximately 75% of the folate in mixed U.S. and Canadian diets is present in the form of polyglutamates (Butterworth *et al.* 1963; U.S. N.R.C. 1977). The ingested folate polyglutamates are deconjugated before being absorbed and utilized in higher organisms (Reisenauer *et al.* 1977; Wang *et al.* 1985; Halsted *et al.* 1986). Following the hydrolysis of folate polyglutamates, which appears to be a function of the mucosal cells, folates enter the portal plasma in the monoglutamate form (Hoffbrand and Peters 1969; Baugh *et al.* 1975; Godwin and Rosenberg 1975; Halsted *et al.* 1975). Hence, both free and conjugated folates can be utilized to meet human nutritional requirements.

Metabolic balance studies with radioactive synthetic folate polyglutamates in humans showed that intestinal absorption of heptaglutamyl folate ranged from 50% to 75%, and of triglutamyl folate, >90% (Butterworth *et al.* 1969). Other studies indicate that monoglutamate and polyglutamate folate were absorbed equally well (Rodriguez 1978). Uncertainty still persists whether folate polyglutamate absorbability decreases with increasing chain length. The absorbability of heptaglutamate has been reported to be 70-100% that of PGA (Halsted *et al.* 1978, 1986; Rodriguez 1978; Rosenberg 1981).

Approximately 90% of folate monoglutamate and 50-90% of folate polyglutamate is absorbed when ingested separately from food, but absorption is decreased in the presence of some foods, regardless of whether the folate was derived from or added to the food (Tamura and Stokstad 1973). On the basis of food composition and intestinal absorption data, with both mono- and polyglutamate forms of folate available for absorption, it is reasonable to assume that on the average, approximately 70% of total dietary folate is absorbed (Tamura and Stokstad 1973; Babu and Srikantia 1976).

Fecal excretion of folate (≈ 200 µg daily) is not a reliable indicator of folate intake or absorption because most of it is folate synthesized by bacteria in the colon (Herbert *et al.* 1984). Daily urinary excretion of folate in well-nourished individuals ranges from 5-40 µg (Herbert 1968). The biological half-life of radioactive PGA, ingested by a healthy subject, was found to be 101 days. Fecal and urinary losses were approximately equal (Baker *et al.* 1965). However, the folate content of bile is about five times that of serum, indicating that enterohepatic recirculation tends to conserve the body pool of folate (Steinberg 1984; Weir *et al.* 1985).

Dietary Intake

In Canada, the mean daily folate intake is estimated to be 205 µg/day for men and 149 µg/day for women, or approximately 3 µg/kg of body weight (Canada. Health and Welfare 1977). This permits liver folate concentration to be maintained at normal and similar levels in both sexes. These liver folate values averaged 7.4 ± 2.2 µg/g for males and 7.3 ± 2.9 µg/g for females (Hoppner and Lampi 1980). On this diet, 8% of Canadian men and 10% of Canadian women have red cell folates below 150 µg/L (Cooper 1978). The comparable data (Senti and Pilch 1984) for American men and women was 8% and 13% respectively, and U.S. dietary folate intake was calculated as 227 µg per capita daily. The latter estimate did not account for food wastage or losses during home food preparation (Herbert 1987a). In the U.K. the mean dietary folate intake over a three year period was 210-213 µg daily, and 8% of the U.K. population was found to have red cell folate below 150 µg/L. The low levels were most prevalent in elderly subjects (Sneath *et al.* 1973; Poh Tan *et al.* 1984).

Folate Status

Folate status can be described by three different states:

Folate adequacy — An individual manifests no clinical, hematological or biochemical defects due to lack of folate which have not been corrected by folate supplementation. There is normal blood and marrow morphology. Liver folate concentration exceeds 3.0 µg/g wet weight and red cell folate exceeds 150 µg/L. The urinary formiminoglutamic acid (FIGLU) excretion would be expected to be less than 17 mg in eight hours after an oral dose of 15 mg of L-histidine. In such individuals, without ingesting dietary folate, stores would last for more than 100 days (Herbert 1962a,b, 1987b).

Impending folate deficiency — Impending folate deficiency is indicated by low serum levels (<3 ng/mL) and reduced stores (red cell folate <150 ng/mL). The excretion of FIGLU is greater than 35 mg in eight hours (Luhby and Cooperman 1964) in otherwise healthy individuals. This situation occurs in approximately 9% of non-pregnant adults consuming North American diets. There are no reserves to meet increased requirements, nor is there prolonged deprivation (Herbert 1987a).

Overt folate deficiency — This stage is characterized by the presence of megaloblasts in the bone marrow and their progeny in the blood: macro-ovalocytes, hypersegmented granulocytes and giant platelets. Serum folates are <3 ng/mL, red blood cell folates <100 ng/mL and liver folate <1.0 µg/g (Herbert 1987b). FIGLU excretion exceeds 100 mg in eight hours (Luhby and Cooperman 1964). Pregnant women deficient in folate may give birth to folate deficient infants (Luhby *et al.* 1967).

Requirements

The minimum daily or basal adult folate requirement has been described as the amount of folate required to sustain biochemical normality (normal DNA synthesis) in the absence of increased and sustained metabolic demands (Herbert 1987a,b).

There are data available on folate loss from the liver in human subjects on very low intakes, but little is known about losses from extra-hepatic tissues, except the red cells. Red cell folate levels are depleted at a rate equal to that of hepatic folate (Wu *et al.* 1975; Herbert 1977). It is assumed that the same is true for other tissues except the brain (Herbert and Colman 1979).

There is no accurate measurement of the total folate pool of which liver folate is a major part (Chanarin 1979). Among 560 livers assayed from autopsies in Canada, only two had a folate content of <3 µg/g of liver (Hoppner and Lampi 1980). The mean levels of folate plateaued at 8.8 µg/g between the ages of 11 and 20 and then gradually decreased. Loss of folate from the liver in patients with neoplastic disease on an intake of 2 µg folate daily, as assessed by liver biopsies, varied from 35 to 47 µg daily (Gailani *et al.* 1970). Assuming that extra-hepatic stores are approximately half those in the liver, total daily folate losses in an adult averages 60 µg. In such adults, morphologic evidence of folate deficiency in bone marrow and peripheral blood does not appear until liver folate levels fall below 1 µg/g (Gailani *et al.* 1970).

An oral intake of 50 µg of folic acid has been shown to sustain serum and red cell concentrations in normal young women (Herbert 1962a,b), and to reverse uncomplicated folate deficiency anemia (Zalusky and Herbert 1961). In another study (Banerjee *et al.* 1975), folate deficiency was produced in healthy volunteers by feeding a low folate diet supplying 15 µg daily. The amount of folate was increased every one to three weeks in the same subjects but insufficient time was allowed for the folate to raise the red cell levels. Under these conditions, the minimal or basal requirement appeared to be about 75 µg per day.

From the various experimental approaches, the average basal requirement is about 60 µg per day.

Toxicity

At the doses of folate discussed in this report, no toxicity has been reported. Very large doses of folic acid may precipitate convulsions in persons whose epilepsy is controlled by phenytoin (Colman and Herbert 1979). In patients with drug-induced megaloblastic anemia, folate doses of 1 mg or more have precipitated status epilepticus (Chanarin *et al.* 1960).

Recommendations

Adults

The recommended intake is based on observations of dietary folate intake and bioavailability in populations without clinical folate deficiency.

In Canada the mean daily folate intake for ages 12-65 years is 205 µg/d for men and 149 µg/d for women or about 3 µg/kg/day. This diet permits maintenance of normal liver folate levels in both sexes (Canada. Health and Welfare 1977; Hoppner and Lampi 1980). Red cell folate levels reflect those in liver fairly closely and the daily intake correlates significantly with red cell levels (Wu *et al.* 1975; Herbert 1977; Chanarin 1979; Bates *et al.* 1982). In the Canadian population about 9% of individuals had red cell folate levels below 150 ng/mL, and could presumably have inadequate stores (Cooper 1978). U.S. and British figures are similar (Sneath *et al.* 1973; Poh Tan *et al.* 1984; Senti and Pilch 1984; Herbert 1987a,b). Forty adult males, living in a metabolic ward on a strictly controlled diet containing 200 ± 68 µg/day, had normal serum and red cell folate levels after six months (Milne *et al.* 1983). In another study, it was determined that a daily intake of 200-250 µg of dietary folate appears to meet the folate requirement of non-pregnant adult women (Sauberlich *et al.* 1987).

Since folate from an average Canadian diet is sufficient to sustain adequate liver stores in most of the population, and in view of the above considerations, the recommended dietary intake is 3.1 µg/kg body weight. This equals a daily intake of 217 µg for a 70 kg man and 170 µg for a 55 kg woman.

This recommendation appears to provide an adequate margin for storage in the liver against periods of negative folate balance. A smaller intake is not recommended because of the possibility of an acute drain on stores, as occurs during pregnancy.

The Elderly

The elderly are considered in the same category as other adults with respect to folate requirements (Rosenberg *et al.* 1982; Suter and Russell 1987). Reported folate intakes have varied between 50-200 µg of dietary folate daily (Rosenberg *et al.* 1982; Suter and Russell 1987). The frequency of low serum and erythrocyte folate is similar to other adults, but folate nutritional status may vary with health and socioeconomic status and institutionalization (Rosenberg *et al.* 1982; Suter and Russell 1987).

There are no consistently demonstrated age-related changes in folate metabolism and/or absorption. Age-related changes in pteroylpolyglutamyl hydrolase activity are uncertain (Rosenberg *et al.* 1982; Suter and Russell 1987), but a recent study (Baily *et al.* 1984) showed no reduction in activity due to age. It has been reported that elderly subjects with atrophic gastritis malabsorb PGA due to a rise in pH in the proximal gastrointestinal tract (Elsborg 1976). This may be compensated for by the folate synthesized by the bacterial overgrowth that occurs in the upper intestinal tract in the absence of gastric acid (Russell *et al.* 1986). Conclusions from several studies indicate that folate absorption does not change with age alone (Suter and Russell 1987).

Infants

Folate deficiency is the most common cause of megaloblastic anemia in infants and children (FAO/WHO 1970; Rodriguez 1978). Despite higher than maternal serum levels at birth, body folate stores are small and rapidly depleted by the requirements for growth. This is especially the case in small premature infants with poor folate stores (Shojania and Gross 1964). It was found that premature infants required 65 µg folate per day to maintain serum and red cell folate levels (Strelling *et al.* 1979). An appropriate maintenance dose to prevent folate deficiency in a premature infant is 50-100 μg/day and is adequate to prevent the folate deficiency that occurs with childhood hemolytic anemias (Herbert 1981). A study of 20 infants aged 2-11 months showed that diets providing 3.6 μg folate/kg body weight daily for 6- to 9-month periods were nutritionally adequate (Asfour *et al.* 1977).

The needs of infants are adequately met by human or cow's milk, which contains 50-60 μg/L of folate. Goat's milk has a much lower folate content (FAO/WHO 1970; U.S.D.A. 1976). If the diet consists of goat's milk, a folate supplement is necessary, unless the milk contains added folate. Boiling, or the preparation of evaporated milk, destroys an average of 50% of the folate in cow's milk (WHO 1968). Infants receiving such prepared formulas should be given additional folate to insure an adequate intake (Ghitis 1966).

Dietary folate megaloblastic anemia is rare in children who drink vegetable or fruit juice or eat some fresh uncooked fruits and vegetables every day (Rodriguez 1978). Up to two years of age, 3.5 μg of dietary folate per kg of body weight appears to be adequate (Waslien 1977).

From the above considerations a recommended daily intake of 4.0 μg dietary folate per kg body weight is adequate and also compatible with the folate content of human milk.

Children and Adolescents

Folate stores in young and adolescent Canadians appear to be satisfactory, with an average daily dietary intake of 3 μg folate/kg body weight (Hoppner and Lampi 1980). Similar or higher intakes were recently reported for adolescent females (Clark *et al.* 1987). Although a high incidence of low serum and erythrocyte folate among the 103 subjects was reported, all the girls appeared to be healthy throughout the study.

From the recommendations for infants and young adults, the recommended daily intake of folate for children and adolescents is interpolated to be 3.5 μg/kg body weight.

Pregnancy

Pregnancy increases the risk and incidence of folate deficiency, particularly among populations with low or marginal intakes of the vitamin (Giles 1966; Lawrence and Klipstein 1967; Colman *et al.* 1975a). In general, pregnancy is associated with evidence of a negative folate balance and often with subclinical folate deficiency. The increased requirement for folate in pregnancy arises from the markedly accelerated cell multiplication involved in the enlargement of the uterus, development of the placenta, expansion of blood volume and growth of the fetus.

Baumslag *et al.* (1970), showed that folate, added to an iron supplement, increased birthweight and reduced the incidence of prematurity in folate deficient African women, but had no effect when given to well-nourished Caucasian women. These observations were confirmed by later studies (Iyengar and Rajalakshmi 1975; Rolschau *et al.* 1979; Tchernia *et al.* 1982), which also demonstrated that placental weights increased significantly when folate supplements were used, suggesting that the beneficial effect on birthweight was due to improved nutrition. Folate supplements did not improve infant weight in well-nourished population groups in Australia and London (Fletcher *et al.* 1971; Giles *et al.* 1971).

There is particular interest in folate intake before conception and in early pregnancy, in view of the reported possible relationship between folate and the occurrence of neural tube defects in the newborn (Laurence *et al.* 1981; Elwood 1983; Smithells *et al.* 1983). Initial findings in a group of women with significantly lower red cell folate levels in the first trimester of pregnancy showed that supplements given before conception reduced the frequency of neural tube defects. The data have been criticized and a large controlled trial on pre-pregnancy folate supplementation in susceptible women is underway (Elwood 1983).

The frequency of megaloblastic haemopoiesis in bone marrow samples from women in late pregnancy ranges from 24% to 60% in the absence of folate supplementation. Prevalency figures of megaloblastosis in marrow samples in pregnancy are reported to range around 25% in Texas, USA, Canada, UK and South Africa; 30% in Ireland and Nigeria; and 54-60% in India (Chanarin 1985).

Studies have been carried out to assess the size of the folate supplement needed to maintain the status quo in pregnancy. PGA supplements ranging from 100-1000 μg/day have been recommended by different investigators in addition to the folate available from a good quality mixed diet (Chanarin *et al.* 1968; Colman *et al.* 1974, 1975 a,b). In 100 pregnant women consuming a usual diet in Britain, a supplement of 100 μg PGA daily produced a rise in the mean red cell folate in the first trimester, and thereafter remained unchanged (Chanarin *et al.* 1968). In 100 women not given the supplement, the mean red cell folate continued to decline throughout pregnancy. In Sweden, a daily supplement of 50 μg PGA did not sustain serum or red cell folate in pregnancy, while 100 μg daily did, and 200 μg or more daily produced large increases in mean red cell folate during pregnancy (Hansen and Rybo 1967). In 35 women receiving only iron supplements at 12, 24, 36 weeks and puerperium the red cell folate levels declined. Near term, 24-32% of women were found to have low red cell levels (Chanarin and Rothman 1971). Since these studies dealt with the mean red cell concentration of groups of women, the required supplement needed to maintain normal red cell folate in all pregnant women is greater than 100 μg/day. In women who start pregnancy with moderate folate stores, all symptoms of deficiency could probably be prevented by diets containing the equivalent of 300 μg PGA per day (Herbert 1977). In a study of women with poor stores, who received essentially no other dietary folate, the progression of deficiency was as effectively prevented by administering 300 μg PGA per day in a food that impaired availability by 44% as it was by higher doses or more efficient vehicles (Colman *et al.* 1975a). Studies in Australia and Denmark did not show any fall in red cell folate levels during normal pregnancies (Giles *et al.* 1971; Ek and Manus 1981), probably reflecting the well-nourished status of a middle-class population. Most other studies in less well-endowed populations report a fall in red cell folate.

When the diet is inadequate, normal pregnancy leads to a negative folate balance, as shown by falling red cell folate levels and increased folate clearance. The amount of folate supplement required on average to maintain red cell folate levels is 100 μg daily. However, in order to meet the needs of all women, including those with below average dietary intakes and poor folate stores, the supplement needs to be of the order of 200-300 μg PGA daily. The daily folate intake should therefore be no less than 370 μg or 7 μg/kg body weight.

Lactation

The added strain of lactation on maternal folate stores was estimated to be 20 μg/day based on 850 mL daily production of milk with an average folate content (Matoth *et al.* 1965). However, maternal milk folate content may be as high as 50-60 μg/L, suggesting a need for daily supplementation in that range for lactating women with marginal reserves (FAO/WHO 1970). It has been reported that supplementation was not necessary in middle-class women in Sweden (Ek 1983).

Based on a daily production of 750 mL of maternal milk and an estimate of 70% absorption a daily supplement of 100 μg is recommended. Therefore, the daily recommended intake for folate during lactation is 270 μg (3.1 μg/kg + 100 μg) or about 5 μg/kg body weight.

References

Antony, A.C., Kane, M.A., Portillo, R.M., Elwood, P.C. and Kolhouse, J.F. 1985. Studies of the role of a particulate folate-binding protein in the uptake of 5-methyltetrahydrofolate by cultured human KB cells. J. Biol. Chem. 260:14911-14917.

Asfour, R., Wahbeh, N., Waslien, C.I., Guindi, S. and Darby, W.J. 1977. Folacin requirements of children. III. Normal infants. Am. J. Clin. Nutr. 30:1098-1105.

Babu, S. and Srikantia, S.C. 1976. Availability of folates from some foods. Am. J. Clin. Nutr. 29:376-379.

Bailey, L.B., Cerda, J.J., Bloch, B.S., Busby, M.J., Vargas, L., Chandler, C.J. and Halsted, C.H. 1984. Effect of age on poly- and monoglutamyl folacin absorption in human subjects. J. Nutr. 114:1770-1776.

Baker, S.J., Kumar, S. and Swaminathan, S.P. 1965. Excretion of folic acid in bile. Lancet 1:685.

Banerjee, D.K., Maitra, A., Basu, A.K. and Chatterjea, J.B. 1975. Minimal daily requirement of folic acid in normal Indian subjects. Indian J. Med. Res. 63:45-53.

Bates, C.J., Black, A.E., Phillips, D.R., Wright, A.J.A. and Southgate, D.A.T. 1982. The discrepancy between normal folate intakes and the folate RDA. Hum. Nutr.: Appl. Nutr. 36A:422-429.

Baugh, C.M. and Krumdieck, C.L. 1971. Naturally occurring folates. Ann. N.Y. Acad. Sci. 186:7-28.

Baugh, C.M., Krumdieck, C.L., Baker, H.J. and Butterworth, C.E., Jr. 1975. Absorption of folic acid poly-γ-glutamates in dogs. J. Nutr. 105:80-89.

Baumslag, N., Edelstein, T. and Metz, J. 1970. Reduction of incidence of prematurity by folic acid supplementation in pregnancy. Br. Med. J. 1:16-17.

Butterworth, C.E., Jr., Santini, R., Jr. and Frommeyer, W.B., Jr. 1963. The pteroylglutamate components of American diets as determined by chromatographic fractionation. J. Clin. Invest. 42:1929-1939.

Butterworth, C.E., Jr., Baugh, C.M. and Krumdieck, C. 1969. A study of folate absorption and metabolism in man utilizing carbon-14-labelled polyglutamates synthesized by the solid phase method. J. Clin. Invest. 48:1131-1142.

Canada. Health and Welfare. Nutrition Canada. Health Protection Branch. Bureau of Nutritional Sciences. 1977. Food consumption patterns report. Ottawa.

Chanarin, I. 1979. The megaloblastic anaemias. 2nd ed. Blackwell Scientific, Oxford.

Chanarin, I. 1985. Folate and cobalamin. Clin. Haematol. 14:629-641.

Chanarin, I. and Perry, J. 1969. Evidence for reduction and methylation of folate in the intestine during normal absorption. Lancet 2:776-778.

Chanarin, I. and Rothman, D. 1971. Further observations on the relation between iron and folate status in pregnancy. Br. Med. J. 2:81-84.

Chanarin, I., Laidlaw, J., Loughridge, L.W. and Mollin, D.L. 1960. Megaloblastic anemia due to phenobarbitone. The convulsant action of therapeutic doses of folic acid. Br. Med. J. 1:1099-1102.

Chanarin, I., Rothman, D., Ward, A. and Perry, J. 1968. Folate status and requirement in pregnancy. Br. Med. J. 2:390-394.

Chanarin, I., Deacon, R., Lumb, M., Muir, M. and Perry, J. 1985. Cobalamin-folate interrelations: a critical review. Blood 66:479-489.

Clark, A.J., Mossholder, S. and Gates, R. 1987. Folacin status of adolescent females. Am. J. Clin. Nutr. 46:302-306.

Colman, N. and Herbert, V. 1979. Dietary assessments with special emphasis on prevention of folate deficiency. *In* Folic acid in neurology, psychiatry and internal medicine. Botez, M.I. and Reynolds, E.H., eds. Raven Press, New York, pp. 23-33.

Colman, N. and Herbert, V. 1980. Abnormal lymphocyte deoxyuridine suppression test: a reliable indicator of decreased lymphocyte folate levels. Am. J. Hematol. 8:169-174.

Colman, N., Barker, M., Green, R. and Metz, J. 1974. Prevention of folate deficiency in pregnancy by food fortification. Am. J. Clin. Nutr. 27:339-344.

Colman, N., Larsen, J.V., Barker, M., Barker, E.A., Green, R. and Metz, J. 1975a. Prevention of folate deficiency by food fortification. III. Effect in pregnant subjects of varying amounts of added folic acid. Am. J. Clin. Nutr. 28:465-470.

Colman, N., Barker, E.A., Barker, M., Green, R. and Metz, J. 1975b. Prevention of folate deficiency by food fortification. IV. Identification of target groups in addition to pregnant women in an adult rural population. Am. J. Clin. Nutr. 28:471-476.

Cooper, B.A. 1978. Reassessment of folic acid requirements. *In* Nutrition in transition: proceedings Western Hemisphere Nutrition Congress V. White, P.L. and Selvey, N., eds. American Medical Association, Munro, WI. pp. 281-288.

Ek, J. 1983. Plasma, red cell and breast milk folacin concentrations in lactating women. Am. J. Clin. Nutr. 38:929-935.

Ek, J. and Manus, E.M. 1981. Plasma and red blood cell folate during normal pregnancies. Acta Obstet. Gynecol. Scand. 60:247-251.

Elwood, J.M. 1983. Can vitamins prevent neural tube defects? Can. Med. Assoc. J. 129:1088-1092.

Elsborg, L. 1976. Reversible malabsorption of folic acid in the elderly with nutritional folate deficiency. Acta Haematol. 55:140-147.

FAO/WHO. 1970. Requirements of ascorbic acid, vitamin D, vitamin B_{12}, folate, and iron. Report of a joint FAO-WHO Expert Group. W.H.O. Tech. Rep. Ser. 452:1-75.

Fletcher, J., Gurr, A., Fellingham, F.R., Prankerd, T.A., Brant, H.A. and Menzies, D.N. 1971. The value of folic acid supplements in pregnancy. J. Obstet. Gynaecol. Br. Commonw. 78:781-785.

Gailani, S.D., Carey, R.W., Holland, J.F. and O'Malley, J.A. 1970. Studies of folate deficiency in patients with neoplastic diseases. Cancer Res. 30:327-333.

Ghitis, J. 1966. The labile folate of milk. Am. J. Clin. Nutr. 18:452-457.

Giles, C. 1966. An account of 335 cases of megaloblastic anemia of pregnancy and puerperium. J. Clin. Pathol. 19:1-11.

Giles, P.F.H., Harcourt, A.G. and Whiteside, M.G. 1971. The effect of prescribing folic acid during pregnancy on birthweight and duration of pregnancy. A double-blind trial. Med. J. Aust. 2:17-21.

Godwin, H.A. and Rosenberg, I.H. 1975. Comparative studies of the intestinal absorption of [^{3}H]pteroylmonoglutamate and [^{3}H]pteroylheptaglutamate in man. Gastroenterology 69:364-373.

Halsted, C.H., Baugh, C.M. and Butterworth, C.E., Jr. 1975. Jejunal perfusion of simple and conjugated folates in man. Gastroenterology 68:261-269.

Halsted, C.H., Reisenauer, A.M., Shane, B., and Tamura, T. 1978. Availability of monoglutamyl and polyglutamyl folates in normal subjects and in patients with coeliac sprue. Gut 19:886-891.

Halsted, C.H., Beer, W.H., Chandler, C.J., Ross, K., Wolfe, B.M., Baily, L. and Cerda, J.J. 1986. Clinical studies of intestinal folate conjugases. J. Lab. Clin. Med. 107:228-232.

Hansen, H. and Rybo, G. 1967. Folic acid dosage in profylactic treatment during pregnancy. Acta Obstet. Gynecol. Scand. 46 (Suppl. 7): 107-112.

Herbert, V. 1962a. Minimal daily adult folate requirement. Arch. Intern. Med. 110:649-652.

Herbert, V. 1962b. Experimental nutritional folate deficiency in man. Trans. Assoc. Am. Physicians 75:307-320.

Herbert, V. 1968. Nutritional requirements for vitamin B_{12} and folic acid. Am. J. Clin. Nutr. 21:743-752.

Herbert, V. 1977. Folic acid requirements in adults (including pregnant and lactating females) and Summary of the workshop. *In* Folic acid: biochemistry and physiology in relation to the human nutrition requirement. Food and Nutrition Board, National Research Council, National Academy of Sciences, Washington, D.C. pp. 247-255, 277-293.

Herbert, V. 1981. Nutritional anaemias of childhood — folate, B_{12}: the megaloblastic anemias. *In* Textbook of pediatric nutrition. Suskind, R.M., ed. Raven Press, New York, pp. 133-144.

Herbert, V. 1985. Biology of disease: megaloblastic anemias. Lab. Invest. 52:3-19.

Herbert, V. 1986. Folate status and folate requirements. *In* Proceedings of the XIII International Congress of Nutrition. Taylor, T.G. and Jenkins, N.K., eds. John Libbey, London, pp. 443-447.

Herbert, V. 1987a. Recommended dietary intakes (RDI) of folate in humans. Am. J. Clin. Nutr. 45:661-670.

Herbert, V. 1987b. Making sense of laboratory tests of folate status: folate requirements to sustain normality. Am. J. Hematol. 26:199-207.

Herbert, V. and Colman, N. 1979. Hematological aspects of folate deficiency. *In* Folic acid in neurology, psychiatry, and internal medicine. Botez, M.I. and Reynolds, E.H., eds. Raven Press, New York, pp. 63-74.

Herbert, V., Drivas, G., Manusselis, C., Mackler, B., Eng, J. and Schwartz, E. 1984. Are colon bacteria a major source of cobalamin analogues in human tissues? Twenty-four-hour human stool contains only about 5 µg of cobalamin but about 100 µg of apparent analogue (and 200 µg of folate). Trans. Assoc. Am. Physicians 97:161-171.

Hoffbrand, A.V. and Peters, T.J. 1969. The subcellular localization of pteroyl polyglutamate hydrolase and folate in guinea pig intestinal mucosa. Biochim. Biophys. Acta 192:479-485.

Hoppner, K. and Lampi, B. 1980. Folate levels in human livers from autopsies in Canada. Am. J. Clin. Nutr. 33:862-864.

Iyengar, L. and Rajalakshmi, K. 1975. Effect of folic acid supplement on birth weights of infants. Am. J. Obstet. Gynecol. 122:332-336.

Laurence, K.M., James, N., Miller, M.H., Tennant, G.B. and Campbell, H. 1981. Double-blind randomized controlled trial of folate treatment before conception to prevent recurrence of neural-tube defects. Br. Med. J. 282:1509-1511.

Lawrence, C. and Klipstein, F.A. 1967. Megaloblastic anemia of pregnancy in New York City. Ann. Intern. Med. 66:25-34.

Luhby, A.L. and Cooperman, J.M. 1964. Folic acid deficiency in man and its interrelationship with vitamin B_{12} metabolism. Adv. Metab. Disord. 1:263-334.

Luhby, A.L., Feldman, R., Gordon, M. and Cooperman, J.M. 1967. Folic acid deficiency in infants of mothers with folate deficiency during pregnancy. Am. J. Clin. Nutr. 20:362.

Matoth, Y., Pinkas, A. and Sroka, C. 1965. Studies on folic acid in infancy. III. Folates in breast fed infants and their mothers. Am. J. Clin. Nutr. 16:356-359.

Milne, D.B., Johnson, L.K., Mahalko, J.R. and Sandstead, H.H. 1983. Folate status of adult males living in a metabolic unit: possible relationships with iron nutriture. Am. J. Clin. Nutr. 37:768-773.

O'Broin, J.D., Temperley, I.J., Brown, J.P., and Scott, J.M. 1975. Nutritional stability of various naturally occurring monoglutamate derivatives of folic acid. Am. J. Clin. Nutr. 28:438-444.

Poh Tan, S., Wenlock, R.W. and Buss, D.H. 1984. Folic acid content of the diet in various types of British Household. Human Nutr.: Appl. Nutr. 38A:17-22.

Reisenauer, A.M., Krumdieck, C.L. and Halsted, C.H. 1977. Folate conjugase: two separate activities in human jejunum. Science 198:196-197.

Rodriguez, M.S. 1978. A conspectus of research of folacin requirements of man. J. Nutr. 108:1983-2075.

Rolschau, J., Date, J. and Kristoffersen, K. 1979. Folic acid supplement and intrauterine growth. Acta Obstet. Gynecol. Scand. 58:343-346.

Rosenberg, I.H. 1981. Intestinal absorption of folate. *In* Physiology of the gastrointestinal tract. Vol. 2. Johnson, L.R., ed. Raven Press, New York, pp. 2:1221-1230.

Rosenberg, I.H., Bowman, B.B., Cooper, B.A., Halsted, C.H. and Lindenbaum, J. 1982. Folate nutrition in the elderly. Am. J. Clin. Nutr. 36:1060-1066.

Russell, R.M., Krasinski, S.D., Samloff, I.M., Jacob, R.A., Hartz, S.C. and Brovender, S.R. 1986. Folic acid malabsorption in atrophic gastritis: possible compensation by bacterial synthesis. Gastroenterology 91:1476-1482.

Sauberlich, H.E., Kretsch, M.J., Skala, J.H., Johnson, H.L. and Taylor, P.C. 1987. Folate requirement and metabolism in non-pregnant women. Am. J. Clin. Nutr. 46:1016-1028.

Scrimgeour, K.G. 1986. Biosynthesis of polyglutamates of folates. Biochem. Cell Biol. 64:667-674.

Senti, F.R. and Pilch, S.M., eds. 1984. Assessment of the folate nutritional status of the US population based on data collected in the second national health and nutrition examination survey, 1976-1980. Life Science Research Office. Federation of American Societies for Experimental Biology, Bethesda, Md.

Shane, B. and Stokstad, E.L.R. 1985. Vitamin B_{12}-folate interrelationships. Annu. Rev. Nutr. 5:115-141.

Shojania, A. and Gross, S. 1964. Folic acid deficiency and prematurity. J. Pediatr. 64:323-329.

Smithells, R.W., Nevin, N.C., Seller, M.J., Sheppard, S., Harris, R., Read, A.P., Fielding, D.W., Walker, S., Schorah, C.J. and Wild, J. 1983. Further experience of vitamin supplementation for prevention of neural tube defect recurrences. Lancet 1:1027-1031.

Sneath, P., Chanarin, I., Hodkinson, H.M., McPherson, C.K. and Reynolds, E.H. 1973. Folate status in a geriatric population and its relation to dementia. Age Ageing 2:177-182.

Steinberg, S.E. 1984. Mechanisms of folate homeostasis. Am. J. Physiol. 246(9):G319-324.

Steinberg, S.E., Fonda, S., Campbell, C.L. and Hillman, R.S. 1983. Cellular abnormalities of folate deficiency. Br. J. Haematol. 54:605-612.

Strelling, M.K., Blackledge, D.G. and Goodall, H.B. 1979. Diagnosis and management of folate deficiency in low birth weight infants. Arch. Dis. Child. 54:271-277.

Suter, P.M. and Russell, R.M. 1987. Vitamin requirements of the elderly. Am. J. Clin. Nutr. 45:501-512.

Tamura, T. and Stokstad, E.L.R. 1973. The availability of food folate in man. Br. J. Haematol. 25:513-532.

Tchernia, G., Blot, I., Rey, A., Kaltwasser, J.P., Zittoun, J. and Papiernik, E. 1982. Maternal folate status, birthweight and gestational age. Dev. Pharmacol. Ther. 4 (Suppl. 1): 58-65.

U.S. Department of Agriculture. 1976. Composition of foods. Dairy and egg products. Raw, processed, prepared. Agriculture Handbook No. 8-1. Agriculture Research Service, Washington, D.C.

U.S. National Research Council. 1977. Folic acid: biochemistry and physiology in relation to the human nutrition requirement. Proceedings of a workshop on human folate requirements, June 2-3, 1975. Food and Nutrition Board, National Academy of Sciences, Washington, D.C.

Wang, T., Reisenauer, A.M. and Halsted, C.H. 1985. Comparisons of folate conjugase activities in human, pig, monkey and rat intestine (abst.). Clin. Research 33:40A.

Waslien, C.I. 1977. Folacin requirements of infants. *In* Folic acid: biochemistry and physiology in relation to the human nutrition requirement. Food and Nutrition Board, National Research Council, National Academy of Sciences, Washington, D.C., pp. 232-246.

Weir, D.G., McGing, P.G. and Scott, J.M. 1985. Folate metabolism, the enterohepatic circulation and alcohol. Biochem. Pharmacol. 34:1-7.

WHO. 1968. Nutritional anaemias. Report of a WHO Scientific Group. W.H.O. Tech. Rep. Ser. 405:1-37.

Wu, A.I., Chanarin, I., Slavin, G. and Levi, A.J. 1975. Folate deficiency in the alcoholic — its relationship to clinical and haematological abnormalities, liver disease, and folate stores. Br. J. Haematol. 29:469-478.

Zalusky, R. and Herbert, V. 1961. Megaloblastic anemia in scurvy with response to 50 microgm. of folic acid daily. N. Engl. J. Med. 265:1033-1038.

Vitamin B_{12}

Cobalamins are characterized by a corrin ring with a central cobalt atom, to which is attached the nucleotide 5,6-dimethylbenzimidazole. The term vitamin B_{12} covers those cobalamin compounds which can be converted in man to methyl- or 5′-deoxyadenosyl cobalamin. By convention, the reference compound is cyanocobalamin (relative molecular mass 1357).

A number of vitamin B_{12}-dependent reactions are known in the intermediary metabolism of bacteria, but only two have been identified with certainty in man: methylcobalamin acts as coenzyme with methionine synthase (Sauer et al. 1973; Taylor 1982) and 5′-deoxyadenosyl cobalamin acts as coenzyme with methylmalonyl CoA mutase (Contreras and Giorgio 1972). The function of the latter as coenzyme for L-leucine-2,3-aminomutase remains unconfirmed (Poston 1977).

Deficiency of vitamin B_{12} in man is manifested by changes in many bodily functions, the most clinically important ones being megaloblastic anemia and neurological disorders.

Chemically defined cyanocobalamin has been synthesized and is relatively simple to quantitate (United States Pharmacopeia 1985). Quantitation of cobalamin in food and other biological samples is more difficult. The vitamin B_{12} content of these is based on microbiological or radioisotopic dilution assays which respond differently to different forms of the vitamin and other compounds. There are also differences in extraction procedures which may incompletely release the vitamin from its bound form, or may chemically alter the molecule (Nexo and Olesen 1982; Pratt and Woldring 1982; Gimsing and Nexo 1983).

In man, the majority of vitamin B_{12} is in the liver, which may contain up to 80% of the total in the body (Cooperman 1972). At birth the full term infant has 25-30 µg (18-22 nmol) of the vitamin in the liver (Ross and Mollin 1957), or a total body content of about 30-40 µg (22-30 nmol) (Grasbeck *et al.* 1958; Adams *et al.* 1970). As the individual grows, the vitamin is accumulated so that the total vitamin B_{12} content of the body, in omnivorous adults, has been estimated by several methods to be in the range of 2-5 mg (1500-3700 nmol) (Grasbeck *et al.* 1958; Adams *et al.* 1970). In vegetarians, the body content of vitamin B_{12} is much lower and is probably similar to that of partially treated subjects with vitamin B_{12} malabsorption. In a group of patients with pernicious anemia in remission, who were hematologically normal and who had serum vitamin B_{12} concentrations greater than 130 pg/mL (96 pM) but below 200 pg/mL (150 pM), the concentration of vitamin B_{12} in liver averaged 0.38 µg/g (280 nmol/kg) and total body content was estimated at 525 µg (390 nmol) (Anderson 1965). In another group of patients with pernicious anemia in whom peripheral blood and bone marrow showed morphological evidence of mild deficiency of vitamin B_{12}, the serum vitamin B_{12} concentrations were between 80 and 130 pg/mL (60-96 pM), liver vitamin B_{12} concentration averaged 0.16 µg/g (120 nmol/kg), and total body content was estimated at 250 µg (180 nmol).

Vitamin B_{12} is excreted into the bile (Grasbeck *et al.* 1958; Chanarin 1979) bound to haptocorrin (R binder, transcobalamin 0, I or III). In the normal subject, the majority of this vitamin B_{12} is reabsorbed. In subjects with pernicious anemia, or those with other defects of vitamin B_{12} absorption, it is likely that reabsorption of biliary cobalamin is decreased. In presumably well-nourished Americans, the excretion of vitamin B_{12} in bile averaged 0.45 µg (0.33 nmol) per 700 mL (average 24-hour volume of bile) or 0.01% of the presumed total body content. If biliary excretion decreases as body content of vitamin B_{12} decreases, in individuals with a total body content of 500 µg (370 nmol) there would be an extra daily loss of 0.05 µg (.037 nmol).

The majority of body vitamin B_{12} (more than 99%) can be considered as forming a single, rapidly equilibrating pool (Reizenstein *et al.* 1966; Adams *et al.* 1968). Loss from this pool is via the feces, urine, and skin. Loss occurs in an exponential fashion at a rate of 0.05% to 0.2% of the pool per day, irrespective of pool size.

The sole source of vitamin B_{12} in nature is synthesis by bacteria, fungi and algae. Cereals, vegetables and fruits do not contain measurable amounts of cobalamin unless contaminated by microorganisms. All higher animals require vitamin B_{12} and store it in their tissues, which, in turn, become the chief dietary sources for man in the form of meat, liver, fish, eggs, milk, and milk products, etc. (Herbert and Colman 1988).

Vitamin B_{12} is ingested from animal products and released from its protein binders by cooking and proteolysis. It usually binds to salivary haptocorrin (R binder) in the mouth and stomach, enters the gut where the haptocorrin is digested by trypsin and the vitamin binds to the gastric intrinsic factor (IF), which is manufactured and stored in gastric parietal cells. The complex of intrinsic factor and vitamin B_{12} (IF-B_{12} complex) binds to specific receptors on the ileal brush border, the vitamin B_{12} is transferred to transcobalamin II (TC2) synthesized in the gut wall, and this complex slowly enters the portal venous plasma (Seetharam and Alpers 1982).

When a physiological dose of vitamin B_{12} is given by mouth, normal subjects absorb a mean of 72% of 0.5 μg (0.37 nmol), and 56% of 1 μg (0.74 nmol). The absolute amount absorbed is dependent on intrinsic factor and intestinal receptor number, but the maximum absorption from a single bolus is about 6 μg (4.44 nmol) (Baker and Mollin 1955). When two doses of cyanocobalamin labelled with different isotopes were administered five hours apart, the absorption of both doses was similar (Heyssel *et al.* 1966), indicating that absorption from three daily meals would not be affected by vitamin B_{12} fed at a previous meal.

The complex of transcobalamin II and vitamin B_{12} (TC2-B_{12}) binds to receptors on cell membranes, is incorporated into lysosomes where the TC2 is digested, and the vitamin B_{12} enters the cytoplasm of the cell. Intracellular cobalamin (Cob (III)alamin) appears to be reduced to cobalamin containing divalent cobalt (Cob(II)alamin), and either enters the mitochondria to form 5′-deoxyadenosyl cobalamin, or binds to cytoplasmic methionine synthase to form methylcobalamin (Cooper and Rosenblatt 1987).

As indicated, vitamin B_{12} is found only in animals and is absent from plants. Strict vegetarians are thus deprived of a source of the vitamin. Vegetarian animals obtain dietary vitamin by direct or indirect coprophagy. Vegetarian monkeys and bats develop deficiency of vitamin B_{12} when fed diets which are scrupulously cleansed of fecal or insect contamination.

Physiological requirements may be estimated from the following considerations:

Estimated Dietary Intake in Replete and Deficient Populations

Dietary intake of vitamin B_{12} varies depending on the animal content of the diet, ranging from 2.7 to 31.6 μg/day (2-23 nmol) (Chung *et al.* 1961) in the USA, estimated to be 4-7 μg/day in most industrialized nations, and averaging less than 0.5 μg/day in Bangladesh, India, and some subgroups in Africa (FAO/WHO 1988). The intake by vegetarians ranges from 0.25 to 0.5 μg/day depending on the strictness of the vegetarianism (Armstrong *et al.* 1974).

The effects of cooking on vitamin B_{12} are complex, since it increases bioavailability by denaturing binding proteins, but may destroy some of the vitamin (Banerjee and Chatterjea 1963; Heyssel *et al.* 1966). Under most cooking conditions, however, 90% of the vitamin B_{12} survives cooking.

The vitamin B_{12} content of breast milk parallels the maternal serum concentration, and varies from about 0.4 μg (0.29 nmol) per litre in mothers ingesting a mixed diet to about 0.05 μg (0.037 nmol) per litre in vegetarian mothers (Baker *et al.* 1962). Cow's milk contains more vitamin B_{12} than does human milk, average 6 μg (4.4 nmol) per litre. Boiling milk reduces the vitamin B_{12} content by about 30%, and drying results in loss of up to 90% of the vitamin B_{12} (Chapman *et al.* 1957).

In two studies (Armstrong *et al.* 1974; Abdulla *et al.* 1981) of vegetarians, mean dietary intake of vitamin B_{12} among 431 subjects was 0.26 ± 0.23 μg/day, and ranged from 0.3 to 0.4 μg/day in six subjects. Serum vitamin B_{12} levels were in the deficient range in only 21 of the former group, none of whom developed other manifestations of vitamin B_{12} deficiency.

Infants of vegetarian mothers who developed nutritional megaloblastic anemia while receiving 0.05 μg (0.037 nmol) or less of vitamin B_{12} in the breast milk recovered when their intake was increased to 0.12-0.15 μg (0.088-0.11 nmol) per day (Srikantia and Reddy 1967).

Quantities of Vitamin B_{12} Required to Correct Clinical Deficiency

Several studies have demonstrated that in patients with megaloblastic anemia, the hemopoietic response to daily injections of 0.1 μg (0.074 nmol) or 0.25 μg (0.18 nmol) of cyanocobalamin was inadequate, but that optimal response was observed to injections of greater quantities (0.5 to 2 μg (0.37-1.44 nmol) per day) (Darby *et al.* 1958; Adams *et al.* 1968; Baker and Mathan 1981). These studies demonstrate that to correct deficiency requires between 0.5 and 1 μg of absorbed vitamin B_{12} daily. A small number of reports have described responses to oral therapy in patients with deficiency of vitamin B_{12} on a nutritional basis. In these, optimal response usually (but not always) required more than 0.5 μg (0.37 nmol) of vitamin B_{12} per day.

Calculations of Daily Turnover of Vitamin B_{12}

If the body content of normal subjects is 5 mg (3700 nmol) (Anderson 1965), and loss occurs exponentially at a rate of 0.05 to 0.2% per day, then 2.5 to 10 μg (1.8 to 7.4 nmol) will be required daily to maintain this level of sufficiency. No clinical manifestations of deficiency can be found in subjects with stores estimated as 500 μg (370 nmol). To maintain this level of body store, which is about twice that estimated in subjects with mild clinical deficiency of vitamin B_{12}, would require 0.25 to 1 μg (0.18-0.74 nmol) per day.

It is apparent that normal stores of vitamin B_{12} are maintained by ingesting 3 μg (0.74 nmol) per day, and that clinical manifestations of deficiency apparently are prevented by daily intake of more than 0.5 μg (0.37 nmol). Whether prolonged limitation of intake to the smaller level would eventually result in clinical illness is unknown. Many residents of India, Pakistan, parts of Africa and Latin America, and many vegetarians in other countries appear to have chronic intakes of vitamin B_{12} in this range, but the impact of supplements of vitamin B_{12} on their health has not been adequately studied.

As indicated, some infants receiving 0.05 µg (0.037 nmol) of vitamin B_{12} daily in breast milk have developed megaloblastic anemia. This was corrected when more than 0.1 µg (0.074 nmol) of vitamin B_{12} per day was ingested.

During the last two trimesters of pregnancy, the needs of the fetus drain an average of 0.1 to 0.2 µg (0.074-0.15 nmol) per day from the mother (Roberts *et al.* 1973). Maternal vitamin requirement is consequently increased by this quantity during pregnancy and during lactation by the quantity of vitamin lost into the milk (0.14 µg or 0.1 nmol per day) (Collins *et al.* 1951).

Recommendations

Intake should not be permitted to fall below the following values:

Normal Adults: 1 µg per day of vitamin B_{12}.

Pregnancy: 1.2 µg (0.89 nmol) per day

Lactation: 1.2 µg (0.89 nmol) per day

Infants: 0.1 µg (0.074 nmol) per day in breast milk or added to cow's milk.

Children: graded intake with body weight. Intake should approximate 0.04 µg (0.029 nmol) per kg of body weight to a maximum of 1 µg.

References

Abdulla, M., Andersson, I., Asp, N-G., Berthelsen, K., Birkhed, D., Dencker, I., Johannsson, C-G., Jagerstad, M., Kolar, K., Nair, B.M., Nilsson-Ehle, P., Norden, A., Rassner, S., Akesson, B. and Ockerman, P-R. 1981. Nutrient intake and health status of vegans. Chemical analyses of diets using the duplicate portion sampling technique. Am. J. Clin. Nutr. 34:2464-2477.

Adams, J.F., Hume, R., Kennedy, E.H., Pirrie, T.G., Whitelaw, J.M. and White, A.M. 1968. Metabolic responses to low doses of cyanocobalamin in patients with megaloblastic anaemia. Br. J. Nutr. 22:575-582.

Adams, J.F., Tankel, H.I. and MacEwan, F. 1970. Estimation of the total body vitamin B_{12} in the live subject. Clin. Sci. 39:107-113.

Anderson, B.B. 1965. Investigations into the Euglena method of assay of vitamin B_{12}: the results obtained in human serum and liver using an improved method of assay. Ph.D. Thesis, University of London.

Armstrong, B.K., Davis, R.E., Nicol, D.J., Van Merwyk, A.J. and Larwood, C.J. 1974. Hematological vitamin B_{12} and folate studies on Seventh Day Adventist vegetarians. Am. J. Clin. Nutr. 27:712-718.

Baker, S.J. and Mollin, D.L. 1955. The relationship between intrinsic factor and the intestinal absorption of vitamin B_{12}. Br. J. Haematol. 1:46-51.

Baker, S.J. and Mathan, V.I. 1981. Evidence regarding the minimal daily requirement of dietary vitamin B_{12}. Am. J. Clin. Nutr. 34:2423-2433.

Baker, S.J., Jacob, E., Rajan, K.T. and Swaminathan, S.P. 1962. Vitamin B_{12} deficiency in pregnancy and the puerperium. Br. Med. J. 1:1658-1661.

Banerjee, D.K. and Chatterjea, J.B. 1963. Vitamin B_{12} content of some articles of Indian diets and effect of cooking on it. Br. J. Nutr. 17:385-389.

Chanarin, I. 1979. The megaloblastic anaemias. 2nd ed. Blackwell Scientific Publications, Oxford.

Chapman, H.R., Ford, J.E., Kon, S.K., Thompson, S.Y., Rowland, S.J., Crossley, E.L. and Rothwell, J. 1957. Further studies of the effect of processing on some vitamins of the B complex in milk. J. Dairy Res. 24:191-197.

Chung, A.S.M., Pearson, W.N., Darby, W.J., Miller, O.N. and Goldsmith, G.A. 1961. Folic acid, vitamin B_6, pantothenic acid and vitamin B_{12} in human dietaries. Am. J. Clin. Nutr. 9:573-582.

Collins, R.A., Harper, A.E., Schreiber, M. and Elvehjem, C.A. 1951. The folic acid and vitamin B_{12} content of the milk of various species. J. Nutr. 43:313-321.

Contreras, E. and Giorgio, A.J. 1972. Leukocyte methylmalonyl-CoA mutase. I. Vitamin B_{12} deficiency. Am. J. Clin. Nutr. 25:695-702.

Cooper, B.A. and Rosenblatt, D.S. 1987. Inherited defects of vitamin B_{12} metabolism. Annu. Rev. Nutr. 7:291-320.

Cooperman, J.M. 1972. Distribution of radioactive and non-radioactive vitamin B_{12} in normal and malignant tissues of an infant with neuroblastoma. Cancer Res. 32:167-172.

Darby, W.J., Bridgforth, E.B., Le Brocquy, J., Clark, S.L., De Oliviera, J.D., Kevany, J., McGanity, W.J. and Perez, C. 1958. Vitamin B_{12} requirement of adult man. Am. J. Med. 25:726-732.

FAO/WHO 1988. Report of a joint FAO/WHO expert consultation. Requirements of vitamin A, iron, folate and vitamin B_{12}. FAO Food and Nutrition Series, no. 23.

Gimsing, P. and Nexo, E. 1983. The forms of cobalamin in biological materials. Methods Hematol. 10:7-30.

Grasbeck, R., Nyberg, W. and Reizenstein, P. 1958. Biliary and fecal vitamin B_{12} excretion in man. An isotope study. Proc. Soc. Exp. Biol. Med. 97:780-784.

Herbert, V.D. and Colman, N. 1988. Folic acid and vitamin B_{12}. *In* Modern nutrition in health and disease. 7th ed. Shils, M.E. and Young, V.R., eds. Lea & Febiger, Philadelphia, pp. 388-416.

Heyssel, R.M., Bozian, R.C., Darby, W.J. and Bell, M.C. 1966. Vitamin B_{12} turnover in man. The assimilation of vitamin B_{12} from natural foodstuff by man and estimates of minimal daily requirements. Am. J. Clin. Nutr. 18:176-184.

Nexo, E. and Olesen, H. 1982. Quantitation of cobalamins in human serum. *In* B_{12}: biochemistry and medicine. Vol. 2. Dolphin, D., ed. Wiley, New York, pp. 87-104.

Poston, J.M. 1977. Leucine 2,3-aminomutase; a cobalamin-dependent enzyme present in bean seedlings. Science 195:301-302.

Pratt, J.J. and Woldring, M.G. 1982. Radioassay of vitamin B_{12} and other corrinoids. Methods Enzymol. 84:369-406.

Reizenstein, P.G., Ek, G. and Matthews, C.M.E. 1966. Vitamin B_{12} kinetics in man. Implications on total body B_{12} determinations, human requirements, and normal and pathological cellular B_{12} uptake. Phys. Med. Biol. 11:295-306.

Roberts, P.D., James, H., Petrie, A., Morgan, J.O. and Hoffbrand, A.V. 1973. Vitamin B_{12} status in pregnancy among immigrants to Britain. Br. Med. J. 3:67-72.

Ross, G.I.M. and Mollin, D.L. 1957. Vitamin B_{12} in tissues in pernicious anaemia and other conditions. *In* Vitamin B_{12} and intrinsic factor. 1. Europäisches symposium. Heinrich, H.C., ed. Enke, Stuttgart, pp. 437-443.

Sauer, H., Wilms, K., Wilmanns, W. and Jaenicke, L. 1973. Die aktivitat der methionin-synthetase (5-methyl-5,6,7,8-tetrahydrofolsaure: homocystein methyltransferase) als proliferationsparameter in wachsenden zellen. [(GE) activity of methionine synthetase (5-methyl-5,6,7,8)-tetrahydrofolate-homocysteine methyltransferase as an indicator for proliferation tendency of a cell population]. Acta Haematol. 49:200-210.

Seetharam, B. and Alpers, D.H. 1982. Absorption and transport of cobalamin (vitamin B_{12}). Annu. Rev. Nutr. 2:343-369.

Srikantia, S.G. and Reddy, V. 1967. Megaloblastic anaemia of infancy and vitamin B_{12}. Br. J. Haematol. 13:949-953.

Taylor, R.T. 1982. B_{12}-dependent methionine biosynthesis. *In* Biochemistry and medicine. Vol. 2. Dolphin D., ed. Wiley, New York, pp. 307-355.

United States Pharmacopeia. 1985. 21st ed. 3.7.1. Cobalamin radiotracer assay. United States Pharmacopeial Convention, Rockville, MD, pp. 1197-1198.

Biotin

Biotin performs its principal metabolic role as the prosthetic group of several carboxylases, propionyl CoA carboxylase, pyruvate carboxylase, beta methylcrotonyl CoA carboxylase and acetyl CoA carboxylase. Nonprosthetic group functions for biotin in the synthesis of growth factors have also been reported (Dakshinamurti and Chauhan In Press).

Ingested biotin is rapidly absorbed from the gastrointestinal tract, and excess is excreted in the urine. Mammals cannot degrade the ring system of biotin, and urinary excretion of the vitamin is essentially in the form of biotin with minor amounts of its metabolites, bisnorbiotin and biotin sulphoxide. The absorption of biotin from the intestinal tract is saturable at physiological concentrations of less than 40 nM. At higher concentrations absorption occurs by passive diffusion. Normal levels of biotin in plasma are in the range of 330-722 ng/L (Sweetman and Nyhan 1986).

Biotin is found in low concentrations in food of both animal and plant origin and in yeast; liver and dairy products are particularly good sources. Usual intakes are sufficient to satisfy requirement, and biotin deficiency has been observed only under special circumstances. Deficiency has been induced by raw eggs which contain the biotin-binding protein, avidin (Sydenstricker *et al.* 1942). The symptoms of deficiency, which included glossitis, anorexia dermatosis, nausea, somnolence, loss of taste and panic, disappeared following daily dosage with 150 µg of biotin.

Biotin deficiency may also accompany chronic hemodialysis due to loss of free biotin in the dialysate (Yatzidis *et al.* 1981). Treatment has consisted of 10 mg biotin per day for three months. Anticonvulsant drugs (phenytoin, primidone, phenobarbital and carbamazepine) can also induce biotin deficiency (Krause *et al.* 1982).

Toxicity due to biotin has not been reported in man despite administration of large doses for periods of up to six months (Miller and Hayes 1982).

While no definite estimate of biotin requirement can yet be made, an intake of 1.5 µg/kg of body weight has been suggested for all age groups. The resulting intake for adults would be about 100 µg which is in the upper range of usual intakes (Bonjour 1977; Williams 1942). This amount easily meets the estimated daily urinary loss of the vitamin (Bonjour 1977). Part of the biotin requirements are provided by intestinal bacteria synthesis, with biotinidase cleavage, for human use. Biotin is recycled and thus conserved in subjects with normal biotinidase activity (Bonjour 1985). Human milk contains 7-13 µg per litre (Sweetman and Nyhan 1986) so that an infant consuming an average amount of breast milk would receive 5-10 µg/day. There is no indication that this amount is inadequate.

References

Bonjour, J.P. 1977. Biotin in man's nutrition and therapy — a review. Int. J. Vitam. Nutr. Res. 47:107-118.

Bonjour, J.P. 1985. Biotin in human nutrition. Ann. N.Y. Acad. Sci. 447:97-104.

Dakshinamurti, K. and Chauhan, J. In Press. Biotin. Vitam. Horm. (N.Y.)

Krause, K.H., Berlit, P. and Bonjour, J.P. 1982. Impaired biotin status in anticonvulsant therapy. Ann. Neurol. 12:485-486.

Miller, D.R. and Hayes, K.C. 1982. Vitamin excess and toxicity. *In* Nutritional toxicity. Vol. 1. Hathcock, J.N., ed. Academic Press, New York, pp. 81-133.

Sweetman, L. and Nyhan, W.L. 1986. Inheritable biotin-treatable disorders and associated phenomena. Ann. Rev. Nutr. 6:317-343.

Sydenstricker, V.P., Singal, S.A., Briggs, A.P., DeVaughn, N.M. and Isbell, H. 1942. Observation on the "egg white injury" in man. J. Am. Med. Assoc. 118:1199-1200.

Williams, R.J. 1942. The approximate vitamin requirements of human beings. J. Am. Med. Assoc. 119:1-3.

Yatzidis, H., Koutsicos, D., Alaveras, A.G., Papastephanidis, C. and Frangos-Plemenos, M. 1981. Biotin for neurologic disorders of uremia. N. Engl. J. Med. 305:764.

Pantothenic Acid

Pantothenic acid is a viscous oil which is produced commercially as the white, crystalline salt D(+)-calcium pantothenate. It occurs mainly in the form of the thioester 4'- phosphopantotheine, a component of two coenzymes: coenzyme A and acyl carrier protein. Coenzyme A has a central role in metabolism as a cofactor for enzymes involved in the oxidation of fatty acids, and in the utilization of acetate derived from glucose, amino acid and fatty acid catabolism for energy production. It is also required for the utilization of acetate in the synthesis of cholesterol, steroid hormones and numerous other compounds. As a component of acyl carrier protein of the fatty acid synthase complex, 4'-phosphopantotheine functions in the assembly of acetate units into longer chain fatty acids.

Distribution

All foods of plant and animal origin contain pantothenic acid, but it is especially high in organ meats, whole grain cereals, yeast and legumes. A double-enzyme treatment with intestinal phosphatase and pigeon liver extract has been widely used for the release of pantothenic acid from its bound forms, and analytical data obtained prior to the introduction of this treatment are suspect. Liver extract has, in some recent analyses, been replaced by purified pantotheinase because it may contain endogenous pantothenate. Values for the pantothenic acid content of foods obtained using this procedure have been assembled by Orr (1969), and by Paul and Southgate (1978), and are summarized in U.S.D.A. Handbook No. 8 (1976). The pantothenic acid content of 75 processed and cooked foods has been reported by Walsh *et al.* (1980). Processing causes moderate losses of pantothenic acid in food products made from refined grains, fruit, extended meats and fish.

Dietary Intake

A composite diet formulated on the basis of the apparent per capita consumption of foods in Canada in 1978 provided 6.1 mg of pantothenic acid per day (Hoppner *et al.* 1978). This value is similar to an estimate of 5.8 mg per day derived from food consumption data for the average U.S. diet (Tarr *et al.* 1981). Calculated pantothenic acid intake by a sample of U.S. women consuming self-selected diets averaged 6.7 mg per day. The estimated average intake of a subsample of low-income women was 4-5 mg per day (Johnson and Nitzke 1975). Pantothenate intakes are subject to marked daily fluctuations. Day to day intakes ranging from 1.1 to 7.2 mg per day have been reported in U.S. girls (Cohenour and Calloway 1972), 1.3 to 16.9 mg in adults (mean 5.4 mg), and 4.0-7.9 mg (mean 5.6 mg) in adolescents (Kathman and Kies 1984). Four-day dietary records on 63 male and female U.S. adolescents indicated that their pantothenic acid intakes ranged from 1.7 to 12.7 mg per day (Eissenstat *et al.* 1986). The average intake was 4.1 mg per day in females and 6.2 mg per day in males. Whole blood levels of pantothenate (412 ± 103 and 345 ± 114 ng/mL, respectively) (Mean $\pm$ SD) were similar to those found by other investigators, and indicate that blood levels are relatively uniform despite large variations in daily intake. Serum contains mainly free pantothenic acid, which is a poor indicator of chronic intake (Eissenstat *et al.* 1986). The pantothenate intake of a sample of institutionalized elderly U.S. subjects was similar to that of free-living elderly (5.9 mg/day or 2.9 mg/1000 kcal) (Srinivasan *et al.* 1981). The availability of pantothenic acid in an average U.S. mixed diet, assessed by comparing its urinary excretion by healthy male volunteers consuming the vitamin in food with that of controls consuming a similar amount in purified form, ranged from 40% to 61% with a mean of 50% (Tarr *et al.* 1981).

Deficiency Symptoms

Pantothenic acid deficiency has not been clearly identified in humans consuming a diet of natural foodstuffs. This is attributable to the widespread distribution of the vitamin in foods. Young, male volunteers given a semi-purified diet lacking pantothenic acid by stomach tube developed deficiency symptoms after about six weeks that included malaise, vomiting, abdominal distress, burning cramps progressing to tenderness in the heels, fatigue, headache, irritability and tremors (Hodges *et al.* 1958). There was also a loss of eosinopenic response to ACTH, impaired antibody production against tetanus, and increased sensitivity to insulin. These symptoms were aggravated in subjects receiving the antagonist omega-methyl pantothenic acid.

Nutritional Status

There is no satisfactory index of pantothenate status. Several studies have been conducted on the relationship between the intake of pantothenic acid and its urinary excretion. Girls 7-9 years of age consuming 2.8-5.0 mg of pantothenic acid per day excreted 1.3-2.9 mg in the urine (Pace *et al.* 1961). The excretion in adolescents averaged 3.74 mg/g creatinine at an average intake of 5.5 mg/day (Kathman and Kies 1984). Adolescent males excreted 3.32 mg and females 4.49 mg/g creatinine/day (Eissenstat *et al.* 1986). Pantothenate excretion in elderly institutionalized and free-living subjects was 7.5 and 5.9 mg/g creatinine, respectively (Srinivasan *et al.* 1981). While these studies reveal the expected correlation between pantothenic acid intake and excretion, they provide little indication of the amount required for adequacy.

Blood serum contains free pantothenic acid, whereas erythrocytes contain primarily bound forms. Serum levels are poorly correlated with whole blood levels. Wide variations in both serum and whole blood levels have been reported (21-118 μg/dL and 20-390 μg/dL, respectively) (Fox 1984). In part, these variations reflect differences in procedures used to liberate the vitamin from its bound forms. The levels indicative of a deficiency are obscure. A sample of U.S. women in late pregnancy and early lactation was found to have a lower mean blood level than a control group of non-pregnant women (Song *et al.* 1985). This difference may reflect an increased requirement for the vitamin during this period or the increase in blood volume.

Toxicity

Large doses of pantothenic acid administrated orally are well tolerated by animals and humans (Miller and Hayes 1982). No symptoms of toxicity, except for occasional diarrhea, were observed in young men who consumed 10-20 g of calcium pantothenate per day for six weeks. The recommended levels of intake therefore pose no risk of toxicity.

Recommendation

In the absence of data on the pantothenic acid requirement, no recommended intake can be formulated on this basis. An intake of 2.3 mg/1000 kcal (2.7 mg/5000 kJ) or 5-7 mg/day appears to prevent signs of deficiency in adults. This level of intake is obtainable from all normal Canadian diets. The central role of pantothenic acid in energy metabolism indicates that the requirement is related to energy intake. Hence the same concentration in the diet is considered adequate to meet the needs of growing children, as well as the increased needs of pregnant and lactating women. From a lack of evidence of deficiency, it is concluded that the pantothenic acid content of the Canadian diet is adequate to meet the needs of all segments of the population.

Values for the pantothenic acid content of mature human milk range from 0.9 to 5.8 mg/L with a median of about 2.0 mg/L (Altman 1961). The intake of pantothenic acid by nursing infants, calculated on the basis of the median value (1.5 mg in 750 mL of milk) is similar, when expressed on an energy basis (2.3 mg/1000 kcal or 2.7 mg/5000 kJ) to the estimated intake of adults. Higher levels of pantothenic acid reported for cow's milk (3.5 mg/L) (Altman 1961) may reflect the synthesis of this vitamin by rumen bacteria. Pantothenic acid in milk is stable to pasteurization at neutral pH. The amount provided by the normal consumption of human or cow's milk appears to be adequate to meet the requirements of all infants.

Claims that pantothenic acid is effective in the prevention of greying hair, neuropathology, alopecia, salicylate toxicity and various other conditions have not been corroborated by experimental or clinical research.

References

Altman, P.L. 1961. Blood and other body fluids. Federation of American Societies for Experimental Biology, Washington, D.C., pp. 458-461.

Cohenour, S.H. and Calloway, D.H. 1972. Blood, urine and dietary pantothenic acid levels of pregnant teenagers. Am. J. Clin. Nutr. 25:512-517.

Eissenstat, B.R., Wyse, B.W. and Hansen, R.G. 1986. Pantothenic acid status of adolescents. Am. J. Clin. Nutr. 44:931-937.

Fox, H.M. 1984. Pantothenic acid. *In* Food Science. Vol. 13. Handbook of vitamins: nutritional, biochemical and clinical aspects. Machlin, L.J., ed. Marcel Dekker, New York, pp. 437-457.

Hodges, R.E., Ohlson, M.A. and Bean, W.B. 1958. Pantothenic acid deficiency in man. J. Clin. Invest. 37:1642-1657.

Hoppner, K., Lampi, B. and Smith, D.C. 1978. An appraisal of the daily intakes of vitamin B_{12}, pantothenic acid and biotin from a composite Canadian diet. Can. Inst. Food Sci. Technol. J. 11:71-74.

Johnson, N.E. and Nitzke, S. 1975. Nutritional adequacy of diets of a selected group of low-income women: identification of some related factors. Home Econ. Res. J. 3:241-248.

Kathman, J.V. and Kies, C. 1984. Pantothenic acid status of free-living adolescent and young adults. Nutr. Res. 4:245-250.

Miller, D.R. and Hayes, K.C. 1982. Vitamin excess and toxicity. F. Pantothenic acid. *In* Nutritional toxicology. Vol. I. Hathcock, J.N., ed. Academic Press, New York, pp. 111-112.

Orr, M.L. 1969. Pantothenic acid, vitamin B_6 and vitamin B_{12} in foods. Home Economics Research Report No. 36, United States Department of Agriculture, Washington, D.C.

Pace, J.K., Stier, L.B., Taylor, D.D. and Goodman, P.S. 1961. Metabolic patterns in pre-adolescent children. V. Intake and urinary excretion of pantothenic acid and of folic acid. J. Nutr. 74:345-351.

Paul, A.A. and Southgate, D.A.T. 1978. McCance and Widdowson's The composition of foods. 4th rev. ed. of MRC Special Report No. 297. Elsevier/North-Holland Biomedical, Amsterdam.

Song, W.O., Wyse, B.W. and Hansen, R.G. 1985. Pantothenic acid status of pregnant and lactating women. J. Am. Diet. Assoc. 85:192-198.

Srinivasan, V., Christensen, N., Wyse, B.W. and Hansen, R.G. 1981. Pantothenic acid nutritional status in the elderly — institutionalized and noninstitutionalized. Am. J. Clin. Nutr. 34:1736-1742.

Tarr, J.B., Tamura, T. and Stokstad, E.L.R. 1981. Availability of vitamin B_6 and pantothenate in an average American diet in man. Am. J. Clin. Nutr. 34:1328-1337.

United States Department of Agriculture. Human Nutrition Information Service. 1976. Composition of foods. Agriculture handbooks 8-1 to 8-16. U.S. Government Printing Office, Washington, D.C.

Walsh, J.H., Wyse, B.W. and Hansen, R.G. 1980. A comparison of microbiological and radioimmunoassay methods for the determination of pantothenic acid in foods. J. Food Biochem. 3:175-189.

Minerals

Calcium and Phosphorus

Calcium

The distribution of calcium in the body is marked by its concentration in the skeletal tissues, and its distribution in the Western diet by its concentration in dairy foods. Ninety-nine percent of the calcium in the body is located in the bones and teeth, and three-quarters of the calcium in the Canadian food supply is furnished by foods of dairy origin. The 1% of body calcium located in the soft tissues has a pervasive involvement in metabolic processes, including enzyme activation, nerve transmission, membrane transport, blood clotting, muscle contraction and hormone function. These functions are affected by the concentration of calcium in the serum, which is self-regulated within a narrow physiological range. Any substantial deviation from this range can have serious metabolic consequences. About half of the calcium in the serum is ionized and physiologically active.

Calcium Absorption

The amount of calcium absorbed by adults is a curvilinear function of intake, responding actively to intakes up to about 10 mg/kg of body weight per day but only moderately to higher intakes (Wilkinson 1976). Conversely, the percentage true absorption (intake minus fecal excretion corrected for calcium of endogenous origin expressed as a percent of intake) decreases rapidly up to 10 mg/kg per day, then slowly at greater intakes. At an intake of 15 mg/kg per day about 11 mg of calcium are excreted in the feces (2 mg of endogenous origin) and 4 mg in the urine. Approximately 7 mg/kg are absorbed, of which 3 mg represent reabsorbed digestive juice calcium (Wilkinson 1976). The true absorption of dietary calcium by adults at this intake is approximately 40%. The efficiency of calcium absorption is enhanced during growth, pregnancy and lactation and declines during aging.

Calcium Deficiency

Simple calcium deficiency is not a recognized clinical entity in human subjects. Although rickets and osteomalacia occur in animals fed diets deficient in calcium, phosphorus or vitamin D, in humans these conditions are associated only with vitamin D deficiency. Beyond weaning age, children and adults of various countries and food cultures subsist on diets differing markedly in calcium content. These differences in calcium intake, which are due mainly to the relative strengths of the dairy industry, have not been demonstrated to have any consequences for nutritional health.

Requirement of Adults

Defining the adult requirement for calcium, upon which a recommended nutrient intake is usually based, has proved to be one of the most difficult problems in the history of human nutrition. The main difficulty in defining the calcium requirement stems from a capacity to adapt to a range of calcium intakes. The mechanism of this adaptation involves hormonal regulation of calcium absorption from the intestine and excretion in the urine. A decrease in calcium intake results in a mild depression of serum calcium, which activates the synthesis of parathyroid hormone. This hormone stimulates the reabsorption of calcium from the renal tubules, thereby reducing its loss in the urine, and the renal synthesis of 1,25-dihydroxyvitamin D (calciferol), the hormonal form of vitamin D. This hormone activates expression of a gene in the nucleus of the epithelial cells of the intestine, which is coded for the synthesis of a protein necessary for the active absorption of calcium from the diet (Henry and Norman 1984). These appear to be the main events in a complex adaptive process which enables calcium needs to be met over a wide range of intakes. However, the limits of adaptation are poorly defined and vary among individuals (Malm 1958). Other hormones involved in calcium metabolism include estrogen, which has a homeostatic effect on bone, and enhances calcium absorption by a vitamin D-mediated process, and calcitonin, a hypocalcemic thyroid hormone which modulates the action of parathyroid hormone on bone and possibly other tissues.

Calcium and Osteoporosis

A study indicating that a relationship exists between calcium intake and bone loss after the menopause (Heaney *et al.* 1978) recently has created interest in the possible value of a high calcium intake in the prevention of osteoporosis, the primary bone disease of postmenopausal women. Linear extrapolation from data for calcium intake by a group of 41 postmenopausal women (mean intake 659 mg/day) indicated that calcium balance could be attained (i.e. postmenopausal bone loss prevented) at an intake of 1500 mg per day. However, several subsequent studies have led to the conclusion that neither dietary calcium intake nor calcium supplementation has a significant influence on the rate of change in bone mineral content in the perimenopausal period (Riggs *et al.* 1987). These findings, together with evidence that osteoporotic bone fractures are, if anything, less frequent among women living in countries with a food supply furnishing less calcium (Hegsted 1986), indicate that the Canadian diet is capable of meeting the calcium needs of postmenopausal women.

It cannot be assumed, however, that the low calcium intake of women living in countries with a cereal-based food economy (400-500 mg/day) is necessarily adequate for women consuming a Western diet. The oxidation of excess sulfur amino acids in the high-protein Western diet generates endogenous acid, the excretion of which results in an acidic urine. The efficiency of the parathyroid hormone-dependent renal reabsorption of calcium from the filtered urine decreases with increasing acidity. Unless this tendency toward an increased urinary loss of calcium is counteracted by other factors, it can result in a negative calcium balance (i.e. in bone loss) (Johnson *et al.* 1970).

Urinary calcium is also affected by the intake of phosphorus. Excess dietary phosphate produces a mild depression in serum calcium similar to that produced by a low calcium intake. The consequent rise in serum parathyroid hormone induces an analogous increase in mobilization of calcium from the skeleton, and renal reabsorption of calcium from the urine. However, there does not appear to be a compensating increase in the efficiency of calcium absorption such as occurs following a decrease in dietary calcium. The stimulus to bone resorption has been shown to result in bone loss in several species of animals, but human adults appear to be able to adapt (i.e. to maintain calcium balance) at phosphorus intakes within the normal range. This adaptation apparently involves an increase in the rate of bone formation, which compensates for the increase in bone resorption.

A strong correlation between the protein and phosphorus contents of foods means that diets high in one are likely to be high in the other. The calciuric effect of excess dietary protein, therefore, is counteracted, at least in part, by the parathyroid-mediated hypocalciuric effect of excess dietary phosphorus. Hence high protein diets apparently increase the phosphorus requirement for the maintenance of calcium homeostasis (Yuen *et al.* 1984).

Whether the counteracting effects of excess dietary protein and phosphorus on urinary calcium consistently result in bone homeostasis is unknown. Recent evidence that the increased parathyroid activity associated with a low intake of calcium has no effect on bone mineral content in perimenopausal women (Riggs *et al.* 1987) lends some assurance that the same is true of parathyroid stimulation caused by excess dietary phosphate. Nevertheless, it is noteworthy that a rapid rate of bone loss has been recorded in adults consuming a high protein, high phosphorus, low calcium diet (Mazess and Mather 1975). The modest intake of calcium recommended for adults by the World Health Organization (400-500 mg/day) (FAO/WHO Expert Group 1962) may not be adequate for adults consuming this type of diet.

Calcium and Blood Pressure

Several epidemiological surveys and experimental studies on humans and animals have provided evidence for an inverse relationship between calcium intake and blood pressure in adults (McCarron and Morris 1986). Research at the cellular level has yielded supportive evidence for a favourable effect of calcium on vascular smooth muscle function, and thereby the resistance of the peripheral vasculature. Although these interesting observations suggest a possible role of dietary calcium in the prevention of hypertension, the evidence is currently inadequate to be a factor in the recommended calcium intake.

Recommendations

Adults

Despite a preponderance of evidence indicating that postmenopausal bone loss is unaffected by calcium intake, the recommended intake for women beyond 50 years of age is maintained at parity with that of men (800 mg/day). This recommendation recognizes the decline in calcium absorption with aging, the likelihood of greater variance in the calcium requirement among the elderly, evidence for a marginal vitamin D status in some postmenopausal women, and the possibility that a liberal calcium intake may moderate bone loss in some instances.

The recommended intake can be met by consuming a balanced diet of ordinary foodstuffs including, if they are preferred, fermented dairy products. Food disappearance data indicate that in 1986 there were 857 mg of calcium per capita per day available for consumption in the Canadian food supply (Robbins 1986), and that an average of 1160 mg was available from the foods purchased, estimated from the Family Food Expenditure Survey (Canada. Agriculture Canada 1986). The higher figure for foods purchased was attributable mainly to calcium added to baked goods as baking powders and sodas, which was not included in the disappearance data. In 1982 the mean calcium intake of a sample of 100 middle class premenopausal women living in the Guelph area was estimated from three-day diet records to be 943 mg per day (Scythes *et al.* 1982). Similar records for Montreal women indicated average intakes of 775 mg per day at ages 20-39 years and 747 mg per day at 40-59 years. The values for men at corresponding ages were 939 mg and 909 mg (Mongeau E., personal communication). Calcium intake by low income elderly subjects living alone in Montreal, assessed from 24-h recall, averaged 676 mg for men (mean age 72.4 yr, N=49) and 576 mg for women (mean age 73.7 yr, N=137) (Delvin *et al.* 1988).

Children and Adolescents

The increments in recommended calcium intake during growth reflect increasing requirements for skeletal maintenance and accretion. The requirements of males and females are similar until the earlier pubertal growth spurt in girls temporarily raises their requirement above that of boys. (See Table 20). In recognition of this requirement and of evidence that skeleton mass at maturity, a major factor in predisposition to osteoporosis in later life, may be related to calcium intake during growth and development (Matkovic *et al.* 1979), the recommended calcium intake of girls 10-12 has been increased by 100 mg/day to a total of 1100 mg/day and that of girls 13-15 years by 200 mg/day to 1000 mg/day.

Infants

Breast milk satisfies the calcium needs of term infants up to six months of age, but contains insufficient calcium to sustain bone mineralization in preterm infants (Chance *et al.* 1977). Based on evidence that breast milk contains sufficient calcium for term infants, their recommended intake is the 250 mg of calcium per day, provided by an average daily milk production of 750 mL. However, to compensate for the hypocalcemic action of excess phosphate in cow's milk formula, a higher intake of calcium is recommended for formula-fed infants. For example, a typical formula containing 275 mg phosphorus per 750 mL should provide 375 mg calcium. A typical formula based on cow's milk protein contains about 1.3 and 2.6 times as much calcium and phosphorus, respectively, as breast milk. The amount of calcium retained by infants receiving formula and breast milk is similar (Chan *et al.* 1982).

Pregnancy and Lactation

An additional calcium intake of 500 mg/day is recommended.

Phosphorus

Like calcium, phosphorus is a major structural element of the bones and teeth, but 20% is present in major classes of macromolecules including proteins, nucleic acids and phospholipids. Phosphorylation reactions play a critical role in many synthetic and degradative processes. The high energy bonds in adenosine triphosphate and other phosphate compounds provide the energy necessary to drive most metabolic processes.

A natural association of phosphorus and protein in foods and the widespread use of phosphate additives render negligible the risk of phosphorus deficiency in persons consuming the Western diet. Food disappearance data indicate that in 1986 there were 1412 mg of phosphorus per person per day available for consumption by Canadians (Robbins 1986). This figure does not include phosphorus present as additives. The amount of phosphorus present in foods purchased, estimated from family food expenditure data, was 1596 mg per capita per day (Canada. Agriculture Canada 1986). A sample of premenopausal urban Ontario women surveyed in 1982 was estimated from three-day diet records to consume an average of 1398 mg of phosphorus per day (Scythes *et al.* 1982). A similar survey on Montreal women yielded estimates of 1168 mg for premenopausal women and 1154 for postmenopausal women (Mongeau E., personal communication). The Ontario subjects consumed more calcium as well as phosphorus.

During rapid growth, when calcium and phosphorus requirements are determined mainly by the needs for these elements in the formation of bone mineral, the requirement for calcium exceeds that for phosphorus. With skeletal maturation, the requirement for calcium decreases more rapidly on a body weight basis than that for phosphorus. However, there is an decrease in the requirement for both elements which eliminates, for practical purposes, the possibility of a phosphorus deficiency.

Recommendations

A typical output of 750 mL of mature breast milk contains 105 mg of phosphorus, which is enough to meet the requirement of the nursing infant. There is little information on the phosphorus requirement for growth or for maintenance, pregnancy and lactation in adults. Based on evidence that the requirement of adult animals is slightly in excess of that for calcium, and that the phosphorus requirement is increased by consumption of a high protein diet, phosphorus intakes of at least 1000 mg/day for men and 850 mg/day for women are recommended. Smaller increments in the intake of phosphorus than of calcium are recommended during pregnancy and lactation, because of the greater efficiency with which phosphorus is absorbed by adults (approximately 70% versus 40%) (Wilkinson 1976). The recommended amounts are readily available from all normal diets.

References

Canada. Agriculture Canada. 1986. Nutrient assessment program. Family food expenditure survey component. Ottawa (computer data base).

Chan, G.M., Roberts, C.C., Folland, D. and Jackson, R. 1982. Growth and bone mineralization of normal breast-fed infants and the effects of lactation on maternal bone mineral status. Am. J. Clin. Nutr. 36:438-443.

Chance, G.W., Radde, I.C., Willis, D.M., Roy, R.N., Park, E. and Ackerman, I. 1977. Postnatal growth of infants of less than 1.3 kg birth weight: effects of metabolic acidosis, of caloric intake, and of calcium, sodium, and phosphate supplementation. J. Pediatr. 91:787-793.

Delvin, E.E., Imbach, A. and Copti, M. 1988. Vitamin D nutritional status and related biochemical indices in an autonomous elderly population. Am. J. Clin. Nutr. 48:373-378.

FAO/WHO Expert Group. 1962. Calcium requirements. W.H.O. Tech. Rep. Ser. 230.

Heaney, R.P., Recker, R.R. and Saville, P.D. 1978. Menopausal changes in calcium balance performance. J. Lab. Clin. Med. 92:953-963.

Hegsted, D.M. 1986. Calcium and osteoporosis. J. Nutr. 116:2316-2319.

Henry, H.L. and Norman, A.W. 1984. Vitamin D: metabolism and biological actions. Annu. Rev. Nutr. 4:493-520.

Johnson, N.E., Alcantara, E.N. and Linkswiler, H. 1970. Effect of level of protein intake on urinary and fecal calcium and calcium retention of young adult males. J. Nutr. 100:1425-1430.

McCarron, D.A. and Morris, C.D. 1986. Metabolic considerations and cellular mechanism related to calcium's antihypertensive effects. Fed. Proc. 45:2734-2738.

Malm, O.J. 1958. Calcium requirement and adaptation in adult men. Oslo University Press, Oslo.

Matkovic, V., Kostial, K., Simonovic, I., Buzina, R., Brodarec, A. and Nordin, B.E.C. 1979. Bone status and fracture rates in two regions of Yugoslavia. Am. J. Clin. Nutr. 32:540-549.

Mazess, R.B. and Mather, W.E. 1975. Bone mineral content in Canadian Eskimos. Human Biol. 47:44-63.

Riggs, B.L., Wahner, H.W., Melton, L.J., III, Richelson, L.S., Judd, H.L. and O'Fallon, W.M. 1987. Dietary calcium intake and rates of bone loss in women. J. Clin. Invest. 80:979-982.

Robbins, L. 1986. The nutritive value of food available for consumption in Canada. Food Markets Analysis Division, Policy Planning and Economics Branch, Agriculture Canada. Ottawa.

Scythes, C.A., Gibson, R.S. and Draper, H.H. 1982. Dietary calcium and phosphorus intakes of a sample of Canadian pre-menopausal women consuming self-selected diets. Nutr. Res. 2:385-396.

Wilkinson, R. 1976. Absorption of calcium, phosphorus and magnesium. *In* Calcium, phosphate and magnesium metabolism: clinical physiology and diagnostic procedures. Nordin, B.E.C., ed. Churchill Livingstone, Edinburgh, pp. 36-112.

Yuen, D.E., Draper, H.H. and Trilok, G. 1984. Effect of dietary protein on calcium metabolism in man. Nutr. Abstr. Rev. 54:447-459.

Magnesium

Function and Action

Magnesium is the fourth most abundant cation in the human body and the second most common in intracellular fluid. The magnesium content of the human body ranges from 11.4 to 17.5 mmol/kg of wet weight. Thus, the body of an adult man contains a total of approximately 1 mole of magnesium. Bone contains approximately 60% of total body magnesium with the remainder distributed equally between muscle and non-muscular soft tissue. Only 1% of the total body content of the mineral is extracellular. This level remains remarkably constant in healthy individuals. One-third of the extracellular magnesium is bound non-specifically to plasma protein, while the remaining two-thirds is ionized and diffusible. This portion appears to be the biologically active component (Aikawa 1980). Normal serum magnesium levels in adults aged 18-74 years, reported in the NHANES I survey, ranged from 0.75 to 0.95 mmol/L (Lowenstein and Stanton 1986).

Magnesium plays a key role in many fundamental enzymatic reactions, including the transfer of phosphate groups (phosphokinases), the acylation of coenzyme A in the initiation of fatty acid oxidation (thiokinases), the hydrolysis of phosphate and pyrophosphate (phosphatases and pyrophosphatases) and the activation of amino acids (amino acid acyl synthetases) (Shils 1984). Magnesium is also required for ribosome aggregation, binding of RNA to ribosomes, and the synthesis and degradation of DNA. The element is essential for the formation of adenosine 3': 5'- cyclic monophosphate (cyclic AMP) and other second messengers, and plays an important role in neuromuscular transmission (Shils 1984).

Approximately 60% to 70% of ingested magnesium is excreted in the stools. Normal absorption is affected by total magnesium intake, intestinal transit time, and the rate of water absorption. Two separate transport systems participate in the absorption of magnesium. The first is thought to be a carrier-mediated system which functions at low intraluminal concentrations. The second is simple diffusion and occurs at higher intraluminal concentrations when the carrier-mediated system is saturated (Shils 1984).

Magnesium homeostasis is maintained by the gastrointestinal tract, bone and kidney (Quamme 1986). The kidneys are extremely efficient in maintaining the body magnesium concentration. When the magnesium intake by human subjects was restricted to 0.5 mmol/day, urinary and fecal losses each dropped to 0.5 mmol/day in approximately a week. When a normal intake was resumed, urinary excretion increased once a normal plasma level was attained, thus demonstrating the homeostatic control exerted by the kidneys (Barnes *et al.* 1960; Shils 1969). Renal handling of magnesium is a filtration-reabsorption process. The ultrafiltrability of magnesium is unaffected by magnesium deficiency, magnesium excess or an elevation in plasma calcium concentration, while reabsorption is dependent on the intraluminal concentration (Quamme 1986). During magnesium deficiency, fractional reabsorption is increased throughout the tubule, with the greatest augmentation occurring in the ascending limb of the loop of Henle (Quamme 1986).

Because of the remarkable ability of the kidney to conserve magnesium, primary depletion by dietary means in healthy individuals is extremely rare (Shils 1984; Quamme 1986). Symptomatic deficiency is observed only in individuals with predisposing or complicating disease states such as severe malabsorption, chronic alchoholism, prolonged infusion of magnesium-free parenteral fluids, renal dysfunction due to disease or secondary to drugs, childhood malnutrition, familial disorders of renal or intestinal conservation, hyperaldosteronism and hyperparathyroidism (Shils 1984; Whang 1984; Berkelhammer and Bear 1985; Lieber 1988). Clinical manifestations of magnesium deficiency are related to its critical role as a cofactor in the enzymes requiring adenosine triphosphate (ATP), in generating cyclic AMP and in regulating neurotransmitters. Deficiency impairs the activity of the sodium-potassium pump (Berkelhammer and Bear 1985; Fischer and Giroux 1987). A decrease in magnesium-dependent adenyl cyclase generation of cAMP leads to a decreased release of parathyroid hormone, which leads to hypocalcemia (Berkelhammer and Bear 1985). Other symptoms are increased vascular smooth muscle tone leading to spasm and hypertension (Altura *et al.* 1983; Altura and Altura 1987), neuromuscular manifestations, and personality changes (Berkelhammer and Bear 1985).

It is extremely difficult to obtain toxic levels of magnesium from the diet. The most common cause of hypermagnesemia is impaired renal function (Aikawa 1980). Elevations in serum levels to about 1.5-2.5 mmol/L are associated with symptoms such as hypotension and drowsiness. Higher levels result in depression of deep tendon reflexes, weakness, atonia and slurred speech (Aikawa 1980).

The average intakes of magnesium by Canadians, based on the Nutrition Canada Food Consumption Data, have been calculated (Table 14) (Shah, B.G., personal communication). These intakes were similar to those reported in the U.S. (323 and 234 mg/day for 20-53-year-old men and women respectively) (Lakshmanan *et al.* 1984). The principal dietary sources of magnesium reported in the Canadian study were cereals (27%), fruits and vegetables (27%) and dairy products (17%). A much higher proportion of the children's magnesium intake came from dairy products (Shah, B.G., personal communication). Lower intakes were reported in the Montreal area in which men and women, aged 20-39 years, had a magnesium intake (mg/day) of 232 and 174 respectively, and those 40-59 had intakes of 254 and 164 (Mongeau, E., personal communication).

Table 14.
Average Intakes of Magnesium by Canadians[a]

Age	Sex	Intake(mg/day)
1 - 4		201
5 - 11		259
12 - 19	males	324
	females	235
20 - 39	males	303
	females	205
40 - 64	males	259
	females	188
>65	males	201
	females	173
	Pregnant women	255

a. Nutrition Canada Food Consumption Patterns

Disease

The results of several studies have suggested an association between dietary magnesium deficiency and sudden death ischemic heart disease (Anderson *et al.* 1975; Johnson *et al.* 1979; Turlapaty and Altura 1980; Karppanen 1981). Epidemiological studies in Finland and in Canada have indicated that individuals residing in soft-water areas have a higher incidence of sudden death ischemic heart disease than people living in hard-water areas (Anderson *et al.* 1975; Karppanen 1981). The myocardial magnesium concentration in accident victims from cities with soft water was 7% lower than in individuals from cities with hard water. Magnesium was the only mineral whose concentration was significantly different between cities (Anderson *et al.* 1975). In the study by Johnson *et al.* (1979), the myocardial magnesium concentration of men dying of myocardial infarction was significantly lower than that of age-matched controls dying of trauma. The lowest myocardial magnesium concentrations in the study were observed in three men with a history of angina (Johnson *et al.* 1979). Turlapaty and Altura (1980) showed that withdrawal of magnesium increased the basal tone of isolated dog coronary arteries and the addition of the mineral caused relaxation. They hypothesized that magnesium deficiency produces coronary artery spasms leading to sudden death ischemic heart disease. There is also some circumstantial evidence connecting magnesium deficiency to the development of atherogenic lesions (Iseri 1984).

Some recent reports have associated sub-optimal magnesium status with hypertension (Dyckner and Wester 1983; Altura *et al.* 1984; Resnick *et al.* 1984; Joffres *et al.* 1987; Motoyama *et al.* 1987; Altura 1988). Altura (1988) suggested that vasoconstriction, leading to hypertension, is caused by the excess entry of Ca^{2+} into vascular cells at low free magnesium ion concentrations. Dyckner and Wester (1983) showed that both systolic and diastolic pressures dropped when patients receiving long term diuretic treatment for hypertension were also given magnesium supplements. Erythrocyte free magnesium ion concentrations were inversely correlated with both systolic and diastolic blood pressure (Resnick *et al.* 1984). Recently, the association between blood pressure and 61 dietary variables, assessed by 24-hour recalls, was investigated in Hawaiian men of Japanese origin. It was found that magnesium had the strongest inverse correlation (Joffres *et al.* 1987). There was, however, a high intercorrelation among many nutrients, making it difficult to separate the effect of magnesium from that of other variables. Magnesium supplementation in patients with essential hypertension resulted in an increase in their erythrocyte ouabain-sensitive ^{22}Na efflux rate constant and a decrease in blood pressure (Motoyama *et al.* 1987). Another group (Cappuccio *et al.* 1985), using a double blind randomized crossover design, also gave patients with mild to moderate essential hypertension magnesium supplements. Despite a significant increase in plasma magnesium concentration and urinary magnesium excretion, no fall in blood pressure could be detected.

Magnesium sulphate has a well-defined role in the treatment of preeclampsia, leading some investigators to suggest that magnesium deficiency may play a role in the pathogenesis of this disease (Ryzen *et al.* 1987). The mononuclear cell magnesium content and serum magnesium concentration of women with preeclampsia, however, were not significantly different from that of normal women. This suggests that this disease is not associated with magnesium deficit and that the efficacy of magnesium therapy in its treatment may be related to a pharmacological action rather than to repletion of low stores (Ryzen *et al.* 1987). A recent study showed that supplementation with magnesium was associated with significantly fewer maternal hospitalizations, a reduction in preterm delivery and less frequent referral of the newborn to the neonatal intensive care unit when compared to women receiving placebo (Spätling and Spätling 1988).

In many of the diseases whose etiology has been related to magnesium depletion, there may actually be a redistribution of magnesium in the body as part of the disease process. Thus, decreased body stores would not be related to onset of the disease. For example, myocardial infarction results in a generalized significant lowering of the magnesium level in the heart ventricles (Speich *et al.* 1988). This rapid loss of myocardial magnesium leads to the subsequent intracellular loss of potassium, and arrhythmias (Iseri 1984). The fall in serum magnesium in acute myocardial infarction may be due to the formation of soap in fat cells undergoing catecholamine-induced lipolysis (Flink *et al.* 1981; Iseri 1984). In patients admitted to a coronary care unit, no significant differences could be found between the plasma magnesium levels of patients with acute myocardial infarction and those whose chest pains were due to other causes (Ellis and Walmsley 1988). In a Canadian study, the serum magnesium levels of patients admitted to a coronary care unit was measured (Kafka *et al.* 1987). Hypomagnesemia was found in only 4% of the patients, although it was more common in those with myocardial infarction than those without (6% vs 3%). Major ventricular arrhythmias occurred more frequently in patients with acute myocardial infarction and hypomagnesemia. The 4% incidence of hypomagnesemia was similar to that reported in an Australian study (4.5%) in which plasma magnesium levels were measured (Croker and Walmsley 1986). This study found that many cases of hypomagnesemia are transient and require no treatment. Those that were not transient had a clinical disorder known to cause magnesium deficiency. In another study of elderly nursing home patients, only three of 75 were found to have mild hypomagnesemia. This was associated with poor eating habits (Dave *et al.* 1987).

In conclusion, although much information appears in the literature suggesting that magnesium deficiency is associated with a number of diseases, no definite proof has been presented. In light of the extremely efficient homeostatic mechanism present in the healthy individual, it is difficult to understand how hypomagnesemia could occur with the ingestion of a normal Canadian diet.

Recommendations

Adults

The majority of studies designed to determine magnesium requirements used the balance method. These studies have shown great variability. Increasing the magnesium intake to 800 mg/day from 200 to 300 mg/day did not improve the balance in adequately nourished subjects (Spencer 1986). In the study by Lakshmanan *et al.* (1984), magnesium balance was determined in men and women consuming self-selected diets. Daily balances of -32 mg and -25 mg respectively were reported. If these individuals were truly in prolonged negative balance, the men would have lost 14 g, or 53% of their total body stores in the course of a year. The women would have lost 11 g or 52% of their stores. This was clearly not the case, and demonstrates that it is inappropriate to use balance data to determine magnesium requirements. This paradox, demonstrated by the balance study of Lakshmanan *et al.* (1984), is typical of other studies in which subjects consumed usual amounts of magnesium. In a review of 251 balance periods with intakes of less than 4 mg/kg/day, Seelig (1981) reported that 83% were negative for men and 73% for women, assuming a sweat loss of 15 mg/day. With intakes between 4 and 5 mg/kg/day, the average daily balance was -28 mg for men and -2 mg for women (Seelig 1981; Wester 1987).

Physiological evidence suggests that the body can adapt to a wide range of magnesium intakes, due to the efficient homeostatic control by the kidneys. Under conditions of extremely low intakes, the kidney can conserve all but 0.5 mmol (12 mg) of magnesium/day (Barnes *et al.* 1960; Shils 1969). If this is combined with reported dermal losses of approximately 15 mg/day (Schroeder *et al.* 1969), the actual requirement might be less than 50 mg/day during adapted conditions. There is some evidence that a renal threshold exists for excretion of magnesium at a value close to the lower limit of the normal plasma level (Aikawa 1980). This level is approximately 0.5 mmol/L (Lowenstein and Stanton 1986). If it is assumed that 75% of plasma magnesium is ultrafiltrable (Quamme 1986), 0.55 mmol/L passes through the kidneys. The median glomerular filtration rate for adult Canadians is 130 mL/min for men and 100 mL/min for women, based on an average of 70 mL/min/M^2 and a surface area of 1.87 M^2 for men and 60 mL/min/M^2 and a surface area of 1.62 M^2 for women (Canada 1980; Merck Manual 1987, p. 1561.). Thus 4.3 and 3.3 mmol would be filtered per hour by the kidneys of men and women respectively. With a reabsorption rate of 97% (Aikawa 1980), the amount excreted would be 3.1 and 2.38 mmol/day (75 mg and 58 mg/day) respectively. If 15 mg in dermal losses are added to this, the total would be 90 mg for men and

72 mg for women. When a 40% absorption factor is applied to the losses, the requirements to maintain a normal plasma level, assuming adequate pre-existing stores, would be 220 mg/day for men and 180 mg/day for women. Thus intakes of 250 and 200 mg/day are recommended for men and women respectively, assuming adequate pre-existing stores. This is equivalent to 3.4 mg/kg and is consistent with the amount currently obtained from the mixed Canadian diet.

Children

The requirement for growing children is greater, since for every kg of increased body weight, 300 mg of magnesium in excess of obligatory losses is required (Schroeder *et al.* 1969). This is equivalent to an increased requirement of about 0.23 mg/kg/day, assuming a 40% absorption factor. Thus the recommendation for growing children and adolescents is 3.7 mg/kg/day. The magnesium concentration of human milk is approximately 30 µg/mL (Vaughan *et al.* 1979). This amount does not change with the length of lactation. Thus, based on milk volumes of 500 mL at one month, 800 mL at three months and 850 mL at six months (Whitehead and Paul 1981), recommended intakes for infants 0-4 months are 20 mg/day and 5-12 months, 32 mg/day.

Pregnancy and Lactation

During pregnancy, in order to provide sufficient magnesium for the increase in fetal and maternal tissue of approximately 1.5 kg during the first trimester, 5 kg during the second trimester and 5 kg during the last trimester (Gibbs and Seitchik 1980), at 300 mg/kg, an extra 12 mg/day during the first trimester and 40 during the second and third are required, assuming a 40% absorption factor. Thus an additional 15 mg during the first trimester and 45 mg during the second and third trimesters are recommended. Since the magnesium concentration of human milk is approximately 30 µg/mL, an additional 23 mg are lost per day during lactation, assuming a milk volume of 750 mL. With a fractional absorption of 40%, an additional intake of 58 mg/day would be required. Thus the recommendation for lactating women is for an additional intake of 65 mg/day.

References

Aikawa, J.K. 1980. Magnesium: its biological significance. CRC Press, Boca Raton, Fla.

Altura, B.M. 1988. Ischemic heart disease and magnesium. Magnesium 7:57-67.

Altura, B.T. and Altura, B.M. 1987. Cardiovascular actions of magnesium: importance in etiology and treatment of high blood pressure. Magnesium-Bull. 9:6-21.

Altura, B.M., Altura, B.T. and Carella, A. 1983. Magnesium deficiency-induced spasms of umbilical vessels: relation to preeclampsia, hypertension, growth retardation. Science 221:376-378.

Altura, B.M., Altura, B.T., Gebrewold, A., Ising, H. and Günther, T. 1984. Magnesium deficiency and hypertension: correlation between magnesium-deficient diets and microcirculatory changes in situ. Science 223:1315-1317.

Anderson, T.W., Neri, L.C., Schreiber, G.B., Talbot, F.D.F. and Zdrojewski, A. 1975. Ischemic heart disease, water hardness and myocardial magnesium. Can. Med. Assoc. J. 113:199-203.

Barnes, B.A., Cope, O. and Gordon, E.B. 1960. Magnesium requirements and deficits: an evaluation in two surgical patients. Ann. Surg. 152:518-533.

Berkelhammer, C. and Bear, R.A. 1985. A clinical approach to common electrolyte problems: 4. Hypomagnesemia. Can. Med. Assoc. J. 132:360-368.

Canada. Health and Welfare. Nutrition Canada. Health Protection Branch. Bureau of Nutritional Sciences. 1980. Anthropometry report: height, weight and body dimensions. Ottawa.

Cappuccio, F.P., Markandu, N.D., Beynon, G.W., Shore, A.C., Sampson, B. and MacGregor, G.A. 1985. Lack of effect of oral magnesium on high blood pressure: a double blind study. Br. Med. J. 291:235-238.

Croker, J.W. and Walmsley, R.N. 1986. Routine plasma magnesium estimation: a useful test? Med. J. Aust. 145:71-76.

Dave, D.M., Katz, P.R. and Gutman, S. 1987. Serum magnesium levels in nursing home patients. Nutr. Res. 7:981-984.

Dyckner, T. and Wester, P.O. 1983. Effect of magnesium on blood pressure. Br. Med. J. 286:1847-1849.

Ellis, V.M. and Walmsley, R.N. 1988. A comparison of plasma magnesium values in patients with acute myocardial infarction and patients with chest pain due to other causes. Med. J. Aust. 148:14-16.

Fischer, P.W.F. and Giroux, A. 1987. Effects of dietary magnesium on sodium-potassium pump action in the heart of rats. J. Nutr. 117:2091-2095.

Flink, E.B., Brick, J.E. and Shane, S.R. 1981. Alterations of long-chain free fatty acid and magnesium concentrations in acute myocardial infarction. Arch. Intern. Med. 141:441-443.

Gibbs, C.E. and Seitchik, J. 1980. Nutrition in pregnancy. *In* Modern nutrition in health and disease. 6th ed. Goodhart, R.S. and Shils, M.E., eds. Lea & Febiger, Philadelphia, pp. 743-752.

Iseri, L.T. 1984. Magnesium in coronary artery disease. Drugs 28(Suppl. 1):151-160.

Joffres, M.R., Reed, D.M. and Yano, K. 1987. Relationship of magnesium intake and other dietary factors to blood pressure: the Honolulu heart study. Am. J. Clin. Nutr. 45:469-475.

Johnson, C.J., Peterson, D.R. and Smith, E.K. 1979. Myocardial tissue concentrations of magnesium and potassium in men dying suddenly from ischemic heart disease. Am. J. Clin. Nutr. 32:967-970.

Kafka, H., Langevin, L. and Armstrong, P.W. 1987. Serum magnesium and potassium in acute myocardial infarction. Influence on ventricular arrhythmias. Arch. Intern. Med. 147:465-469.

Karppanen, H. 1981. Epidemiological studies on the relationship between magnesium intake and cardiovascular disease. Artery 9:190-199.

Lakshmanan, F.L., Rao, R.B., Kim, W.W. and Kelsay, J.L. 1984. Magnesium intakes, balances, and blood levels of adults consuming self-selected diets. Am. J. Clin. Nutr. 40:1380-1389.

Lieber, C.S. 1988. The influence of alcohol on nutritional status. Nutr. Rev. 46:241-254.

Lowenstein, F.W. and Stanton, M.F. 1986. Serum magnesium levels in the United States, 1971-1974. J. Am. Coll. Nutr. 5:399-414.

Merck manual of diagnosis and therapy. 1987. 15th ed. Berkow, R., ed. Merck and Co., Rahway, NJ.

Motoyama, T., Sano, H., Suzuki, H., Kawaguchi, K., Saito, K., Furuta, Y. and Fukuzaki, H. 1987. Oral magnesium treatment and the erythrocyte sodium pump in patients with essential hypertension. J. Hypertens. 4(Suppl. 6):S682-S684.

Quamme, G.A. 1986. Renal handling of magnesium: drug and hormone interactions. Magnesium 5:248-272.

Resnick, L.M., Gupta, R.K. and Laragh, J.H. 1984. Intracellular free magnesium in erythrocytes of essential hypertension: relationship to blood pressure and serum divalent cations. Proc. Nat. Acad. Sci. U.S.A. 81:6511-6515.

Ryzen, E., Greenspoon, J.S., Diesfield, P. and Rude, R.K. 1987. Blood mononuclear cell magnesium in normal pregnancy and preeclampsia. J. Am. Coll. Nutr. 6:121-124.

Schroeder, H.A., Nason, A.P. and Tipton, I.H. 1969. Essential metals in man. Magnesium. J. Chronic Dis. 21:815-841.

Seelig, M.S. 1981. Magnesium requirements in human nutrition. Magnesium-Bull. 3:26-47.

Shils, M.E. 1969. Experimental human magnesium depletion. Medicine 48:61-85.

Shils, M.E. 1984. Magnesium. *In* Nutrition Review's present knowledge in nutrition. 5th ed. Nutrition Foundation, Washington, pp. 422-438.

Spätling, L. and Spätling, G. 1988. Magnesium supplementation in pregnancy. A double-blind study. Br. J. Obstet. and Gynecol. 95:120-125.

Speich, M., Gelot, S., Robinet, N., Arnaud, P. and Nguyen, V.G. 1988. Movements of magnesium, zinc, calcium, potassium, cholesterols and creatine kinase in men and women during the twelve days following acute myocardial infarction. Correlation and regression studies. Magnesium-Bull. 10:2-8.

Spencer, H. 1986. Minerals and mineral interactions in human beings. J. Am. Diet. Assoc. 86:864-867.

Turlapaty, P.D.M.V. and Altura, B.M. 1980. Magnesium deficiency produces spasms of coronary arteries: relationship to etiology of sudden death ischemic heart disease. Science 208:198-200.

Vaughan, L.A., Weber, C.W. and Kemberling, S.R. 1979. Longitudinal changes in the mineral content of human milk. Am. J. Clin. Nutr. 32:2301-2306.

Wester, P.O. 1987. Magnesium. Am. J. Clin. Nutr. 45:1305-1312.

Whang, R. 1984. Magnesium deficiency - causes and clinical implications. Drugs 28(Suppl. 1):143-150.

Whitehead, R.G. and Paul, A.A. 1981. Infant growth and human milk requirements: a fresh approach. Lancet 2:161-163.

Iron

The iron-containing compounds hemoglobin, myoglobin and enzymes such as cytochrome oxidase, catalase, ribonucleotide reductase and xanthine oxidase, serve a variety of metabolic functions. These include transport and storage of oxygen, mitochondrial electron transport, catecholamine metabolism and DNA synthesis. Depending on the stage of development, these compounds account for 25 to 55 mg of iron/kg body weight, more than 80% of which is located in hemoglobin. Iron storage compounds include ferritin and hemosiderin in the liver, spleen and bone marrow. These compounds represent 5 to 25 mg of iron/kg body weight (Dallman *et al.* 1980; Cook and Lynch 1986). The amounts of myoglobin and iron-containing enzymes in the tissues are roughly proportional to body weight in both sexes. The loss of iron through menstruation usually leads to lower iron stores in women.

Iron absorption is variable and its efficiency is dependent on the iron status of an individual. Iron-depleted persons absorb more of the mineral than those who have stores. This variability complicates the setting of requirements.

Iron Deficiency

Severe iron deficiency is usually characterized by microcytic hypochromic anemia. Nonhematological effects include general gastrointestinal malabsorption and abnormalities in host defence, work performance and neurological function (Cook and Lynch 1986). Chronically anemic agricultural workers in the developing world suffer from a dramatic impairment in work capacity and a reduction in productivity (Cook and Lynch 1986). Whereas the effects of iron deficiency on work performance, cell-mediated immunity and neutrophil killing are established, the effects on the incidence and susceptibility to infection are less clear, because of the difficulty in carrying out properly controlled studies (Dallman 1987). Iron therapy may reduce the incidence of mild infections by correcting a defect in cell-mediated immunity. There is, however, some evidence that rapid alleviation of iron deficiency may promote certain bacterial and parasitic infections (Dallman *et al.* 1980).

Deficits in attention span, cognitive development and learning ability in iron-deficient infants, preschool and school-age children have been reported (Webb and Oski 1973; Oski *et al.* 1983). In adults, iron deficiency may cause a perversion of taste (pica) leading to the consumption of non-food items such as ice, dirt and laundry starch. The neurophysiological mechanisms involved in these effects of iron deficiency are still largely speculative. It is, however, known that iron is required for the activity of enzymes, such as tyrosine hydroxylase, tryptophan hydroxylase and monoamine oxidase, that are important in neurotransmitter metabolism (Cook and Lynch 1986).

Hemoglobin levels in the members of the 1976 Canadian Olympic team were found to be lower than those reported in Australian and Dutch teams and also those observed in the general Canadian population (Clement *et al.* 1977). Magnusson *et al.* (1984a,b), who investigated the iron metabolism of Swedish elite runners, concluded that "runner's anemia" is not true anemia, nor is it caused by iron deficiency. They could not satisfactorily explain occasional findings of low iron stores. Low serum ferritin levels, indicative of low iron stores, are not associated with impaired athletic performance, and correction of this condition does not influence indices of fitness in trained athletes (Matter *et al.* 1987).

Iron Excess

Physiologic regulation of iron absorption confers a high degree of protection against iron toxicity. Iron overload due to chronic excessive dietary iron intake has been documented only in the South African Bantu, who consume a home-brewed alcoholic beverage providing as much as 100 mg/day of bioavailable iron in addition to approximately 15 mg of food iron. The exact role played by alcohol in this condition has not been elucidated (Bothwell and Charlton 1982). This level of iron intake is unlikely to be observed in the Canadian population.

Iron toxicity in Canada is most often due to the accidental ingestion by children of large quantities of iron from supplements. Individuals carrying the gene for hemochromatosis are at risk of iron overload. Studies of pedigrees in several countries including Canada indicate a gene frequency of 5-7% for this autosomal recessive disease (Valberg and Ghent 1985). The Canadian estimates of heterozygous and homozygous gene frequencies of 11% and 0.3%, respectively, were obtained from a study of 19 family pedigrees. In heterozygotes, there was no serious deregulation of absorptive mechanisms (Borwein *et al.* 1983). A subsequent assessment of 1105 transferrin saturation and serum ferritin values from the Nutrition Canada Survey (Canada. Health and Welfare 1973) revealed abnormalities in three subjects. This gene frequency (0.27%), without rigorous demonstration of iron overload, agrees with estimates made by Borwein *et al.* (1983). The prolonged oral ingestion of a therapeutic dose of iron can cause hemochromatosis in individuals not carrying the gene for hemochromatosis, but such cases are very rare (Jalihal and Barlow 1984).

Interaction With Other Minerals

Since an increasing number of Canadian women have been using calcium supplements, an effect of calcium on iron absorption would potentially have widespread significance. The inhibiting effect of calcium on iron absorption appears to be caused by salt forms, with calcium phosphate and carbonate having the greatest effect (Cook *et al.* 1981; O'Neill-Cutting and Crosby 1986). This effect was observed in individuals subjected to either an elemental formula diet or to fasting conditions. Whether the effect would be observed in conjunction with a mixed Canadian diet remains to be determined.

Excess dietary iron may have a negative impact on copper and/or zinc bioavailability. For example, copper absorption was depressed in infants fed an iron supplemented formula (10.2 mg/L), compared to that of the same infants receiving a formula containing only 2.5 mg iron/L (Haschke *et al.* 1986). Because of the relatively small difference, the authors did not consider the effect to be clinically significant. Furthermore, Yip *et al.* (1985) failed to observe an effect of supplemental iron on either zinc or copper serum levels in 1-year-old infants.

Supplemental iron has been reported to depress the absorption of zinc sulphate in adults when the iron to zinc ratio is 3:1 (Solomons 1982). Recently, iron-folate supplements (100 mg ferrous iron + 350 µg folate), used during pregnancy, were found to have an adverse effect on the absorption of a zinc sulphate suspension (Simmer *et al.* 1987). Whether the absorption of dietary zinc, which is in the organic form, is also affected by large iron supplements remains to be determined. Present evidence does not warrant a recommendation for zinc supplementation during iron therapy.

Intake

After the publication of the Nutrition Canada Survey (Canada. Health and Welfare 1975), smaller surveys indicated that the average iron intakes of infants were mostly above the recommended intakes (Yeung *et al.* 1982; Canada. Health and Welfare 1983). The daily iron intake of adult men averaged over 14 mg, of which 14% was heme iron (Henderson Sabry and Grief 1982). Premenopausal and postmenopausal women consumed about 12 mg of iron per day, including approximately 12% heme iron (Gibson *et al.* 1984). The food expenditure patterns of the elderly in Canada (1974 to 1982) indicated that the consumption of red meats was decreasing while that of poultry and fish, which are lower in iron, was increasing (Robbins 1986). During the same period, the proportion of the food dollar spent on fruits and vegetables increased. The vitamin C provided by these foods promotes the absorption of non-heme iron (Cook *et al.* 1981). The intake of dietary fibre also increased. Even if the dietary fibre intake were doubled, as recommended by the Expert Advisory Committee on Dietary Fibre, it would not have a deleterious effect on the iron status of adults nor of elderly Canadians, provided they consume a mixed diet (Bunker *et al.* 1984; Canada. Health and Welfare 1985).

The prevalence of frank anemia in Canada was found to be minimal in the Nutrition Canada Survey undertaken in 1970-72. The highest prevalence (2.4%) was observed in males over 65 years. The prevalence of low iron stores was about 12% in children below 10 years, 8% to 10% in all females under 65 years of age and 7% in males over 65 years (Canada. Health and Welfare 1975). Similar observations were made subsequently from the analysis of storage iron in liver specimens taken at autopsy from accident victims in different parts of Canada (Shah and Belonje 1976). Recently it has been suggested that the hematologic standards used for young adults are not appropriate for the elderly (Yip *et al.* 1984). If so, the prevalence of anemia in elderly males was over-estimated. It can be concluded that the iron intake of the general population approximates the amount needed to prevent signs of iron deficiency.

The prevalence of anemia or low iron status may be high among new vegetarians and even among individuals who are accustomed to a predominantly lacto-ovo vegetarian diet (Bindra and Gibson 1986; Helman and Darnton-Hill 1987). This may be attributed to a high intake of dietary fibre, phytate and tannins, which have an adverse effect on iron absorption (Cook *et al.* 1981).

Obligatory Losses

Estimates of iron requirements are based on obligatory losses, which include those from exfoliation of cells from internal and external surfaces, urine, sweat and menstrual fluids, in addition to the iron needed for growth. Measurements of iron losses are difficult and inaccurate. Data from twelve Americans revealed daily iron losses of 0.95 ± 0.3 mg/day, with a coefficient of variation of 32% (Green *et al.* 1968).

A more recent study of eleven healthy Swedish men supported a modest contribution of 22.5 ± 7.6 µg of iron/L of sweat to total obligatory iron losses (Brune *et al.* 1986). In this case, the coefficient of variation (34%) was similar to that of Green *et al.* (1968). These limited data suggest that the coefficient of variation for obligatory iron losses may be higher than the 15% which has been previously used.

Absorption

Dietary iron is composed of heme and non-heme iron, the former being better absorbed. It has been estimated that 15% of the iron in the Canadian diet is in the heme form (Henderson Sabry and Grief 1982; Gibson *et al.* 1984) and that 20-30% of heme iron would be absorbed in iron-replete individuals. The absorption of non-heme iron is highly variable, ranging from 1% to 40%. It is enhanced by concurrent ingestion of meat, poultry, seafood and ascorbic acid, and inhibited by tea, coffee and egg yolk, as well as by bran, which contains both fibre and phytate (Bothwell *et al.* 1979). In the most recent FAO/WHO monograph on iron requirements, meals are categorized into low, intermediate and high iron bioavailability, with a conservative estimate of absorption of 5%, 10% and 15% respectively, by an individual with no iron stores but normal iron transport. The typical Canadian meal would rank in the "high bioavailability" category, which is defined as "a diversified diet containing generous quantities of meat, poultry, fish or foods containing high amounts of ascorbic acid" (FAO/WHO 1988).

It is difficult to agree upon one number to define iron absorption, because absorption increases with decreasing stores (Cook *et al.* 1974; Disler *et al.* 1975; Walters *et al.* 1975; Charlton *et al.* 1977; Heinrich *et al.* 1977; Bezwoda *et al.* 1979). It was shown in Swedish men that absorption increased from 21% to 74% as bone marrow hemosiderin decreased (Magnusson *et al.* 1981). Similarly, in nondepleted men, mean absorption was 49% when serum ferritin values were somewhat low (24 µg/L), compared to 21% when ferritin levels were high (79 µg/L) (Magnusson *et al.* 1981). Thus absorption is variable, depending on the iron status of the population studied.

Although there are no studies that detail iron absorption from typical Canadian meals, a group of iron-replete British adult males showed absorption rates of 12.7% when provided with a typical Gambian meal, compared to 32.9% in Gambian men given the same meal (Fairweather-Tait *et al.* 1987). These authors suggested that the 12.7% absorption was typical for the British men on a mixed British diet. Iron absorption from a typical Canadian diet, using the model of Monsen *et al.* (1978) that predicts average iron absorption from single meals, would be 10% for adult males and postmenopausal women. An absorption of 12.5% was selected as being typical of the Canadian adult population and was used in formulating the current recommendations for this age group.

Growing children and adolescents require additional iron beyond that needed to replace obligatory losses and to maintain stores. Despite this, there is no evidence supporting a different fractional absorption in this group, compared to adults, if stores are adequate. Thus, an absorption factor of 12.5% was also used in calculating the recommendations for children and adolescents. In iron-deficient children, absorption increases two to three times (Schulz and Smith 1958). Although there is controversy around this issue, the elderly may have a decreased absorption of iron (Freiman *et al.* 1963; Jacobs and Owen 1969; Marx 1979; Bunker *et al.* 1984). There is, however, insufficient evidence to assign a different absorption factor for this group. There is more than a two-fold increase in iron absorption during the second and third trimester of pregnancy (Hahn *et al.* 1951; Heinrich *et al.* 1968; Apte and Iyengar 1970; Heinrich 1970). Thus, an absorption factor of 25% was used to calculate the recommended iron intake during the last two-thirds of pregnancy.

Infants

The average iron content of human milk is 0.35 mg/L (Vuori *et al.* 1980; Stolley *et al.* 1981; Fransson *et al.* 1984; Fransson and Lönnerdal 1984; Lönnerdal *et al.* 1984). Based on an average milk intake of 750 mL/day during the first months of life, the iron intake would be 0.26 mg/day. Assuming that 50% of the iron in human milk is absorbed (McMillan *et al.* 1976), the amount of absorbed iron would be 0.13 mg/day. Smith and Rios (1974) have estimated that obligatory iron losses in the first six months of life amount to 0.04 mg/kg/24 h. This amount includes measured intestinal losses and estimates for skin and urine losses.

Soon after birth, there is a significant decrease in total body iron stores. Although the body weight of the infant has approximately doubled by four months, the total amount of iron in the body is equal to that at birth. Thus, the iron requirement for growth and stores during the first four months after birth is zero. Obligatory iron losses during this time average 0.24 mg/day. Breast milk, however, provides only 50% of the iron necessary to replace these losses, resulting in a depletion of stores deposited during fetal development. Thus, it is currently recommended by the Canadian Paediatric Society Nutrition Committee (1979) that additional iron-containing foods, eg. iron fortified infant cereals, be started at between four to six months of age.

Menstruating Women

Menstrual losses of iron do not follow a normal distribution, but are skewed upward. Among a large group of Swedish women, 10% lost more than 84 mL of blood, equivalent to approximately 1.3 mg of iron per day (Hallberg *et al.* 1966). The mean and the median iron losses were 0.6 and 0.4 mg per day respectively. The menstrual loss of adolescent girls was somewhat lower. In Canadian women, the median iron loss was 0.44 mg per day (Beaton *et al.* 1970). Brazilian and Mexican women showed an average menstrual iron loss of 0.5 mg per day (Shaw *et al.* 1980; Pedron *et al.* 1982). Women whose menstrual loss is greater than the average are likely to increase their efficiency of absorption. Since the recommended iron intakes were calculated from an average absorption factor, the average menstrual loss of 0.5 mg per day for adolescent girls and 0.7 mg per day for women was used to arrive at the values given in Table 15.

Table 15.
Derivation of Recommended Iron Intake

Age	Sex	Wt kg	Obligatory Iron Losses mg/day	Iron Accretion Growth + Stores mg/day	Menstrual Loss mg/day	Total Iron Requirement mg/day	Dietary Intake mg/day
Months 0-4	M/F	6[a]	0.24[b]	0.0[c]		0.24	0.26[d]
5-12	M/F	9	0.37	0.34		0.7	7.0
Years 1-2	M/F	11	0.44	0.29		0.7	6.0[e]
3-5	M/F	16	0.48[f]	0.23		0.7	6.0
6-11	M/F	27	0.64	0.35		1.0	8.0
12-15	M	46	0.71	0.49		1.2	10
	F	47	0.72	0.41	0.5	1.6	13
16-18	M	64	0.90	0.33		1.2	10
	F	53	0.78	0.16	0.5	1.4	12
19+	M	72	0.95[g]	0.1		1.1	9.0
	F	59	0.85	0.1	0.7	1.7	13
Post-menopausal		59	0.85	0.1		1.0	8.0
65+	M/F		0.85	0.1		1.0	8.0

a. Canada. Health and Welfare 1983.

b. Estimated from Smith and Rios 1974 at 0.04 mg/kg/day.

c. Calculated from data by Smith and Rios 1974.

d. The average iron content of human milk is 0.35 mg/L. Based on an average milk intake of 750 mL/day, the iron intake would be 0.26 mg/day. Assuming 50% absorption from human milk, intake will not meet requirement.

e. Assumes 12.5% absorption.

f. Estimated from Smith and Rios 1974.

g. Green *et al.* 1968.

Pregnancy and Lactation

The requirement of the pregnant woman merits special attention. Iron is transferred, during the latter half of gestation, to the growing fetus and placenta. Although menstruation ceases during pregnancy, iron is lost in blood and lochia at delivery. A summary of iron requirements during pregnancy is shown in Table 16.

During pregnancy, about 450 mg of iron is required for red cell expansion (Bothwell *et al.* 1979). Over the last two trimesters, this amounts to 2.4 mg/day (Table 16) (Bothwell *et al.* 1979). The additional need for iron can be met from iron stores if they are present before pregnancy. Restoration of maternal iron stores depends on the amount of blood lost during the delivery of the infant, and on the contraction of the red blood cell mass after delivery. There is about 75 mg of iron/kg body weight in the full-term infant (Widdowson and Spray 1951). Thus approximately 260 mg of iron is also required during pregnancy for the growing fetus. The placenta contains an additional 75 mg of iron, which at parturition is lost from the mother (McCoy *et al.* 1961). For the woman with no iron stores, therefore, the total iron requirements during the second and third trimesters of pregnancy are 4.6 and 5.7 mg/day, respectively. Based on an absorption rate of 25% during pregnancy (Hahn *et al.* 1951; Heinrich *et al.* 1968; Apte and Iyengar 1970; Heinrich 1970), dietary intake alone cannot meet the total recommended intake of 18 and 23 mg/day for the last two trimesters. An iron supplement is recommended on the assumption that pre-pregnant stores are inadequate. With normal iron stores a supplement is unnecessary.

The requirement for lactation is derived from a weighted average of 0.35 mg of iron/L of milk and a daily production of 750 mL (Vuori *et al.* 1980; Stolley *et al.* 1981; Fransson and Lönnerdal 1984; Fransson *et al.* 1984; Lönnerdal *et al.* 1984). Accordingly, daily iron losses in milk are about 0.3 mg. During early lactation, menstruation is unlikely to occur; thus iron loss in milk is counterbalanced by an absence of menstrual losses. An iron supplement during lactation, therefore, is not necessary (Table 16).

Table 16.
Iron Requirement During Pregnancy and Lactation (mg/day)

	Obligatory Losses	Red Cell Expansion	Fetus + Placenta	Total Requirement	Recom. Intake Diet	+ Supplement
1st Trimester	0.85	0.1 (stores)		1.0	8[a,b]	—
2nd Trimester	0.85	2.4	1.0 + 0.3	4.6	13[c]	5[d]
3rd Trimester	0.85	2.4	1.9 + 0.5	5.7	13[c]	10[d]
Lactation	0.85	0.4[g]		1.3	10[ef]	—

a. Assumes 12.5% absorption.

b. The value of 8 mg/day is less than the recommended iron intake of females over age 19 yrs. because during pregnancy, there are no menstrual losses. To replete stores, the usual intake for the non-pregnant female (13 mg/day) may be maintained.

c. Assumes 25% absorption.

d. An iron supplement is recommended on the assumption that pre-pregnant iron stores are inadequate. With normal iron stores, a supplement is unnecessary because storage iron will be used to meet iron needs.

e. Assumes 12.5% absorption.

f. The value, 10 mg/day, is less than the recommended iron intake of non-pregnant adult females because during lactation, no (or minimal) menstrual iron is lost. To replete stores, the usual intake for the non-pregnant female (13 mg/day) may be maintained.

g. The value of 0.4 mg is composed of 0.3 mg secreted in milk and 0.1 mg for stores.

Recommendations

In Recommended Nutrient Intakes for Canadians (Canada. Health and Welfare 1983), iron requirements were calculated using mean values for both obligatory losses (Green *et al.* 1968) and growth (Hawkins 1964). A coefficient of variation of 15% was assumed and the mean was increased by 30% (two standard deviations) to account for biologic variability. To calculate the recommended iron intake, absorption was taken to be 15% and 20% for men and menstruating women respectively, and 15% for children. The present recommendation did not employ an identical method because, as outlined above, neither the figure used to account for biologic variability nor the absorption values was judged to be appropriate. An overriding factor in arriving at the current recommendation was the adaptive increase in iron absorption in response to declining iron stores. Since iron absorption is homeostatically balanced by need, the recommended iron intakes are based on average requirements. These recommended intakes are summarized in Table 15 and are supported by specific comments on certain physiological groups.

References

Apte, S.V. and Iyengar, L. 1970. Absorption of dietary iron in pregnancy. Am. J. Clin. Nutr. 23:73-77.

Beaton, G.H., Thein, M., Milne, H. and Veen, M.J. 1970. Iron requirements of menstruating women. Am. J. Clin. Nutr. 23:275-283.

Bezwoda, W.R., Bothwell, T.H., Torrance, J.D., MacPhail, A.P., Charlton, R.W., Kay, G. and Levin, J. 1979. The relationship between marrow iron stores, plasma ferritin concentrations and iron absorption. Scand. J. Haematol. 22:113-120.

Bindra, G.S. and Gibson, R.S. 1986. Iron status of predominantly lacto-ovo vegetarian East Indian immigrants to Canada: a model approach. Am. J. Clin. Nutr. 44:643-652.

Borwein, S.T., Ghent, C.N., Flanagan, P.R., Chamberlain, M.J. and Valberg, L.S. 1983. Genetic and phenotypic expression of hemochromatosis in Canadians. Clin. Invest. Med. 6:171-179.

Bothwell, T.H. and Charlton, R.W. 1982. A general approach to the problems of iron deficiency and iron overload in the population at large. Semin. Hematol. 19:54-67.

Bothwell, T.H., Charlton, R.W., Cook, J.D. and Finch, C.A. 1979. Iron metabolism in man. Blackwell Scientific Publications, Oxford, pp. 7-43.

Brune, M., Magnusson, B., Persson, H. and Hallberg, L. 1986. Iron losses in sweat. Am. J. Clin. Nutr. 43:438-443.

Bunker, V.W., Lawson, M. and Clayton, B.E. 1984. Uptake and excretion of iron by healthy elderly subjects. J. Clin. Path. 37:1353-1357.

Canada. Health and Welfare. Nutrition Canada. 1973. Nutrition: a national priority. National survey. Ottawa.

Canada. Health and Welfare. Nutrition Canada. Health Protection Branch. Bureau of Nutritional Sciences. 1975. The Ontario survey report. Ottawa.

Canada. Health and Welfare. Health Protection Branch. Bureau of Nutritional Sciences. 1983. Recommended nutrient intakes for Canadians. Ottawa.

Canada. Health and Welfare. Health Protection Branch. 1985. Report of the Expert Advisory Committee on Dietary Fibre. Ottawa.

Canadian Paediatric Society. Nutrition Committee. 1979. Infant feeding. Can. J. Public Health 70:376-385.

Charlton, R.W., Derman, D., Skikne, B., Lynch, S.R., Sayers, M.H., Torrance, J.D. and Bothwell, J.M. 1977. Iron stores, serum ferritin and iron absorption. *In* Proteins of iron metabolism. Brown, E.B., Aisen, P., Fielding, J. and Crichton, R.R., eds. Grune & Stratton, New York, pp. 387-392.

Clement, D.B., Asmundson, R.C. and Medhurst, C.W. 1977. Hemoglobin values: comparative survey of the 1976 Canadian Olympic team. Can. Med. Assoc. J. 117:614-616.

Cole, S.K. 1972. Haematological characteristics and menstrual blood losses. J. Obstet. Gynaecol. Br. Commonw. 79:994-1001.

Cole, S.K., Billewicz, W.Z. and Thomson, A.M. 1971. Sources of variation in menstrual blood loss. J. Obstet. Gynaecol. Br. Commonw. 78:933-939.

Cook, J.D. and Lynch, S.R. 1986. The liabilities of iron deficiency. Blood 68:803-809.

Cook, J.D., Lipschitz, D.A., Miles, L.E.M. and Finch, C.A. 1974. Serum ferritin as a measure of iron stores in normal subjects. Am. J. Clin. Nutr. 27:681-687.

Cook, J.D., Morck, T.A., Skikne, B.S. and Lynch, S.R. 1981. Biochemical determinants of iron absorption. *In* Nutrition in health and disease and international development: symposia from the XII International Congress of Nutrition. Harper, A.E. and Davis, G.K., eds. A.R. Liss, New York, pp. 323-331.

Dallman, P.R. 1987. Iron deficiency and the immune response. Am. J. Clin. Nutr. 46:329-334.

Dallman, P.R., Siimes, M.A. and Stekel, A. 1980. Iron deficiency in infancy and childhood. Am. J. Clin. Nutr. 33:86-118.

Disler, P.B., Lynch, S.R., Charlton, R.W., Torrance, J.D., Bothwell, T.H., Walker, R.B. and Mayet, F. 1975. The effect of tea on iron absorption. Gut 16:193-200.

Fairweather-Tait, S.J., Minski, M.J. and Singh, J. 1987. Nonradioisotopic method for measuring iron absorption from a Gambian meal. Am. J. Clin. Nutr. 46:844-848.

FAO/WHO 1988. Report of a joint FAO/WHO expert consultation. Requirements of vitamin A, iron, folate and vitamin B_{12}. FAO Food and Nutrition Series, no. 23.

Fransson, G.B and Lonnerdal, B. 1984. Iron, copper, zinc, calcium and magnesium in human milk fat. Am. J. Clin. Nutr. 39:185-189.

Fransson, G.B., Gebre-Medhin, M. and Hambraeus, L. 1984. The human milk contents of iron, copper, zinc, calcium and magnesium in a population with a habitually high intake of iron. Acta Paediatr. Scand. 73:471-476.

Freiman, H.D., Tauber, S.A. and Tulsky, E.G. 1963. Iron absorption in the healthy aged. Geriatrics 18:716-720.

Gibson, R.S., Martinez, O. and MacDonald, A.C. 1984. Available dietary iron intakes of a selected sample of pre- and post-menopausal Canadian women. Nutr. Res. 4:315-323.

Green, R., Charlton, R., Seftel, H., Bothwell, T., Mayet, F., Adams, B., Finch, C. and Layrisse, M. 1968. Body iron excretion in man. Am. J. Med. 45:336-353.

Hahn, P.F., Carother, E.L., Darby, W.J., Martin, M., Sheppard, C.W., Cannon, R.O., Beam, A.S., Densen, P.M. and Peterson, J.C. 1951. Iron metabolism in human pregnancy as studied with the radioactive isotope Fe^{59}. Am. J. Obstet. Gynecol. 61:477-486.

Hallberg, L., Hogdahl, A.M., Nilsson, L. and Rybo, G. 1966. Menstrual blood loss — a population study. Variation at different ages and attempts to define normality. Acta Obstet. Gynecol. Scand. 45:320-351.

Haschke, F., Ziegler, E.E., Edwards, B.B. and Fomon, S.J. 1986. Effect of iron fortification of infant formula on trace mineral absorption. J. Pediatr. Gastroenterol. Nutr. 5:768-773.

Hawkins, W.W. 1964. Iron, copper and cobalt. *In* Nutrition: a comprehensive treatise. Vol. 1. Beaton, G.H. and McHenry, E.W., eds. Academic Press, London, pp. 309-372.

Heinrich, H.C. 1970. Intestinal iron absorption in man — methods of measurement, dose relationship, diagnostic and therapeutic applications. *In* Iron deficiency: pathogenesis, clinical aspects, therapy. Colloquia Geigy. Hallberg, L., Harwerth, H.G. and Vannotti, A., eds. Academic Press, New York, pp. 213-296.

Heinrich, H.C., Bartels, H., Heinisch, B., Hausmann, K., Kuse, R., Humke, W. and Mauss, H.J. 1968. Intestinale ^{59}Fe-Resorption und prälatenter Eisenmangel während der Gravidität des Menschen. [Intestinal ^{59}Fe resorption and prelatent iron deficiency during human pregnancy]. Klin. Wochenschr. 46:199-202.

Heinrich, H.C., Bruggemann, J., Gabbe, E.E. and Glaser, M. 1977. Correlation between diagnostic $^{59}Fe^{2+}$ absorption and serum ferritin concentration in man. Z. Naturforsch. (C) 32:1023-1025.

Helman, A.D. and Darnton-Hill, I. 1987. Vitamin and iron status in new vegetarians. Am. J. Clin. Nutr. 45:785-789.

Henderson Sabry, J. and Grief, H. 1982. Calculated available iron, heme iron and non-heme iron in diets of a group of men. J. Can. Diet. Assoc. 43:132-136,154.

Jacobs, A.M. and Owen, G.M. 1969. The effect of age on iron absorption. J. Gerontol. 24:95-96.

Jalihal, S.S. and Barlow, A.M. 1984. Haemochromatosis following prolonged oral iron ingestion. J. Roy. Soc. Med. 77:690-692.

Lönnerdal, B., Keen, C.L., Glazier, C.E. and Anderson, J. 1984. A longitudinal study of Rhesus monkey (Macaca mulatta) milk composition: trace elements, minerals, protein, carbohydrate and fat. Pediatr. Res. 18:911-914.

Magnusson, B., Bjorn-Rasmussen, E., Hallberg, L. and Rossander, L. 1981. Iron absorption in relation to iron status. Scand. J. Haematol. 27:201-208.

Magnusson, B., Hallberg, L., Rossander, L. and Swolin, B. 1984a. Iron metabolism and "sports anemia". I. A study of several iron parameters in elite runners with differences in iron status. Acta. Med. Scand. 216:149-155.

Magnusson, B., Hallberg, L., Rossander, L. and Swolin, B. 1984b. Iron metabolism and "sports anemia". II. A hematological comparison of elite runners and control subjects. Acta. Med. Scand. 216:157-164.

Marx, J.J.M. 1979. Normal iron absorption and decreased red cell iron uptake in the aged. Blood 53:204-211.

Matter, M., Stittfall, T., Graves, J., Myburg, K., Adams, B., Jacobs, P. and Noakes, T.D. 1987. The effect of iron and folate therapy on maximal exercise performance in female marathon runners with iron and folate deficiency. Clin. Sci. 72:415-422.

McCoy, B.A., Bleiler, R. and Ohlson, M.A. 1961. Iron content of intact placentas and cords. Am. J. Clin. Nutr. 9:613-615.

McMillan, J.A., Landaw, S.A. and Oski, F.A. 1976. Iron sufficiency in breast-fed infants and the availability of iron from human milk. Pediatr. 58:686-691.

Monsen, E.R., Hallberg, L., Layrisse, M., Hegsted, D.M., Cook, J.D., Mertz, W. and Finch, C.A. 1978. Estimation of available dietary iron. Am. J. Clin. Nutr. 31:134-141.

O'Neil-Cutting, M.A. and Crosby, W.H. 1986. The effect of antacids on the absorption of simultaneously ingested iron. JAMA, J. Am. Med. Assoc. 255:1468-1470.

Oski, F.A., Honig, A.S., Helu, B. and Howanitz, P. 1983. Effect of iron therapy on behavior performance in nonanemic, iron-deficient infants. Pediatrics 71:877-880.

Pedron, N., Gallegos, A.J., Lozano, M. and Aznar, R. 1982. Menstrual blood loss estimates in women using Copper 7 and Multiload-250 intrauterine devices. Contraception 26:475-485.

Robbins, L.G. 1986. The food expenditure patterns of the elderly in Canada, 1974-82. Food Market Comment. 8:29-43.

Schulz, J. and Smith, N.J. 1958. A quantitative study of the absorption of food iron in infants and children. AMA J. Dis. Child. 95:109-119.

Shah, B.G. and Belonje, B. 1976. Liver storage iron in Canadians. Am. J. Clin. Nutr. 29:66-69.

Shaw, S.T., Jr., Andrade, A.T.L., Paixao de Souza, J., Macauley, L.K. and Rowe, P.J. 1980. Quantitative menstrual and intermenstrual blood loss in women using Lippes Loop and Copper T intrauterine devices. Contraception 21:343-352.

Simmer, K., Iles, C.A., James, C. and Thompson, R.P.H. 1987. Are iron-folate supplements harmful? Am. J. Clin. Nutr. 45:122-125.

Smith, N.J. and Rios, E. 1974. Iron metabolism and iron deficiency in infancy and childhood. Adv. Pediatr. 21:239-280.

Solomons, N.W. 1982. Biological availability of zinc in humans. Am. J. Clin. Nutr. 35:1048-1075.

Stolley, H., Galgan, V. and Droese, W. 1981. Nahr-und Wirkstoffe in Frauenmilch: Protein, Laktose, Mineralien, Spurenelemente und Thiamin. [Nutrient content in human milk: protein, lactose, minerals, trace elements, and thiamin]. Monatsschr. Kinderheilkd. 129:293-297.

Valberg, L.S. and Ghent, C.N. 1985. Diagnosis and management of hereditary hemochromatosis. Annu. Rev. Med. 36:27-37.

Vuori, E., Makinen, S.M., Kara, R. and Kuitunen, P. 1980. The effects of the dietary intakes of copper, iron, manganese, and zinc on the trace element content of human milk. Am. J. Clin. Nutr. 33:227-231.

Walters, G.O., Jacobs, A., Worwood, M., Trevett, D. and Thomson, W. 1975. Iron absorption in normal subjects and patients with idiopathic haemochromatosis: relationship with serum ferritin concentration. Gut 16:188-192.

Webb, T.E. and Oski, F.A. 1973. Iron deficiency anemia and scholastic achievement in young adolescents. J. Pediatr. 82:827-830.

Widdowson, E.M. and Spray, C.M. 1951. Chemical development in utero. Arch. Dis. Child. 26:205-214.

Yeung, D.L., Pennell, M.D., Hall, J. and Leung, M. 1982. Food and nutrient intake of infants during the first 18 months of life. Nutr. Res. 2:3-12.

Yip, R., Johnson, C. and Dallman, P.R. 1984. Age-related changes in laboratory values used in the diagnosis of anemia and iron deficiency. Am. J. Clin. Nutr. 39:427-436.

Yip, R., Reeves, J.D., Lönnerdal, B., Keen, C.L. and Dallman, P.R. 1985. Does iron supplementation compromise zinc nutrition in healthy infants? Am. J. Clin. Nutr. 42:683-687.

Iodine

Function and Action

Iodine is an essential trace element whose sole known function is its role in the synthesis of the thyroid hormones. These hormones are required for normal calorigenesis, thermoregulation, intermediary metabolism, protein synthesis, reproduction, growth, development, hematopoiesis and neuromuscular function (Fisher and Carr 1974).

Iodine is ingested largely in the inorganic form as iodide or iodate salts. Oxidized forms are reduced in the gastrointestinal tract and are rapidly and completely absorbed and distributed throughout the extracellular fluid (Silva 1985). Some of the iodine is actively taken up by the gastric mucosa, the salivary glands and, during lactation, by the mammary glands. During lactation, 10% to 15% of the iodine intake can be excreted in the milk (Silva 1985). The iodine that is concentrated by the gastric mucosa and by the salivary glands is secreted back into the gastrointestinal tract from which it is reabsorbed.

The kidney clears iodine at a relatively constant rate, removing the iodide in 37 mL of plasma/min in adult men and 25 mL/min in adult females (Silva 1985). Thus excretion depends on plasma concentration, which is related to intake and thyroid clearance. During pregnancy, renal clearance is increased and may be important under conditions of limited iodine supply (Silva and Silva 1981).

The thyroid gland takes up iodine by an energy requiring process. The rate of uptake is dependent on the plasma inorganic iodide concentration and on thyroid stimulating hormone (TSH). In the thyroid, the iodide is oxidized by a peroxidase system and is incorporated into mono- and diiodotyrosine residues of thyroglobulin. These residues react in a coupling reaction to form the active thyroxine and triiodothyronine hormones. The iodinated thyroglobulin is taken up by endocytosis into the follicular cells, where the vesicles merge with lysosomes. The lysosomal proteases break down the thyroglobulin, releasing thyroxine and triiodothyronine, as well as iodotyrosine. The latter is stripped of its iodine, which is reutilized, while the hormones pass into the circulation by a passive mechanism (Cavalieri 1980). Although triiodothyronine is released from the thyroid, about 75% of the total circulating hormone is produced peripherally from the 5′-deiodination of thyroxine (Silva 1985). Every step in the biosynthesis of the hormones, from the uptake of iodine to the proteolysis of thyroglobulin, is stimulated by TSH. A fall in the concentration of thyroid hormone results in the release of thyrotropin releasing hormone from the hypothalamus which, in turn, causes release of TSH from the anterior pituitary. Thus, the synthesis of thyroid hormone is under a sensitive negative feedback control (Hershman and Pittman 1971).

Disease

Worldwide, iodine deficiency is one of the most common nutritional disorders, with an estimated 200 million people suffering from goitre, three million from overt cretinism and millions more from intellectual deficit. There is a consensus that 800 million are at risk from living in iodine-deficient environments (Hetzel *et al.* 1987). Goitre is caused by insufficient iodine intake, causing the thyroid to enlarge, as a result of TSH stimulation, so that more of the available iodine can be trapped. Maternal iodine deficiency causes teratogenic effects in the offspring, referred to as endemic cretinism, with symptoms of dwarfism, hypothyroidism, neuromuscular disturbances, deafness and mental retardation (Warkany 1985; Delange 1986).

In Canada, due to the mandatory addition of 76 µg of iodine/g of salt for table and general household use (Canada. Health and Welfare 1986), endemic goitre is no longer a problem. To the contrary, excessive intakes of iodine may now be a cause for concern. Recent evidence has suggested that a single injection of 480 mg of iodine as iodized oil, given intramuscularly to goitrous individuals, resulted in the appearance of thyroid autoantibodies (Boukis *et al.* 1983). Iodized salt, used prophylactically in an endemic goitre region of Argentina, resulted in an increase in lymphoid infiltration of the thyroid (Harach *et al.* 1985). In Britain it has been speculated that the increase in the incidence of thyrotoxicosis seen in the spring and early summer may be related to high milk iodine levels in winter. Intakes from milk of 119 µg/day during the winter and 18 µg/day during the summer were reported by males. The intakes by females were 108 µg and 19 µg/day respectively (Nelson and Phillips 1985). In the American Ten-State Nutrition Survey, the highest prevalence of goitre was found among persons excreting high levels of iodine, suggesting high intakes (Trowbridge *et al.* 1975). In Japan, high intakes of iodine have been associated with a high incidence of chronic lymphocytic thyroiditis in school children (Inoue *et al.* 1975). These studies indicate that both acute (Boukis *et al.* 1983) and chronic exposure (Harach *et al.* 1985) to large amounts of iodine may result in the onset of thyroiditis. Also, they suggest that women are at greater risk of developing thyroiditis than men (Inoue *et al.* 1975; Trowbridge *et al.* 1975; Harach *et al.* 1985). The results of these epidemiological studies have also been supported by data from animal experiments. With rats and chicks, dietary intakes of iodine from 15 times the recommended amount were shown to increase thyroglobulin antibodies and lymphocytic thyroiditis in genetically susceptible strains (Bagchi *et al.* 1985; Allen *et al.* 1986; Fischer at al. 1989).

The iodine intake of Canadians is in excess of 1000 µg/day, based on the analysis of a representative diet, with 60% coming from table salt and 25% from dairy products (Fischer and Giroux 1987a). Cow's milk is a key, and variable, source of iodine. Much of the iodine present in milk comes from ethylenediamine dihydroiodide (EDDI), added to feed to prevent footrot in cattle (Berg and Padgitt 1985), and from the improper use of iodophor sanitizers (Dunsmore and Wheeler 1977). Levels in retail milk samples collected from across Canada varied from <100 to >1300 µg/L (Fischer and Giroux 1987b). For some groups, this can be a very significant source of the element. Children aged 1-4, for instance, consume an average of 660 mL of milk per day (Canada. Health and Welfare 1977). In Ontario, the mean iodine concentration in partially skimmed milk was 380 µg/L. Thus the intake from this source in the above group would be 250 µg/day, or four times their recommended intake. If the samples that contained over 1000 µg/L were consumed routinely, along with high intakes from salt, levels of iodine causing undesirable effects on the thyroid could conceivably be ingested.

Recommendations

Since the publication of Recommended Nutrient Intakes for Canadians (Canada. Health and Welfare 1983), no new studies have been published to indicate that the recommendations require revision. Consequently, the same recommendations are made here. Briefly, they are calculated in the following manner. In order to maintain a normal plasma concentration of 0.15 µg/dL with a high normal renal clearance rate of 55 mL/min, a daily intake of 120 µg of iodine is required. Added to this requirement would be the high normal fecal excretion of 40 µg/day, resulting in a daily required intake of 160 µg/day. Balance studies have found that intakes ranging from 44 to 162 µg/day are sufficient to maintain positive balance. The recommended intake for adolescents and adults is therefore set at 160 µg/day. Mature human milk provides 4-9 µg of iodine/100 kcal, or 5-11 µg/500 kJ, and infant formula sold in Canada must contain 5 µg/100 kcal (6 µg/500 kJ). Since this amount appears to be adequate, the recommendation for infants is set at 5 µg/100 kcal (6 µg/500 kJ). This amount is similar to that recommended for adults and adolescents when expressed in terms of energy requirement. Thus, the recommendation for children is also set at 5 µg/100 kcal (6 µg/500 kJ). For pregnant women, an additional 25 µg/day is recommended (Canada. Health and Welfare 1983). In view of the potential detrimental effects that high intakes of iodine might have on thyroid function, intakes in excess of 1000 µg/day are not recommended.

References

Allen, E.M., Appel, M.C. and Braverman, L.E. 1986. The effect of iodide ingestion on the development of spontaneous lymphocytic thyroiditis in the diabetes-prone BB/W rat. Endocrinology 118:1977-1981.

Bagchi, N., Brown, T.R., Urdanivia, E. and Sundick, R.S. 1985. Induction of autoimmune thyroiditis in chickens by dietary iodine. Science 230:325-327.

Berg, J.N. and Padgitt, D. 1985. Iodine concentrations in milk of dairy cattle fed various levels of iodine as ethylenediamine dihydroiodide (EDDI) (Abst. p.70). J. Dairy Sci. 68 (Suppl. 1):139.

Boukis, M.A., Koutras, A., Souvatzoglou, A., Evangelopoulou, A., Vrontakis, M. and Moulopoulos, S.D. 1983. Thyroid hormone and immunological studies in endemic goiter. J. Clin. Endocrinol. Metab. 57:859-862.

Canada. Health and Welfare Canada. 1986. Departmental consolidation of the Food and Drugs Act and of the Food and Drug Regulations, Part B. Dept. of Supply and Services, Ottawa, B.17.003.

Canada. Health and Welfare. Nutrition Canada. Health Protection Branch. Bureau of Nutritional Sciences. 1977. Food consumption patterns report. Ottawa, pp. 27-43.

Canada. Health and Welfare. Health Protection Branch. Bureau of Nutritional Sciences. 1983. Iodine. *In* Recommended nutrient intakes for Canadians. Ottawa, pp. 136-140.

Cavalieri, R.R. 1980. Trace elements. A. Iodine. *In* Modern nutrition in health and disease. 6th ed. Goodhart, R.S. and Shils, M.E., eds. Lea & Febiger, Philadelphia, pp. 395-407.

Delange, F.M. 1986. Endemic cretinism. *In* Werner's the thyroid: a fundamental and clinical text. 5th ed. Ingbar, S.H. and Braverman, L.E., eds. Lippincott, Philadelphia, pp. 722-734.

Dunsmore, D.G. and Wheeler, S.M. 1977. Iodophors and iodine in dairy products. VIII. The total industry situation. Aust. J. Dairy Technol. 32:166-171.

Fischer, P.W.F. and Giroux, A. 1987a. Iodine content of a representative Canadian diet. J. Can. Diet. Assoc. 48:24-27.

Fischer, P.W.F. and Giroux, A. 1987b. Iodine content of Canadian retail milk samples. Can. Inst. Food Sci. Technol. J. 20:166-169.

Fischer, P.W.F., Campbell, J.S. and Giroux, A. 1989. Effect of dietary iodine on autoimmune thyroiditis in the BB Wistar rat. J. Nutr. 119:502-507.

Fisher, K.D. and Carr, C.J. 1974. Iodine in foods: chemical methodology and sources of iodine in the human diet. Life Sciences Research Office, Federation of American Societies for Experimental Biology, Washington.

Harach, H.R., Escalante, D.A., Onativia, A., Outes, J.L., Day, E.S. and Williams, E.D. 1985. Thyroid carcinoma and thyroiditis in an endemic goitre region before and after iodine prophylaxis. Acta Endocrinol. 108:55-60.

Hershman, J.M. and Pittman, J.A., Jr. 1971. Control of thyrotropin secretion in man. N. Engl. J. Med. 285:997-1006.

Hetzel, B.S., Dunn, J.T. and Stanbury, J.B., eds. 1987. The prevention and control of iodine deficiency disorders. Elsevier, Amsterdam.

Inoue, M., Taketani, N., Sato, T. and Nakajima, H. 1975. High incidence of chronic lymphocytic thyroiditis in apparently healthy school children: epidemiological and clinical study. Endocrinol. Jpn. 22:483-488.

Nelson, M. and Phillips, D.I.W. 1985. Seasonal variations in dietary iodine intake and thyrotoxicosis. Hum. Nutr.: Appl. Nutr. 39A:213-216.

Silva, J.E. 1985. Effects of iodine and iodine-containing compounds on thyroid function. Med. Clin. North Am. 69:881-898.

Silva, J.E. and Silva, S. 1981. Interrelationships among serum thyroxine, triiodothyronine, reverse triiodothyronine, and thyroid-stimulating hormone in iodine-deficient pregnant women and their offspring: effects of iodine supplementation. J. Clin. Endocrinol. Metab. 52:671-677.

Trowbridge, F.L., Hand, K.A. and Nichaman, M.Z. 1975. Findings relating to goiter and iodine in the Ten-State Nutrition Survey. Am. J. Clin. Nutr. 28:712-716.

Warkany, J. 1985. Teratogen update: iodine deficiency. Teratology 31:309-311.

Zinc

Function and Action

Zinc is an essential trace element for both animals and man. It is the sixth most common cation in the body, with a total of 2 to 3 g in adult man. The cation is found in all human tissues, varying in concentration from 10 µg to 200 µg per g wet weight. The highest zinc concentrations occur in the iris, retina and choroid of the eye, and in the prostate, prostatic secretions and spermatozoa (Sandstead 1985). Normal human serum contains a zinc concentration of approximately 120 µg/dL, a level that does not change readily with normal daily alterations in dietary intake (Wada *et al.* 1985).

The main biological function of zinc is its role in metalloenzymes. Over 200 zinc-containing enzymes have been identified (Falchuk and Vallee 1985). The diverse role of zinc in enzymes is demonstrated by the fact that each of the six enzyme categories contains at least one zinc metalloenzyme. Consequently, it plays an important part in the metabolism of proteins, carbohydrates, lipids and nucleic acids (Prasad 1979).

Chronic zinc deficiency in man was first documented in the Middle East in 1963 (Prasad *et al.* 1963). It has since been reported in a number of other developing countries. Deficiencies in these countries have been attributed to the high level of phytate and fibre present in the mainly cereal-based diets (Prasad 1979). Clinical manifestations of chronic zinc deficiency include growth retardation, hypogonadism in males, poor appetite, impaired taste acuity, mental lethargy and skin changes (Prasad 1983).

Marginal zinc intakes associated with low hair zinc levels, poor growth patterns and objective hypogeusia were reported in middle and low-income infants and children in Denver (Hambidge 1977). Recently, in Canada, 4-5 year old males with hair zinc levels of less than 70 µg/g (mean = 103 ± 35 µg/g) had a significantly lower mean height-for-age percentile than those with hair zinc levels greater than 70 µg/g. Using 3-day weighed food records, those male subjects with hair zinc concentrations of less than 70 µg/g and/or a height-for-age percentile of less than 15% consumed less food with readily available zinc, although their average zinc intake was similar to that of boys with hair zinc greater than 70 µg/g and/or a height-for-age percentile greater than 15%. In a zinc supplementation study, it was estimated that 4% of boys in Southern Ontario, aged five to seven years, would show a positive response to zinc supplementation in terms of increased height increment (Gibson, R.S., personal communication). These relationships were not observed for female preschool children in the study (Smit Vanderkooy and Gibson 1987).

Zinc absorption is affected by the amount of zinc in the diet (Wada *et al.* 1985), age (Turnlund *et al.* 1986) and the presence of interfering substances such as phosphate, fibre, iron and phytate, especially in the presence of high calcium intakes (Forbes and Erdman 1983; Prasad 1983; Solomons 1986). Foods from animal sources enhance the absorption and retention of zinc (Prasad 1979). When there is a decrease in dietary zinc concentration, the apparent efficiency of zinc absorption increases (Wada *et al.* 1985). When extremely low levels of zinc are ingested (0.3 mg/day), urinary excretion decreases (Baer and King 1984). In a 75-day metabolic study of adult men, in which zinc intakes were decreased from 16.5 mg/day to 5.5 mg, urinary zinc, however, did not decrease (Wada *et al.* 1985). In this study, fecal excretion decreased from 14.2 mg to 4.5 mg per day, probably due to a decrease in the unabsorbed zinc remaining in the gut. Another possible reason for the lower fecal excretion may be a decrease in the gastrointestinal secretion of endogenous zinc. The effect of varying intakes of dietary zinc on gastrointestinal zinc secretion has not been tested in humans, but Jackson *et al.* (1984) suggested that this responds quickly to dietary fluctuations, although by a relatively small amount.

The mixed Canadian diet provides approximately 5 mg/1000 kcal (6 mg/5000 kJ), with about one-half derived from meat, fish and poultry (Kirkpatrick and Coffin 1974; Srivastava *et al.* 1977). The zinc intake of 100 pre-menopausal women consuming self-selected diets was 10.1 ± 0.6 mg/day (Gibson and Scythes 1982) and that of 90 post-menopausal women was 7.6 mg/day, based on the analysis of one-day duplicate diet samples, and 10.1 mg/day, based on calculations from three-day dietary records (Gibson *et al.* 1985a). Thirty-six Canadian 22-month-old children were found to have an intake of 6.2 ± 1.7 mg/day (Gibson *et al.* 1985b). Canadian pre-school children, aged 4-5 years, had an intake of 6.9 ± 3.1 mg/day for boys and 6.0 ± 2.4 mg/day for girls. This was an average intake for both the males and females of 4.6 ± 1.0 mg/1000 kcal (Smit Vanderkooy and Gibson 1987). Red meat, liver, egg yolk, shellfish, poultry, milk, cheese and whole grain cereals are good sources of zinc (Murphy *et al.* 1975). Human milk contains between 1.1 and 2.6 µg/mL (Moser and Reynolds 1983), depending on the duration of lactation, while cow's milk contains 4.2 µg/mL (Anon. 1984). Over 90% of the zinc in cow's milk, however, is bound to casein, which is incompletely digested by infants, accounting for its lower bioavailability when compared to human milk (Roth and Kirchgessner 1985).

Disease Prevention

Little is known about the role of zinc in the etiology of chronic disease. There is some evidence to indicate that maternal zinc deficiency before and during pregnancy is associated with idiopathic intrauterine growth retardation and fetal congenital abnormalities (Jameson 1976; Cavdar *et al.* 1980; Mukherjee *et al.* 1984). Some of these malformations were similar to those produced experimentally in zinc-deficient animals (Hurley 1981). It has recently been suggested that the intrauterine growth retardation might occur through disturbed prostaglandin synthesis associated with zinc depletion (Simmer *et al.* 1985). Mothers of small-for-gestational-age infants had lower polymorphonuclear and mononuclear cell zinc content and higher PGE_2:F_{2a} ratios than mothers of appropriate-for-gestational-age babies. PGF_{2a} production and PGE2:F2a ratios were correlated with tissue zinc status (Simmer *et al.* 1985).

Depressed serum zinc concentrations and hyperzincuria were found in both type I and type II diabetes mellitus (Kinlaw *et al.* 1983; Canfield *et al.* 1984; Niewoehner *et al.* 1986). The increased urinary excretion of zinc is positively related to glucose excretion. It is suggested that this hyperzincuria may result in zinc deficiency and is one of the explanations for the fact that some children and adolescents with type I diabetes often display delayed growth and sexual development (Canfield *et al.* 1984). Furthermore, a decrease in taste acuity, one of the symptoms of sub-optimal zinc status, has been noted in some diabetic individuals (Hardy *et al.* 1981). It has been suggested that zinc deficiency also plays a role in abnormal immune function associated with type II diabetes mellitus (Niewoehner *et al.* 1986).

Abnormal zinc intakes have been associated with impaired immune function. Zinc deficiency produces hyperplasia of the thymus, spleen and lymph nodes (Schmidt and Bayer 1987). In children with zinc deficiency and protein energy malnutrition, zinc supplementation was able to reverse thymic atrophy (Golden *et al.* 1978). In marasmic infants, zinc supplementation resulted in a significant increase in serum IgA concentration, associated with an improved host defense mechanism (Castillo-Duran *et al.* 1987). Lymphocyte counts and T-lymphocyte killer cells were reduced in zinc deficiency (Fernades *et al.* 1979; Tapazoglou *et al.* 1985). Also, lymphocytes from zinc-deficient patients exhibited reduced proliferation when challenged with antigens and mitogens. This activity was restored by zinc supplementation (Cunningham-Rundles *et al.* 1979). Zinc is also essential for the phagocytic activity and bactericidal capacities of neutrophils (Briggs *et al.* 1981). Excessive intakes of zinc have also been shown to impair immune response. The ingestion of 150 mg of zinc twice a day for six weeks was associated with a reduction in lymphocyte stimulation response to phytohemagglutinin, as well as chemotaxis and phagocytosis of bacteria by polymorphonuclear leucocytes (Chandra 1984).

High intakes of zinc have been shown to affect copper metabolism in humans. Prasad *et al.* (1978) reported that 150 mg of zinc per day, given to a man suffering from sickle cell anemia, resulted in copper deficiency, marked by low serum copper levels and depressed ceruloplasmin levels. Abdulla (1979) showed that 45 mg of supplemental zinc per day, given to healthy adults, resulted in a 44% drop in serum copper concentrations when compared to controls. Fifty mg of supplemental zinc, given in two equal doses daily for six weeks, significantly reduced the activity of erythrocyte superoxide dismutase, an enzyme whose activity depends on copper status (Fischer *et al.* 1984). Raising the intake of zinc from 12 mg to 15.2 mg per day in adolescent girls caused an increase in the fecal excretion of copper (Greger *et al.* 1978).

In view of the potential detrimental effects of high intakes of zinc on the immune system (Chandra 1984), as well as on copper metabolism (Prasad *et al.* 1978), it is suggested that large supplementary amounts of the element be avoided. There is no scientific evidence to support the ingestion of megadoses of zinc, except in the treatment of Wilson's disease (Brewer *et al.* 1983) and sickle cell anemia (Prasad *et al.* 1978).

Recommendations

Adults

The zinc recommendations are established using the factorial approach whereby the obligatory zinc losses are divided by the fractional absorption to obtain the requirement. The endogenous zinc losses in males and females ingesting a diet providing only 0.3 mg of zinc per day were measured (Hess *et al.* 1977; Baer and King 1984). The sum of fecal, urinary and integumental losses were adjusted by linear regression to account for the decreased excretion seen with such low intakes of zinc. This gave an estimate of the obligatory excretion with normal intakes, which for women was equal to 1.6 mg per day and for men 2.2 mg per day. In women, losses due to menstrual fluids were negligible, while in men, one seminal emission would increase the loss by 0.6 mg per day (Hess *et al.* 1977; Baer and King 1984). In a five day turnover study of 12 females and five males between the ages of 21 and 73, using isotopically labelled zinc, Foster *et al.* (1979) reported an endogenous excretion of 2.7 mg of zinc per day. This value agrees with the endogenous fecal and urinary losses reported for older men, aged 65 to 74. Younger men, aged 22 to 30, had an endogenous loss of 3.8 mg per day (Turnlund *et al.* 1986). The endogenous losses, unlike those reported by Hess *et al.* (1977) and Baer and King (1984), occurred with an intake of 15.4 mg/day and do not represent obligatory losses. In studies attempting to establish the obligatory zinc loss, the coefficient of variation was large. In the study by Hess *et al.* (1977), in which female subjects were used, this coefficient was 44%. In the study of Baer and King (1984) with male subjects, the coefficient of variation was 43%.

In order to establish requirements from values for endogenous losses, the fractional absorption of dietary zinc must be estimated. This is difficult since the fractional absorption varies with the amount of zinc present in the diet, as well as with the dietary source (King 1986). Using stable isotopes to estimate absorption, the fractional absorption from a diet of mixed conventional food providing 16.4 mg of zinc per day was 24.7 ± 5.5%, while it was 52.6 ± 10.7% when the diet provided only 5.5 mg of zinc per day (Wada *et al.* 1985). If one assumes that the relationship between fractional absorption of zinc and dietary zinc concentration is linear, then 40% will be absorbed from a diet providing 10 mg of zinc per day (King 1986). A diet high in fibre and phytate, however, would tend to decrease the fractional absorption. Using radioisotopically labelled zinc, Foster *et al.* (1979) reported a fractional absorption of 37%. Unfortunately, they did not report the details of their diet. Turnlund *et al.* (1986) fed a semi-purified diet, supplemented with selected food items and labelled with stable isotopes of zinc, providing 15 mg of zinc per day to a group of young (age 22-30) and a group of elderly (age 65-74) men. They reported a fractional absorption of 31% and 17% respectively. Zinc balance, however, did not differ between the two groups, since the elderly men had a lower endogenous zinc excretion than the young men. Thus, there may be a lower requirement for absorbed zinc in the elderly.

In view of these data, it is assumed that the requirement to replace obligatory endogenous losses of the element is 2.2 mg per day for men and 1.6 mg per day for women. Since the coefficient of variation was 44% for men and 43% for women, applying a safety factor of 2 standard deviations would make the requirements 4.1 mg per day and 3.0 mg per day respectively. It is assumed that the safety factor is sufficient to provide for zinc losses through seminal emissions in men. Assuming a fractional absorption of 35%, 5% lower than the 40% estimated for a diet providing 10 mg of zinc per day to account for the presence of fibre and phytate, the recommended intake for males over 13 would be 12 mg per day and for females over 13, 9 mg per day.

Infants and Children

Human milk contains 2.6 ± 0.2 µg of zinc per mL at one month, and 1.3 to 0.1 mg/mL at three months (Moser and Reynolds 1983). Assuming that this provides adequate zinc, at an average intake of 750 mL of milk, the requirement for fully breast-fed infants is set at 2.0 mg/day for 0-4 months. The zinc concentration of breast milk decreases as postpartum time increases from 2.6 ± 0.2 µg/mL at one month to 1.1 ± 0.1 µg/mL at six months. Thus, infants older than five or six months may not get adequate zinc from breast milk alone (Moser and Reynolds 1983). It has recently been suggested, however, that the zinc requirements are highest during early infancy and decrease during later infancy due to the decrease in growth velocity (Krebs and Hambidge 1986). If this is the case, exclusively breast-fed infants are likely to get adequate zinc up to at least six months, despite the decrease in milk zinc concentration. The requirement for formula-fed infants is likely to be higher due to the lower zinc bioavailability. For children older than five months, inadequate data exist to allow for the establishment of firm dietary recommendations. However, a linear requirement to weight ratio was assumed for children six months to 13 years.

Pregnancy and Lactation

Schraer and Calloway (1974) calculated that in order to allow for a normal pregnancy weight gain, an additional 1.5 mg of zinc would have to be retained daily throughout pregnancy. Taper *et al.* (1985) showed that intakes of 8.9 ± 3.2 mg/day by pregnant women in their second trimester resulted in a retention of 1.9 ± 3.4 mg daily. This calculation, however, did not account for integumental losses, which are equal to approximately 0.5 mg daily. This would then bring the retention close to the requirement suggested by Schraer and Calloway (1974). Consequently, the recommendation for pregnant women, after applying a safety factor of two standard deviations to the above intake, is 15 mg per day.

If the assumption is made that 750 mL of milk are secreted daily by the lactating mother, providing 0.38 mg of zinc per 100 kcal (0.46 mg/500 kJ), and that human milk provides 67 kcal/dL (281 kJ/dL) (American Academy of Pediatrics 1977), then 1.9 mg of zinc are required daily. Assuming a fractional absorption of 35%, the recommendation for lactating women is an additional 6 mg of zinc daily, or a total of 15 mg per day.

References

Abdulla, M. 1979. Copper levels after oral zinc. Lancet 1:616.

American Academy of Pediatrics. Committee on Nutrition. 1977. Nutritional needs of low-birth-weight infants. Pediatrics 60:519-530.

Anonymous. 1984. Bioavailability of milk zinc in infants. Nutr. Rev. 42:220-222.

Baer, M.T. and King, J.C. 1984. Tissue zinc levels and zinc excretion during experimental zinc depletion in young men. Am. J. Clin. Nutr. 39:556-570.

Brewer, G.J., Hill, G.M., Prasad, A.S. and Cossack, Z.T. 1983. Oral zinc therapy for Wilson's disease. Ann. Intern. Med. 99:314-320.

Briggs, W.A., Pedersen, M., Mahajan, S., Sillix, D., Rabbani, P., McDonald, F. and Prasad, A. 1981. Mononuclear and polymorphonuclear cell function in zinc (Zn) deficient hemodialysis patients (abst.). Am. J. Clin. Nutr. 34:628.

Canfield, W.K., Hambidge, K.M. and Johnson, L.K. 1984. Zinc nutriture in type I diabetes mellitus: relationship to growth measures and metabolic control. J. Pediatr. Gastroenterol. Nutr. 3:577-584.

Castillo-Duran, C., Heresi, G., Fisberg, M. and Uauy, R. 1987. Controlled trial of zinc supplementation during recovery from malnutrition: effects on growth and immune function. Am. J. Clin. Nutr. 45:602-608.

Cavdar, A.O., Arcasoy, A., Baycu, T. and Himmetoglu, O. 1980. Zinc deficiency and anencephaly in Turkey. Teratology 22:141.

Chandra, R.K. 1984. Excessive intake of zinc impairs immune responses. J. Am. Med. Assoc. 252:1443-1446.

Cunningham-Rundles, C., Cunningham-Rundles, S., Garafolo, J., Iwata, T., Incefy, G., Twomey, J. and Good, R.A. 1979. Increased T-lymphocyte function and thymopoietin following zinc repletion in man (abst.). Fed. Proc. 38:1222.

Falchuk, K.H. and Vallee, B.L. 1985. Zinc and chromatin structure, composition and function. *In* Trace elements in man and animals — TEMA 5. Mills, C.F., Bremner, I. and Chesters, J.K., eds. Commonwealth Agricultural Bureaux, Farnham Royal, Slough, U.K., pp. 48-55.

Fernandes, G., Nair, M., Onoe, K., Tanaka, T., Floyd, R. and Good, R.A. 1979. Impairment of cell-mediated immunity functions by dietary zinc deficiency in mice. Proc. Nat. Acad. Sci. U.S.A. 76:457-461.

Fischer, P.W.F., Giroux, A. and L'Abbé, M.R. 1984. Effect of zinc supplementation on copper status in adult man. Am. J. Clin. Nutr. 40:743-746.

Forbes, R.M. and Erdman, J.W., Jr. 1983. Bioavailability of trace minerals. Annu. Rev. Nutr. 3:213-231.

Foster, D.M., Aamodt, R.L., Henkin, R.I. and Berman, M. 1979. Zinc metabolism in humans: a kinetic model. Am. J. Physiol. 237:R340-R349.

Gibson, R.S. and Scythes, C.A. 1982. Trace element intakes of women. Br. J. Nutr. 48:241-248.

Gibson, R.S., Martinez, O.B. and MacDonald, C.A. 1985a. The zinc, copper and selenium status of a selected sample of Canadian elderly women. J. Gerontol. 40:296-302.

Gibson, R.S., Friel, J.K. and Scythes, C.A. 1985b. The zinc, copper, and manganese status of a selected group of Canadian children twenty-two months of age. J. Can. Diet. Assoc. 46:182-185.

Golden, M.H.N., Golden, B.E., Harland, P.S.E.G. and Jackson, A.A. 1978. Zinc and immunocompetence in protein-energy malnutrition. Lancet 1:1226-1228.

Greger, J.L., Zaikis, S.C., Bennett, O.A., Abernathy, R.P. and Huffman, J. 1978. Mineral and nitrogen balances of adolescent females fed two levels of zinc (abst.). Fed. Proc. Fed. Am. Soc. Exp. Biol. 37:254.

Hambidge, K.M. 1977. The role of zinc and other trace metals in pediatric nutrition and health. Pediatr. Clin. North Am. 24:95-106.

Hardy, S.L., Brennand, C.P. and Wyse, B.W. 1981. Taste thresholds of individuals with diabetes mellitus and of control subjects. J. Am. Diet. Assoc. 79:286-289.

Hess, F.M., King, J.C. and Margen, S. 1977. Zinc excretion in young women on low zinc intakes and oral contraceptive agents. J. Nutr. 107:1610-1620.

Hurley, L.S. 1981. Teratogenic aspects of manganese, zinc, and copper nutrition. Physiol. Rev. 61:249-295.

Jackson, M.J., Jones, D.A., Edwards, R.H.T., Swainbank, I.G. and Coleman, M.L. 1984. Zinc homeostasis in man: studies using a new stable isotope-dilution technique. Br. J. Nutr. 51:199208.

Jameson, S. 1976. Zinc and copper in pregnancy. Correlations to fetal and maternal complications. Acta Med. Scand., Suppl. 593:5-20.

King, J.C. 1986. Assessment of techniques for determining human zinc requirements. J. Am. Diet. Assoc. 86:1523-1528.

Kinlaw, W.B., Levine, A.S., Morley, J.E., Silvis, S.E. and McClain, C.J. 1983. Abnormal zinc metabolism in type II diabetes mellitus. Am. J. Med. 75:273-277.

Kirkpatrick, D.C. and Coffin, D.E. 1974. The trace metal content of representative Canadian diets in 1970 and 1971. Can. Inst. Food Sci. Technol. J. 7:56-58.

Krebs, N.F. and Hambidge, K.M. 1986. Zinc requirements and zinc intakes of breast-fed infants. Am. J. Clin. Nutr. 43:288-292.

Moser, P.B. and Reynolds, R.D. 1983. Dietary zinc intake and zinc concentrations of plasma, erythrocytes, and breast milk in antepartum and postpartum lactating and nonlactating women: a longitudinal study. Am. J. Clin. Nutr. 38:101-108.

Mukherjee, M.D., Sandstead, H.H., Ratnaparkhi, M.V., Johnson, L.K., Milne, D.B. and Stelling, H.P. 1984. Maternal zinc, iron, folic acid, and protein nutriture and outcome of human pregnancy. Am. J. Clin. Nutr. 40:496-507.

Murphy, E.W., Willis, B.W. and Watt, B.K. 1975. Provisional tables on the zinc content of foods. J. Am. Diet. Assoc. 66:345-355.

Niewoehner, C.B., Allen, J.I., Boosalis, M., Levine, A.S. and Morley, J.E. 1986. Role of zinc supplementation in type II diabetes mellitus. Am. J. Med. 81:63-68.

Prasad, A.S. 1979. Zinc in human nutrition. CRC Press, Boca Raton, Fla.

Prasad, A.S. 1983. Clinical, biochemical and nutritional spectrum of zinc deficiency in human subjects: an update. Nutr. Rev. 41:197-208.

Prasad, A.S., Miale, A., Jr., Farid, Z., Sandstead, H.H. and Schulert, A.R. 1963. Zinc metabolism in patients with the syndrome of iron deficiency anemia, hepatosplenomegaly, dwarfism and hypogonadism. J. Lab. Clin. Med. 61:537-549.

Prasad, A.S., Brewer, G.J., Schoomaker, E.B. and Rabbani, P. 1978. Hypocupremia induced by zinc therapy in adults. J. Am. Med. Assoc. 240:2166-2168.

Roth, H.P. and Kirchgessner, M. 1985. Utilization of zinc from picolinic acid or citric acid complexes in relation to dietary protein source in rats. J. Nutr. 115:1641-1649.

Sandstead, H.H. 1985. Requirement of zinc in human subjects. J. Am. Coll. Nutr. 4:73-82.

Schmidt, K.H. and Bayer, W. 1987. Interactions of minerals and trace elements with host defense mechanisms - a review article. Trace Elem. Med. 4:35-41.

Schraer, K.K. and Calloway, D.H. 1974. Zinc balance in pregnant teenagers. Nutr. Metab. 17:205-212.

Simmer, K., Punchard, N.A., Murphy, G. and Thompson, R.P.H. 1985. Prostaglandin production and zinc depletion in human pregnancy. Pediatr. Res. 19:697-700.

Smit Vanderkooy, P.D. and Gibson, R.S. 1987. Food consumption patterns of Canadian preschool children in relation to zinc and growth status. Am. J. Clin. Nutr. 45:609-616.

Solomons, N.W. 1986. Competitive interaction of iron and zinc in the diet: consequences for human nutrition. J. Nutr. 116:927-935.

Srivastava, U.S., Nadeau, M.H. and Carbonneau, N. 1977. Mineral intakes of university students. Zinc content. J. Can. Diet. Assoc. 38:302-308.

Tapazoglou, E., Prasad, A.S., Hill, G., Brewer, G.J. and Kaplan, J. 1985. Decreased natural killer cell activity in patients with zinc deficiency with sickle cell disease. J. Lab. Clin. Med. 105:19-22.

Taper, L.J., Oliva, J.T. and Ritchey, S.J. 1985. Zinc and copper retention during pregnancy: the adequacy of prenatal diets with and without dietary supplementation. Am. J. Clin. Nutr. 41:1184-1192.

Turnlund, J.R., Durkin, N., Costa, F. and Margen, S. 1986. Stable isotope studies of zinc absorption and retention in young and elderly men. J. Nutr. 116:1239-1247.

Wada, L., Turnlund, J.R. and King, J.C. 1985. Zinc utilization in young men fed adequate and low zinc intakes. J. Nutr. 115:1345-1354.

Copper

Function and Action

Copper is an essential trace element which occurs in adult man at levels from 70 to 100 mg, with one-third being present in the liver and brain, one-third in the musculature, and one-third dispersed in other tissues (Mason 1979).

The main function of copper is its role in the cuproenzymes that catalyze oxido-reduction reactions. Examples of these are ceruloplasmin (ferroxidase I), Cu,Zn-superoxide dismutase, lysyl oxidase, tyrosinase, cytochrome c oxidase and dopamine β-hydroxylase. Thus, copper is important in erythropoiesis, antioxidant protection, connective tissue formation, pigmentation of the integument, oxidative phosphorylation and catecholamine synthesis.

Manifestations of copper deficiency are related to decreased activities of the cuproenzymes. These include: anemia, due to diminished ferroxidase activity, leading to impaired transport of iron to the erythropoietic sites; skeletal and vascular effects, due to decreased lysyl oxidase activity, which catalyzes the cross-linking in collagen and elastin; achromotrichia, due to impaired melanin synthesis, as a result of lower tyrosinase activity; and CNS disturbances due to myelinization derangements, abnormal catecholamine concentrations associated with diminished dopamine β-hydroxylase activity, and decreased levels of cytochrome c oxidase (Mason 1979). Copper deficiency in man is rare. The first case was reported in 1964 in a marasmic infant exclusively fed a cow's milk diet (Cordano *et al.* 1964). It has also been seen in patients receiving copper-free total parenteral nutrition (Karpel and Peden 1972), in individuals receiving zinc therapy for sickle cell anemia (Prasad *et al.* 1978) and in a woman whose normal diet was supplemented with antacids (Anon. 1984).

Copper absorption takes place mainly in the duodenum (Mason 1979). The copper moves from the intestinal lumen into the mucosal cells by simple diffusion (Fischer and L'Abbé 1985), where it binds to a high molecular weight protein fraction and to metallothionein. The latter acts as an "intestinal block". The synthesis of metallothionein is induced by zinc, and thus, at high zinc intakes, the increased amounts of metallothionein bind copper making it unavailable for serosal transfer. This is the basis for the interaction between zinc and copper (Fischer *et al.* 1983).

Biliary excretion is the major route of copper loss in man, with additional losses occurring through the urine, saliva, gastrointestinal secretions, menses and sweat (Williams 1983). The role that these various excretory pathways play in copper homeostasis is not known.

Since copper is ubiquitous in plants and animals, it is widely distributed in foods. The richest sources are liver and shellfish. Other sources, in descending order of concentration, are nuts, high-protein cereals, dried fruits, poultry, fish, meats, legumes, root vegetables, leafy vegetables, fresh fruits and non-leafy vegetables. Cow's milk is one of the poorest sources in our food supply (Mason 1979).

Disease Prevention

In 1973, based on studies in rats, Klevay (1973, 1975) postulated that a relative or absolute deficiency of copper, characterized by a high dietary zinc to copper ratio, is hypercholesterolemic, and thus, an important risk factor in the etiology of cardiovascular disease. It has been demonstrated in a number of species that feeding a copper deficient diet results in increased serum cholesterol levels (Klevay *et al.* 1984). This effect, to date, however, has been reported in only a single human. A young adult man was fed a diet providing 0.8 mg of copper per day for a period of 105 days. During that time, erythrocyte Cu,Zn-superoxide dismutase activity, ceruloplasmin concentration and plasma copper concentration dropped. Plasma cholesterol increased from 202 to 234 mg/dL. Upon repletion with 4 mg of supplemental copper per day for 39 days, these parameters returned to normal (Klevay *et al.* 1984). Other studies relating copper intakes to serum cholesterol levels in humans gave results that were inconsistent with Klevay's findings (Medeiros *et al.* 1983; Shapcott *et al.* 1985). Recently, a study in which the copper concentration of various tissues removed at autopsy was related to the severity of coronary artery and aortic sclerosis, found a significant inverse relationship between liver copper concentration and sclerosis, thus supporting Klevay's hypothesis (Aalbers and Houtman 1985).

Rats fed a copper deficient diet were shown to have abnormal electrocardiograms (Klevay and Viestenz 1981). In other rat studies, it was shown that severe copper deficiency, leading to sudden death by heart rupture, was reduced when the low copper diets included starch rather than sucrose or fructose (Reiser *et al.* 1983). In a human study, designed to compare the effects of ingesting low copper diets containing either 20% fructose or 20% starch on copper status, four of the 24 subjects exhibited heart-related abnormalities. Three of the four (two exhibiting tachycardia and one a type II, second degree heart block) had ingested the fructose diet for at least four weeks (Reiser *et al.* 1985). Although there may be other reasons to explain these heart-related abnormalities, this study does suggest that low copper intakes might be related to cardiovascular disease.

Since copper is so efficiently metabolized, excesses rarely develop in humans. When they do arise, especially due to acute poisoning, they can be fatal, resulting in ulceration of the intestinal mucosa, hepatic cell necrosis, nausea, vomiting, diarrhea, hemolysis, hemoglobinuria and jaundice (Zelkowitz *et al.* 1980). High intakes, solely from the diet, pose no threat of causing copper toxicity.

Recommendations

Adults

The analyses of representative Canadian diets have shown daily copper intakes of 2.1 and 1.6 mg (Kirkpatrick and Coffin 1974, 1977). The mean daily calculated copper intakes of 100 Canadian pre-menopausal women was 1.9 ± 0.6 mg, based on three day dietary records (Gibson and Scythes 1982). The mean calculated intake of 90 post-menopausal Canadian women, again based on three day dietary records, was 1.9 mg/day (Gibson *et al.* 1985a). Three day dietary records of Canadian children, aged 22 months, indicated a mean intake of 1.1 ± 0.5 mg/day (Gibson *et al.* 1985b). Sixty-two Canadian boys, aged 4 to 5 years, had copper intakes of 1.1 ± 0.4 mg/day and 44 Canadian girls of the same age had an intake of 0.9 ± 0.4 mg/day (Smit Vanderkooy and Gibson 1987). In the U.S., lower intakes of 1.0 ± 0.1 mg/day have been reported (Holden *et al.* 1979). A survey of intakes of American adult males, infants and toddlers from 1974 to 1982 indicates dietary intakes of 1.57, 0.56 and 0.7 mg/day respectively (Pennington *et al.* 1984).

Most attempts to estimate human copper requirements have used balance studies. In 13 men, fed conventional American diets containing 16% protein, 40% fat and 44% carbohydrates, linear regression of balance results (intake minus fecal and urinary excretion) indicated a daily requirement of 1.30 mg of copper (Klevay *et al.* 1980). Surface losses were not included, but in a separate publication were reported to be 0.34 ± 0.24 mg/day (Jacob *et al.* 1981). If it is assumed that copper absorption is approximately 40% (Turnlund *et al.* 1983), then this surface loss will add another 0.85 mg to the daily requirement. Thus, the requirement will be just over 2 mg of copper per day. This seems to be significantly higher than the reported intakes cited above, especially those from the U.S. The discrepancies may be due to the relatively short duration of the balance studies, and clearly indicate the inadequacies of this approach in estimating copper requirements. The study by Klevay *et al.* (1984), using the depletion-repletion approach, is a much better way of establishing requirements. In this study, already discussed above, a male adult was given a diet containing 0.87 mg of copper per day for 105 days, during which time a number of functional indicators of copper status changed. During the 39 day repletion period, these indicators again returned to normal. This suggested that an intake of 0.86 mg/day was insufficient for this individual. More studies of this type must be carried out before a satisfactory estimate of copper requirements can be made. In the meantime, an intake of 2 mg of copper per day for adults seems to be adequate and safe.

Infants and Children

The copper content of human milk is 0.6 ± 0.12 µg/mL on day five of lactation and declines to 0.41 ± 0.04 µg/mL by day 28. The average daily intake of copper by infants from human milk over a one month period was reported to be 0.25 mg (Casey *et al.* 1985). Vuori (1979) reported daily intakes by exclusively breast fed infants of 0.31, 0.26 and 0.25 mg during the first, second, and third month of lactation respectively. The recommended amount of copper for infant formulas is 60 µg/100 kcal (72 µg/500 kJ), which is approximately equal to a daily intake of 0.3 mg (American Academy of Pediatrics 1977). This seems to be an adequate intake, especially since neonates have a proportionally higher copper content in their livers than do adults (Turnlund *et al.* 1983). Balance studies carried out on children aged three to 10 years suggest requirements of from 0.05 to 0.1 mg/kg/day, depending on the study (Mason 1979). As is the case for adults, insufficient data exist to allow the establishment of definite recommendations.

References

Aalbers, T.G. and Houtman, J.P.W. 1985. Relationships between trace elements and atherosclerosis. Sci. Total Environ. 43:255-283.

American Academy of Pediatrics. Committee on Nutrition. 1977. Nutritional needs of low-birth-weight infants. Pediatrics 60:519-530.

Anonymous. 1984. Conditioned copper deficiency due to antacids. Nutr. Rev. 42:319-321.

Casey, C.E., Hambidge, K.M. and Neville, M.C. 1985. Studies in human lactation: zinc, copper, manganese and chromium in human milk in the first month of lactation. Am. J. Clin. Nutr. 41:1193-1200.

Cordano, A., Baertl, J.M. and Graham, G.G. 1964. Copper deficiency in infancy. Pediatrics 34:324-336.

Fischer, P.W.F., Giroux, A. and L'Abbé, M.R. 1983. Effects of zinc on mucosal copper binding and on the kinetics of copper absorption. J. Nutr. 113:462-469.

Fischer, P.W.F. and L'Abbé, M.R. 1985. Copper transport by intestinal brush border membrane vesicles from rats fed high zinc or copper deficient diets. Nutr. Res. 5:759-767.

Gibson, R.S. and Scythes, C.A. 1982. Trace element intakes of women. Br. J. Nutr. 48:241-248.

Gibson, R.S., Martinez, O.B. and MacDonald, A.C. 1985a. The zinc, copper and selenium status of a selected sample of Canadian elderly women. J. Gerontol. 40:296-302.

Gibson, R.S., Friel, J.K. and Scythes, C.A. 1985b. The zinc, copper and manganese status of a selected group of Canadian children twenty-two months of age. J. Can. Diet. Assoc. 46:182-185.

Holden, J.M., Wolf, W.R. and Mertz, W. 1979. Zinc and copper in self-selected diets. J. Am. Diet. Assoc. 75:23-28.

Jacob, R.A., Sandstead, H.H., Munoz, J.M., Klevay, L.M. and Milne, D.B. 1981. Whole body surface loss of trace metals in normal males. Am. J. Clin. Nutr. 34:1379-1383.

Karpel, J.T. and Peden, V.H. 1972. Copper deficiency in long-term parenteral nutrition. J. Pediatr. 80:32-36.

Kirkpatrick, D.C. and Coffin, D.E. 1974. The trace metal content of representative Canadian diets in 1970 and 1971. Can. Inst. Food Sci. Technol. J. 7:56-58.

Kirkpatrick, D.C. and Coffin, D.E. 1977. The trace metal content of a representative Canadian diet in 1972. Can. J. Public Health 68:162-164.

Klevay, L.M. 1973. Hypercholesterolemia in rats produced by an increase in the ratio of zinc to copper ingested. Am. J. Clin. Nutr. 26:1060-68.

Klevay, L.M. 1975. Coronary heart disease: the zinc/copper hypothesis. Am. J. Clin. Nutr. 28:764-774.

Klevay, L.M. and Viestenz, K.E. 1981. Abnormal electrocardiograms in rats deficient in copper. Am. J. Physiol. 240:H185-H189.

Klevay, L.M., Reck, S.J., Jacob, R.A., Logan, G.M., Munoz, J.M. and Sandstead, H.H. 1980. The human requirement for copper. I. Healthy men fed conventional, American diets. Am. J. Clin. Nutr. 33:45-50.

Klevay, L.M., Inman, L., Johnson, L.K., Lawler, M., Mahalko, J.R., Milne, D.B., Lukaski, H.C., Bolonchuk, W. and Sandstead, H.H. 1984. Increased cholesterol in plasma in a young man during experimental copper depletion. Metabolism 33:1112-1118.

Mason, K.E. 1979. A conspectus of research on copper metabolism and requirements of man. J. Nutr. 109:1979-2066.

Medeiros, D., Pellum, L. and Brown, B. 1983. Serum lipids and glucose as associated with hemoglobin levels and copper and zinc intake in young adults. Life Sci. 32:1897-1904.

Pennington, J.A.T., Wilson, D.B., Newell, R.F., Harland, B.F., Johnson, R.D. and Vanderveen, J.E. 1984. Selected minerals in foods surveys, 1974-1981/82. J. Am. Diet. Assoc. 84:771-780.

Prasad, A.S., Brewer, G.J., Schoomaker, E.B. and Rabbani, P. 1978. Hypocupremia induced by zinc therapy in adults. J. Am. Med. Assoc. 240:2166-2168.

Reiser, S., Ferretti, R.J., Fields, M. and Smith, J.C., Jr. 1983. Role of dietary fructose in the enhancement of mortality and biochemical changes associated with copper deficiency in rats. Am. J. Clin. Nutr. 38:214-222.

Reiser, S., Smith, J.C., Jr., Mertz, W., Holbrook, J.T., Scholfield, D.J., Powell, A.S., Canfield, W.K. and Canary, J.J. 1985. Indices of copper status in humans consuming a typical American diet containing either fructose or starch. Am. J. Clin. Nutr. 42:242-251.

Shapcott, D., Vobecky, J.S., Vobecky, J. and Demers, P.P. 1985. Plasma cholesterol and the plasma copper/zinc ratio in young children. Sci. Total Environ. 42:197-200.

Smit Vanderkooy, P.D. and Gibson, R.S. 1987. Food consumption patterns of Canadian preschool children in relation to zinc and growth status. Am. J. Clin. Nutr. 45:609-616.

Turnlund, J.R., Swanson, C.A. and King, J.C. 1983. Copper absorption and retention in pregnant women fed diets based on animal and plant proteins. J. Nutr. 113:2346-2352.

Vuori, E. 1979. Intake of copper, iron, manganese and zinc by healthy, exclusively-breast-fed infants during the first three months of life. Br. J. Nutr. 42:407-411.

Williams, D.M. 1983. Copper deficiency in humans. Semin. Hematol. 20:118-128.

Zelkowitz, M., Verghese, J.P. and Antel, J. 1980. Copper and zinc in the nervous system. *In* Zinc and copper in medicine. Karcioglu, Z.A. and Sarper, R.M., eds. C.C. Thomas, Springfield, Ill., pp. 418-463.

Fluoride

Function and Action

Approximately 99% of the fluoride in the body occurs in bones and teeth. The level of fluoride in human bone increases with age and up to about 2500 µg/g fat-free dry weight, it does not have any harmful effect (Underwood 1977; WHO 1984). Seventy-five percent of the fluoride of blood is in the plasma. The serum or plasma level of fluoride depends on the level in the drinking water. In low fluoride areas where drinking water is fluoridated to 1 mg/L, the serum level ranges from 10 to 15 mg/L. The level is increased approximately five-fold in areas where the natural level of fluoride is about 4 mg/L. Normal levels of fluoride in other soft tissues are less than 1 mg/kg wet weight. Higher levels may be found in the aorta, tendons, cartilage and placenta (WHO 1984).

The requirement for fluoride in man and large animals is specific for the reduction of dental caries. Several attempts to demonstrate its essentiality for growth and reproduction in experimental animals have not been successful (Richmond 1985; Krishnamachari 1987).

The absorption of small amounts of soluble fluoride (such as sodium fluoride) by man is so rapid that maximum blood levels are reached within 1 h, and 20-30% of the absorbed fluoride appears in urine in the succeeding 3-4 h (Krishnamachari 1987). Metabolic studies have shown that the absorption of fluoride from insoluble sources such as fish protein concentrate is slightly less than that from sodium fluoride. High dietary calcium and phosphorus increase the fecal excretion of fluoride, but the fluoride balance remains unaffected. In younger persons, but not in adults, fluoride balance is positive, probably because of rapidly growing bones which have more trabecular bone (Shah and Belonje 1988). Fluoride metabolism in women during early and late pregnancy is not markedly altered, although the balance is slightly positive (Maheshwari *et al.* 1983).

Intake

The fluoride intake of infants in Canada was reported to be 0.25 mg/day in nonfluoridated communities, and 0.47 mg/day in communities with fluoridated water supplies. On a body weight basis the fluoride intakes ranged from 0.02 to 0.18 mg/kg (Dabeka *et al.* 1982). These intakes were within the range recommended by the Nutrition Committee of the Canadian Pediatric Society (1987). The diet of Canadian adults living in fluoridated (1 mg F/L water) areas was found to contain an average of 2.8 mg F/day (40 µg/kg/day), whereas the fluoride intake in nonfluoridated communities (less than 0.2 mg F/L water) was only 0.56 mg/day (8.5 µg/kg/day). The median intakes were about three-quarters of the means. Water and beverages provided 70% and 80% of the total fluoride intake in nonfluoridated and fluoridated communities respectively (Dabeka *et al.* 1987). These intakes are comparable to those reported from the U.S.A., U.K. and some other parts of the world (Subba Rao 1984). Tea, fish products and mechanically deboned meats are high in fluoride, and a variation in the consumption of these foods can appreciably affect the fluoride intake (Walters *et al.* 1983; Smid and Kruger 1985; Dabeka *et al.* 1987). Human milk is very low in fluoride (4-8 ng/mL) because its transfer from plasma to milk is minimal (Ekstrand *et al.* 1984a,b). Cow's milk in Canada contains 40 ng/mL; infant formula manufactured in Canada contains less than 300 ng/mL. There is no placental barrier against fluoride under normal conditions (WHO 1984).

Toxicity

Skeletal fluorosis occurs through long-term exposure to an excess of fluoride, usually because of high natural levels in drinking water (4 mg/L or more) or because of the air around factories producing aluminium, magnesium or superphosphate (WHO 1984). In the Guizhou province of China, however, foods containing abnormally high amounts have been reported to cause skeletal fluorosis. Dental fluorosis due to foodborne fluoride was also observed in Thailand and Vietnam (Krishnamachari 1987). Although exposure to high levels of fluoride in drinking water has been implicated in increased mortality due to cancer, heart disease, intracranial lesions, nephritis, cirrhosis, mongoloid births or total deaths, the evidence is not convincing (Richmond 1985).

Disease Prevention

In temperate areas where the natural fluoride level is low, the fluoridation of drinking water to 1 mg/L reduces the incidence of dental caries in children by 40% to 60%. This protection continues into adulthood (WHO 1984; Richmond 1985). Alternative methods of providing fluoride, such as the fluoridation of salt, flour, or milk, taking fluoride tablets, or the topical application of fluorides have a similar effect, but they are not as successful (WHO 1984). Fluoridation of water to 1 mg/L therefore is strongly recommended. At present, only 39.2% of the Canadian population receives fluoridated water. The proportions in Manitoba and Ontario are high (74% and 63%), whereas they are lowest in British Columbia and Newfoundland (12% and 8% respectively) (Wood, G., personal communication). Fluoride has also been used therapeutically in the treatment of osteoporosis (Shah and Belonje 1988) and osteosclerosis (WHO 1984) but the results are equivocal.

Recommendations

Requirement can only be based on the beneficial effect on dental caries; the optimal level in drinking water for the cariostatic effect in children has been established at 1 mg/L in temperate regions. Moreover, this effect of water fluoridation continues into adulthood. A significant reduction in the prevalence of cemental caries in middle-aged and older people has also been attributed to fluoride ions (WHO 1984). Also, the Joint Public Information Committee of the American Institute of Nutrition and the American Society for Clinical Nutrition (1986) confirmed that the fluoridation of community water supplies to an optimum level, wherever the natural level is less than required, is a safe, economical and effective measure to improve dental health. It is recommended that water contain one part per million of fluoride.

For infants and children there is no need for a fluoride supplement if the drinking water contains more than 0.7 mg/L fluoride. If the level in the drinking water is less than 0.7 mg/L, the recommended fluoride supplement ranges from 0.25 to 1 mg/day depending on the age of the child and the fluoride level in the water (Table 17). Prenatal fluoride supplements are not recommended at present (Canadian Pediatric Society 1987; Canada. Health and Welfare Canada 1988).

Table 17.
Recommended Fluoride Supplements for Children with Different Water Supplies[a]

Fluoride in water supply (mg/L)	> 0.3	0.3-0.7	< 0.7
Age		Supplemental fluoride ion (mg/day)[b]	
0 - 2 years[c]	0.25	0	0
2 - 3 years	0.50	0.25	0
3 - 12 years	1.00	0.50	0

a. Canadian Paediatric Society 1987.
b. 2.21 mg of sodium fluoride provides 1.0 mg of fluoride iron in either fluorine tablets or solution.
c. Start supplements in the first few months of life.

References

Canada. Health and Welfare. Health Services Directorate. 1988. Preventive dental services. 2nd ed. Ottawa.

Canadian Paediatric Society. Nutrition Committee. 1987. Fluoride supplementation. Contemporary Pediatr. (Canada) March/April:50-56.

Dabeka, R.W. and McKenzie, A.D. 1987. Lead, cadmium and fluoride levels in market milk and infant formulas in Canada. J. Assoc. Off. Anal. Chem. 70:754-757.

Dabeka, R.W., McKenzie, A.D., Conacher, H.B.S. and Kirkpatrick, D.C. 1982. Determination of fluoride in Canadian infant foods and calculation of fluoride intakes by infants. Can. J. Public Health 73:188-191.

Dabeka, R.W., McKenzie, A.D. and LaCroix, G.M.A. 1987. Dietary intakes of lead, cadmium, arsenic and fluoride by Canadian adults: a 24-hour duplicate diet study. Food Addit. Contam. 4:89-102.

Ekstrand, J., Hardell, L.I. and Spak, C.J. 1984a. Fluoride balance studies on infants in a 1-ppm-water-fluoride area. Caries Res. 18:87-92.

Ekstrand, J., Spak, C.J., Falch, J., Afseth, J. and Ulvestad, H. 1984b. Distribution of fluoride to human breast milk following intake of high doses of fluoride. Caries Res. 18:93-95.

Joint Public Information Committee of the American Institute of Nutrition and The American Society for Clinical Nutrition. 1986. Special announcement — resolution on fluoridation of drinking water. J. Nutr. 116:176.

Krishnamachari, K.A.V.R. 1987. Fluorine. *In* Trace elements in human and animal nutrition. Vol. 1. 5th ed. Mertz, W., ed. Academic Press, New York, pp 365-415.

Maheshwari, U.R., King, J.C., Leybin, L., Newbrun, E. and Hodge, H.C. 1983. Fluoride balances during early and late pregnancy. JOM, J. Occup. Med. 25:587-590.

Richmond, V.L. 1985. Thirty years of fluoridation: a review. Am. J. Clin. Nutr. 41:129-138.

Shah, B.G. and Belonje, B. 1988. Calcium and bone health of women. Nutr. Res. 8:431-442.

Smid, J.R. and Kruger, B.J. 1985. The fluoride content of some teas available in Australia. Aust. Dent. J. 30:25-28.

Subba Rao, G. 1984. Dietary intake and bioavailability of fluoride. Annu. Rev. Nutr. 4:115-136.

Underwood, E.J. 1977. Fluorine. *In* Trace elements in human and animal nutrition. 4th ed. Academic Press, New York, pp. 347-374.

Walters, C.B., Sherlock, J.C., Evans, W.H. and Read, J.I. 1983. Dietary intake of fluoride in the United Kingdom and fluoride content of some foodstuffs. J. Sci. Food Agric. 34:523-528.

WHO. 1984. Fluorine and fluorides. Environmental Health Criteria 36. Geneva.

Manganese

Function and Action

Manganese is an essential trace element in both animals and man. The total amount of manganese in the body of the adult man has been estimated to be 10-20 mg, with the highest concentration present in those tissues rich in mitochondria, such as liver, pancreas and kidney. Up to 25% of total body manganese is present in the skeleton and is not readily mobilized (Keen *et al.* 1984a).

Manganese functions as both an enzyme activator and as a constituent of metalloenzymes. The first function is a non-specific one. Manganese ions are chemically similar to magnesium ions, and can activate many enzymes, such as kinases, decarboxylases, hydrolases and transferases, enzymes which are also activated by magnesium (Keen *et al.* 1984a). Manganese is a specific activator of the glycosyl transferases, and is therefore required for normal glycosaminoglycan and glycoprotein synthesis. Manganese is an integral constituent of arginase, pyruvate carboxylase and mitochondrial superoxide dismutase (Keen *et al.* 1984a).

Manganese deficiency in animals consuming natural diets is very rare, with the exception of the avian species. When deficiency does occur, however, its main manifestations, seen in all species, but varying with the degree and duration of deficiency and with the stage of development during which the deficiency occurs, are impaired growth, skeletal abnormalities, disturbed reproductive function, ataxia of the newborn and defects in lipid and carbohydrate metabolism (Hurley and Keen 1987). The gross effect of manganese deficiency on the skeletal system can be explained in terms of its effect on mucopolysaccharide synthesis (Hurley and Keen 1987). There have been only two studies reporting manganese deficiency in humans (Doisy 1973; Friedman *et al.* 1987). In the first, an adult male subject was given a purified diet in which manganese was inadvertently omitted. The symptoms thought to be associated with manganese deficiency were loss of weight, transient dermatitis, nausea and vomiting, reddening of hair colour, hypocholesterolemia and a prolonged clotting time. It was postulated that manganese is required for the biosynthesis of glycoproteins involved in clotting, and that it is a cofactor in the synthesis of cholesterol (Doisy 1973). In the second study, five of seven subjects fed a semi-purified diet providing 0.11 mg of manganese per day for 39 days developed transient dermatitis and hypocholesterolemia, symptoms similar to those reported by Doisy (1973) (Friedman *et al.* 1987).

Absorption of manganese appears to occur equally well throughout the length of the small intestine. In the adult human, intestinal absorption has been estimated to range from 3% to 8% (Mena 1981; Sandström *et al.* 1985). The fractional absorption of manganese is independent of dietary concentration (Mena 1981). It can, however, be affected by other dietary factors. Lactose was shown to increase manganese absorption in rats (King *et al.* 1979). Manganese bioavailability is enhanced by ascorbic acid and by meat-containing diets, and is decreased by iron and some dietary fibre sources, including wheat bran and hemicellulose. At high manganese intakes ascorbic acid decreases bioavailability (Kies *et al.* 1987). Although tea contains large amounts of manganese, it is essentially unavailable to humans (Kies *et al.* 1987). The ingestion of ethanol increases the intestinal transport of manganese (Keen *et al.* 1984a). In animal experiments, feeding iron-supplemented milk at a level comparable to that found in iron-fortified infant formula resulted in a significantly lower liver manganese concentration (Keen *et al.* 1984b). The significance of this observation to human infant nutrition remains to be determined. The major route of manganese excretion is through the bile (Mena 1981).

Manganese toxicity in humans results mainly from environmental contamination. The clinical manifestations of toxicity are neuropsychiatric abnormalities characterized by hallucinations, delusions and compulsions, as well as Parkinson's disease-type symptoms (Mena 1981). Toxicity resulting from oral ingestion is extremely rare. In Japan, 16 cases of intoxication were reported as a result of drinking water from a contaminated well (Kawamura *et al.* 1940). One case of toxicity, following prolonged consumption of mineral supplements containing manganese, has also been documented (Banta and Markesbury 1977).

Disease Prevention

It has been suggested that suboptimal manganese intakes in children may be associated with epileptic seizures (Tanaka *et al.* 1977). Dupont *et al.* (1977) reported that a large proportion of children suffering from such seizures had an abnormally low blood manganese concentration. Giving manganese supplements resulted in an increase in blood manganese levels and a decreased number of seizures. Adult epileptics have also been shown to have lower blood manganese levels, with the frequency of seizures directly related to the concentration in their blood (Papavasiliou *et al.* 1979). In a more recent study, however, the blood manganese concentrations of epileptics did not correlate with seizure frequency (Carl *et al.* 1986). These investigators did show that the mean blood manganese concentration of hospitalized epileptic patients whose epilepsy was not the result of trauma was significantly lower than the concentration in those whose seizures resulted from accidents. Both groups had lower blood manganese concentrations than non-epileptic controls. Although blood manganese concentrations appear to be lower in epileptics, there is no evidence that a sub-optimal intake of manganese is related to the etiology of the disease. Experiments with mice have suggested that the decreased blood concentration may be due to a redistribution of manganese to the liver as a result of an increased energy requirement of that organ following a seizure (Papavasiliou and Miller 1983).

Recommendations

Most of the manganese in the diet comes from fruit and grain products (Gibson *et al.* 1985a,b). The mean manganese intake of adult Canadians is estimated to range from 3 to 3.8 mg/day (Kirkpatrick and Coffin 1977; Gibson and Scythes 1982; Gibson *et al.* 1985b). The mean intake of Canadian children, 22 months of age, is approximately 1.5 mg/day (Gibson *et al.* 1985a). Those aged 4-6 years had dietary intakes ranging from 1.9 to 2.3 mg/day (Gibson *et al.* 1983). Intakes by exclusively breast-fed infants were found to be 0.9, 0.6 and 0.5 µg/kg/day for the 1st, 2nd and 3rd month of lactation respectively (Vuori 1979). Vaughan *et al.* (1979) reported breast milk concentrations of 1.98, 2.38 and 2.53 µg/100 mL for 1-3, 4-6 and 7-9 months of lactation. Canadian infant formula contains at least 5 µg/100 kcal (Canada. Health and Welfare. Food and Drugs Act and Regulations 1983).

Most attempts to estimate human manganese requirements have used the balance technique. Freeland-Graves *et al.* (1987) combined all the manganese balance data for adults in which normal mixed diets were used, and in which the manganese was analysed by atomic absorption spectroscopy. Theoretical manganese equilibrium was obtained with an intake of 3.55 mg/day. Recently, Freeland-Graves *et al.* (1988) measured manganese balance in five males, aged 19-20, consuming conventional foods. When obligatory losses, at a theoretical intake of 0 manganese, were combined with integumental losses, and the mean positive retention taken into account, an intake of 3.5 mg/day or 50 µg/kg/day was required to maintain balance. Since no evidence of manganese deficiency in the Canadian population exists, present intakes are deemed to be sufficient. Because of the scarcity of studies on manganese requirements, insufficient data exist to establish firm recommendations.

References

Banta, R.G. and Markesbury, W.R. 1977. Elevated manganese levels associated with dementia and extrapyramidal signs. Neurology 27:213-216.

Canada. Health and Welfare. Food and Drugs Act and Regulations 1983.

Carl, G.F., Keen, C.L., Gallagher, B.B., Clegg, M.S., Littleton, W.H., Flannery, D.B. and Hurley, L.S. 1986. Association of low blood manganese concentrations with epilepsy. Neurology 36:1584-1587.

Doisy, E.A., Jr. 1973. Micronutrient controls on biosynthesis of clotting proteins and cholesterol. *In* Trace substances in environmental health. VI. Proceedings of University of Missouri's 6th annual conference. Hemphill, D.D., ed. University of Missouri, Columbia, pp. 193-199.

Dupont, C., Harpur, E.R., Skoryna, S.C. and Tanaka, Y. 1977. Blood manganese levels in relation to convulsive disorders in children (abst.). Clin. Biochem. 10:P11.

Freeland-Graves, J.H., Bales, C.W. and Behmardi, F. 1987. Manganese requirements of humans. *In* Nutritional bioavailability of manganese. Kies, C., ed. American Chemical Society, Washington, pp. 90-104.

Freeland-Graves, J.H., Behmardi, F., Bales, C.W., Dougherty, V., Lin, P.-H., Crosby, J.B. and Trickett, P.C. 1988. Metabolic balance of manganese in young men consuming diets containing five levels of dietary manganese. J. Nutr. 118:764-773.

Friedman, B.J., Freeland-Graves, J.H., Bales, C.W., Behmardi, F., Shorey-Kutschke, R.L., Willis, R.A., Crosby, J.B., Trickett, P.C. and Houston, S.D. 1987. Manganese balance and clinical observations in young men fed a manganese-deficient diet. J. Nutr. 117:133-143.

Gibson, R.S. and Scythes, C.A. 1982. Trace element intakes of women. Br. J. Nutr. 48:241-248.

Gibson, R.S., Anderson, B.M. and Scythes, C.A. 1983. Regional differences in hair zinc concentrations: a possible effect of water hardness. Am. J. Clin. Nutr. 37:37-42.

Gibson, R.S., Friel, J.K. and Scythes, C.A. 1985a. The zinc, copper, and manganese status of a selected group of Canadian children twenty-two months of age. J. Can. Diet. Assoc. 46:182-185.

Gibson, R.S., Macdonald, A.C. and Martinez, O.B. 1985b. Dietary chromium and manganese intakes of a selected sample of Canadian elderly women. Hum. Nutr.: Appl. Nutr. 39A:43-52.

Hurley, L.S. and Keen, C.L. 1987. Manganese. *In* Trace elements in human and animal nutrition. Vol. 1. 5th ed. Mertz, W., ed. Academic Press, San Diego, pp. 185-223.

Kawamura, R., Ikuta, H. and Fukuzami, T. 1940. On the familial manganese poisoning by drinking water from a well. Jpn. J. Bacteriol. 537:687-710.

Keen, C.L., Lonnerdal, B. and Hurley, L.S. 1984a. Manganese. *In* Biochemistry of the essential ultratrace elements. Frieden, E., ed. Plenum Press, New York, pp. 89-132.

Keen, C.L., Fransson, G.B. and Lonnerdal, B. 1984b. Supplementation of milk with iron bound to lactoferrin using weanling mice. II. Effects on tissue manganese, zinc and copper. J. Pediatr. Gastroenterol. Nutr. 3:256-261.

Kies, C., Aldrich, K.D., Johnson, J.M., Creps, C., Kowalski, C. and Wang, R.H. 1987. Manganese availability for humans: effect of selected dietary factors. *In* Nutritional bioavailability of manganese. Kies, C., ed. American Chemical Society, Washington, pp. 136-145.

King, B.D., Lassiter, J.W., Neathery, M.W., Miller, W.J. and Gentry, R.P. 1979. Manganese retention in rats fed different diets and chemical forms of manganese. J. Anim. Sci. 49:1235-1241.

Kirkpatrick, D.C. and Coffin, D.E. 1977. The trace metal content of a representative Canadian diet in 1972. Can. J. Public Health 68:162-164.

Mena, I. 1981. Manganese. *In* Disorders of mineral metabolism. Vol. I. Trace minerals. Bronner, F. and Coburn, J.W., eds. Academic Press, New York, pp. 233-270.

Papavasiliou, P.S., Kutt, H., Miller, S.T., Rosal, V., Wang, Y.Y. and Aronson, R.B. 1979. Seizure disorders and trace metals: manganese tissue levels in treated epileptics. Neurology 29:1466-1473.

Papavasiliou, P.S. and Miller, S.T. 1983. Generalized seizures alter the cerebral and peripheral metabolism of essential metals in mice. Exp. Neurol. 82:223-236.

Sandström, B., Cederblad, A, Davidsson, L. and Lönnerdal, B. 1985. Manganese absorption from infant formula (abst.). Am. J. Clin. Nutr. 41:842.

Tanaka, Y., Dupont, C. and Harpur, E.R. 1977. Manganese: its neurological and teratological significance in man. Abstr. Pap. Am. Chem. Soc. 174:Biol 130.

Vaughan, L.A., Weber, C.W. and Kemberling, S.R. 1979. Longitudinal changes in the mineral content of human milk. Am. J. Clin. Nutr. 32:2301-2306.

Vuori, E. 1979. Intake of copper, iron, manganese and zinc by healthy, exclusively-breast-fed infants during the first three months of life. Br. J. Nutr. 42:407-411.

Selenium

Inorganic soil selenium is utilized by plants for the synthesis of selenomethionine, which is incorporated into plant proteins. When these proteins are consumed by humans and animals, the selenomethionine released in digestion is used nonspecifically for the synthesis of tissue proteins. Humans and animals also convert selenomethionine to selenocysteine, which is incorporated selectively into the enzyme glutathione peroxidase, the only known metabolically active form of selenium in the body (Stadtman 1987). This enzyme catalyzes the reduction by glutathione of hydrogen peroxide and fatty acid hydroperoxides, thereby preventing the generation of oxygen free radicals which catalyze the oxidative decomposition of polyunsaturated fatty acids in the phospholipids of cell membranes. The function of selenium is related to that of vitamin E, which acts as a scavenger of fatty acid peroxy radicals, and this interrelationship is reflected in a sparing effect of each nutrient on the requirement for the other.

Dietary Sources

Cereals are the most important source of selenium in the Canadian diet (Thompson *et al.* 1975). However, cereals are highly variable in their selenium content, which reflects differences in the selenium content of soils on which they are grown. Meat, dairy and poultry products, the other major dietary sources, are more constant in selenium content because this element is essential in the diet of animals, and is toxic at moderately high concentrations in the tissues. Fruits and vegetables are poor sources of selenium.

Analysis of four composites of 11 food groups purchased in three different cities indicated that a typical Canadian diet provided an average of 197 µg of selenium per day with a range of 113 µg to 220 µg (Thompson *et al.* 1975). This estimate is compatible, after allowance for wastage, with an estimate of 170 µg/day derived from food disappearance data (Jenkins and Hidiroglou 1972). These and similar data for U.S. foods indicate that most North American mixed diets provide between 100 µg and 200 µg of selenium per day.

Selenium Deficiency

Tracer studies have shown that about 80% of dietary selenium is absorbed (Thomson and Robinson 1980). Chronic selenium status is best assessed in terms of whole blood selenium concentration or erythrocyte glutathione peroxidase activity (Thomson and Robinson 1980). The selenium level in serum is strongly influenced by short term intake.

Selenium deficiency, often expressed by a concomitant low intake of vitamin E, is common in animals fed unsupplemented feedstuffs grown in regions where there is a low concentration of selenium in the soil. Such regions may be localized or, as in the case of New Zealand and Finland, comprise much of the national land area. In Canada, the soils of the extensive grain-growing areas of the prairie provinces are adequate in selenium, whereas those in some areas of the central and maritime provinces are too low to prevent a deficiency in livestock fed locally grown feeds. The national distribution of many human foodstuffs, particularly cereals, provides insurance against risk of selenium deficiency arising from consumption of foods produced from plants grown on locally deficient soils.

The presence of glutathione peroxidase in the tissues constituted the only evidence that selenium is an essential nutrient for humans, until the discovery that selenium deficiency is the cause of a severe cardiomyopathy in children living in the Keshan district of China (Yang *et al.* 1984). The occurrence of this syndrome, called Keshan disease, is associated with a diet consisting mainly of cereals grown on local soils with an exceptionally low selenium content. The disease responds rapidly to oral administration of sodium selenite. Selenium-responsive muscle pain associated with a very low plasma selenium level also has been reported in patients maintained for long periods with parenteral solutions lacking this element (van Rij *et al.* 1979).

Selenium Requirement

The selenium requirement of human adults has not been firmly established. Extensive studies on the residents of New Zealand, where the selenium content of the soil, and therefore of cereals, is unusually low, have failed to reveal any adverse effects on health attributable to selenium deficiency in subjects consuming normal diets, despite a selenium intake (28-56 µg/d) and whole blood level (70 ng/mL) less than half those of Canadians (Thomson and Robinson 1980). However, plasma glutathione peroxidase is somewhat lower, suggesting that the selenium intake of some individuals is suboptimal.

Radioisotope studies on New Zealand women indicated that 20-30 µg/d was adequate to maintain selenium balance. A somewhat higher intake was required to reach a plateau in erythrocyte glutathione peroxidase activity. In the United States, young men were estimated to require 70 µg/day to restore their selenium status after a period of depletion, and 54 µg/day to maintain normal plasma levels and body stores (Levander *et al.* 1981). There is evidence of adaptability to a lower intake.

Children with Keshan disease, who have the lowest blood selenium levels reported in free-living persons (≤20 ng/mL), have been estimated to require at least 20 µg selenium per day (Yang *et al.* 1984). This estimate is based on a comparison of the selenium content of maize and rice consumed in affected areas, where these cereals contain an average of 0.005 and 0.007 ppm, respectively, and in unaffected areas, where they contain an average of 0.036 and 0.024 ppm.

Blood levels in infants are low at birth (about 50 ng/mL), decline during the first few weeks, then rise progressively during growth (Thomson and Robinson 1980). The selenium requirement of neonates is not well defined, but in New Zealand infants it has been observed that an intake of less than 5 µg per day is associated with low erythrocyte glutathione peroxidase activity (Thomson and Robinson 1980).

The mature milk of a sample of 241 women residing in 17 urban areas of the U.S. was found to average 0.018 ppm selenium (Shearer and Hadjimarkos 1975), a concentration which would provide 14 µg of selenium per day in a milk flow of 750 mL. Although lower concentrations have been found in the breast milk of women living in low selenium areas, deficiency symptoms in term infants have been seen only in extremely selenium-poor localities in China (Yang *et al.* 1984). Colostrum is higher in selenium than mature milk, whereas cow's milk formula is generally lower, particularly if the milk has been obtained from cows in a low selenium area. Prematures have lower blood levels of selenium and glutathione peroxidase than term infants, and this may be a contributing factor in the greater susceptibility of their erythrocytes to oxidative stress (Lubin and Oski 1972).

Selenium Toxicity

Endemic selenium intoxication arising from consumption of foods grown on seleniferous soils has been well documented in humans and animals. Cereal grains produced on seleniferous alkaline soils may contain several hundred ppm selenium. When fed to farm animals they produce emaciation, loss of hair, incoordination and sloughing of hooves (alkali disease). Foods grown on soil contaminated with high selenium coal and fertilized with lime produce a similar syndrome in Chinese subjects, characterized by loss of hair and nails and lesions of the nervous system (Yang *et al.* 1983). Selenium intakes averaged 5000 µg/day and blood selenium 3200 ng/mL. Selenium intake by asymptomatic residents of seleniferous areas of Venezuela and China have been reported to average 326 µg per day and 750 µg per day, respectively (Yang *et al.* 1983).

Selenium intoxication in laboratory rodents becomes clinically manifest at a concentration of 2 ppm in the diet or 20 times their requirement (U.S. N.R.C. 1978). Subclinical manifestations may occur below this level of intake. This concentration in the diet of human adults would provide an average of about 1000 µg of selenium per day, a level of intake which, as sodium selenite, has been observed to produce definite symptoms of chronic toxicity (Yang *et al.* 1983). Some composite Canadian diets exceed 200 µg/day (Thompson *et al.* 1975).

Selenium and Cancer Prevention

Selenium intakes above the normal range inhibit the development of some cancers induced by administration of chemical carcinogens to experimental animals, possibly by a selective toxicity for cancer cells. Some prospective studies have indicated that serum selenium concentration in humans is inversely related to risk of cancer development in future years (Clark and Combs 1986; Salonen 1986). However, serum selenium level is not a reliable indicator of long term selenium intake, and whether this association is due to differences in dietary selenium or to some other factor(s) is unclear. Most of the evidence for a protective effect of selenium against cancer in humans stems from comparisons between subjects with blood levels in the lowest and highest quintiles of the normal range. Several intervention trials are in progress to evaluate the effect of supplementing low selenium diets to bring them into the upper end of the normal range of selenium intakes (about 200 µg per day). In as much as typical Canadian diets already provide this amount of selenium, supplementation for cancer prevention is unnecessary, and is counterindicated by the narrow margin of safety for this element.

Recommendations

Although selenium intake by the inhabitants of some geographic areas indicates that as little as 25 µg per day may satisfy the requirement of most adults, 50 µg per day appears to be necessary to maintain the selenium status typical of North American adults. This amount is exceeded 2- to 5-fold by all normal diets consumed by Canadians. Further, the concentration of selenium in the Canadian diet (0.15-0.30 ppm) exceeds the concentration required in the diet of experimental and domestic animals (0.1 ppm) (Thompson *et al.* 1973). Supplementation of the diet with either inorganic forms of selenium such as sodium selenite, or organic forms such as selenium-enriched yeast preparations therefore is unnecessary and may entail a risk of toxicity.

References

Clark, L.C. and Combs, G.F., Jr. 1986. Selenium compounds and the prevention of cancer: research needs and public health implications. J. Nutr. 116:170-173.

Jenkins, K.J. and Hidiroglou, M. 1972. A review of selenium/vitamin E responsive problems in livestock: a case for selenium as a feed additive in Canada. Can. J. Anim. Sci. 52:591-620.

Levander, O.A., Sutherland, B., Morris, V.C. and King, J.C. 1981. Selenium balance in young men during selenium depletion and repletion. Am. J. Clin. Nutr. 34:2662-2669.

Lubin, B. and Oski, F.A. 1972. Red cell metabolism in the newborn infant. VI. Irreversible oxidant-induced injury. J. Pediatr. 81:698-704.

Salonen, J.T. 1986. Selenium and cancer. Ann. Clin. Res. 18:18-21.

Shearer, T.R. and Hadjimarkos, D.M. 1975. Geographic distribution of selenium in human milk. Arch. Environ. Health 30:230-233.

Stadtman, T.C. 1987. Specific occurrence of selenium in enzymes and amino acid tRNAs. FASEB J. 1:375-379.

Thompson, J.N., Beare-Rogers, J.L., Erdody, P. and Smith, D.C. 1973. Appraisal of human vitamin E requirement based on examination of individual meals and a composite Canadian diet. Am. J. Clin. Nutr. 26:1349-1354.

Thompson, J.N., Erdody, P. and Smith, D.C. 1975. Selenium content of food consumed by Canadians. J. Nutr. 105:274-277.

Thomson, C.D. and Robinson, M.F. 1980. Selenium in human health and disease with emphasis on those aspects peculiar to New Zealand. Am. J. Clin. Nutr. 33:303-323.

U.S. National Research Council. Committee on Animal Nutrition. 1978. Nutrient requirements of laboratory animals. 3rd rev. ed. National Academy of Sciences, Washington, D.C.

van Rij, A.M., Thomson, C.D., McKenzie, J.M. and Robinson, M.F. 1979. Selenium deficiency in total parenteral nutrition. Am. J. Clin. Nutr. 32:2076-2085.

Yang, G., Wang, S., Zhou, R. and Sun, S. 1983. Endemic selenium intoxication of humans in China. Am. J. Clin. Nutr. 37:872-881.

Yang, G., Chen, J., Wen, Z., Ge, K., Zhu, L., Chen, X. and Chen, X. 1984. The role of selenium in Keshan disease. Adv. Nutr. Res. 6:203-231.

Chromium

Function and Action

Chromium is a component of a circulating organic complex known as the glucose tolerance factor (GTF), of which the exact chemical composition and structure are not precisely known. Conversion of inorganic chromium to a biologically active form is essential for the physiological functioning of chromium (Borel and Anderson 1984). The primary physiological function of chromium is to potentiate the action of insulin; therefore it is involved in carbohydrate metabolism and other insulin-dependent processes such as protein and lipid metabolism.

Chromium is an essential nutrient for animals (Wallach 1985). In man, three cases of chromium deficiency have been reported in individuals receiving total parenteral nutrition without added chromium (Jeejeebhoy *et al.* 1977; Freund *et al.* 1979; Brown *et al.* 1986). The most common deficiency symptoms involve disturbed glucose metabolism as evidenced by hyperglycemia, glucosuria and glucose intolerance requiring insulin therapy. Other symptoms include high free fatty acid levels and abnormalities in nitrogen metabolism (Jeejeebhoy *et al.* 1977). Neuropathy (Jeejeebhoy *et al.* 1977) and encephalopathy (Freund *et al.* 1979) have also been reported, but these symptoms may be later manifestations of the deficiency (Brown *et al.* 1986).

The methodology for the analysis of chromium has undergone vast improvement in recent years. Reported levels of chromium in blood and urine have declined markedly over the last two decades due to improved methods of sampling, prevention of contamination, and improved instrumentation (Wallach 1985).

Chromium is widely distributed, at low concentration, throughout the human body. It is not concentrated in any known tissue or organ (Underwood 1977). Tissue chromium concentrations have been reported to decline with age (Schroeder *et al.* 1970), but this has not been confirmed, using the improved methodology of recent years, nor is it known whether differences are due to the normal aging process or due to prolonged sub-optimal intakes (Peereboom 1985). Two subsequent studies in the elderly have failed to demonstrate significant changes in serum chromium with age (Vir and Love 1978; Abraham *et al.* 1981).

Inorganic chromium is poorly absorbed, with fractional absorption estimated to be only 0.5-1% (Borel and Anderson 1984). In a recent study of individuals consuming a self-selected diet containing varying amounts of chromium (10-40 µg/day), absorption was found to vary with dietary intakes, while urinary excretion remained constant. At an intake of 10 µg/day, chromium absorption was 2% compared to 0.5% when 40 µg/day was consumed (Anderson and Kozlovsky 1985). Absorbed chromium is excreted almost exclusively in the urine, and only small amounts are lost via hair, perspiration and bile. Once chromium is utilized it does not appear to be reabsorbed by the kidneys, but is rapidly excreted in the urine (Anderson 1986).

Disease

Prolonged chromium supplementation has been shown to result in slight improvements in glucose tolerance in glucose-intolerant or diabetic individuals, as well as producing small increases in HDL-cholesterol and decreases in total cholesterol (Wallach 1985). Insulin-dependent diabetics excrete nearly 3-fold more chromium than control subjects (Anderson 1986); however, absorption is also elevated (Doisey *et al.* 1976). Overall, there does not appear to be much evidence that chromium deficiency is involved in diabetes, although the interpretation of results may be complicated by the variety of etiologies in the disease, analytical methodology problems or inadequate methods to assess chromium status. Chromium deficiency has been suggested as a risk factor for cardiovascular disease (Simonoff 1984), since supplemental chromium has been shown in several studies to decrease the total cholesterol to HDL cholesterol ratio, regardless of glucose tolerance (Wallach 1985); however, in other studies, it had no effect (Anderson *et al.* 1983; Rabinowitz *et al.* 1983). Strenuous exercise (Anderson *et al.* 1984) and physical trauma (Borel *et al.* 1984) lead to elevated urinary chromium losses, although the significance of these changes on chromium status has not been determined.

Intake

The Canadian diet, formulated from food disappearance data, provided 282 µg Cr/day (Meranger and Smith 1972) and 136-152 µg/day (Kirkpatrick and Coffin 1974). However, in a more recent study using one day food composites from 84 premenopausal Canadian women, mean chromium intake was 56 µg/day (Gibson and Scythes 1984) and 96 µg/day for elderly women (Gibson *et al.* 1985). These lower intakes are somewhat higher, but comparable to recent estimates obtained from the United States. High intakes of chromium were associated with increased consumption of cheese, dry legumes and nuts (Gibson and Scythes 1984), and with tea consumption in the elderly (Gibson *et al.* 1985). Stainless steel cutlery and utensils may also contribute to chromium intakes.

Recommendation

There is no evidence that adult intakes of chromium fail to meet the requirement of normal, healthy individuals. In a 12-day metabolic study of two subjects consuming 37 µg Cr/day, both individuals were in positive chromium balance (Offenbacher *et al.* 1986). Similarly, equilibrium or positive chromium balance was achieved in free-living individuals, at daily chromium intakes of 20 µg for women and 30 µg for men. Only two individuals out of 22 were in slight negative balance and one in severe negative chromium balance (Bunker *et al.* 1984). Although neither of these studies accounted for the minor losses in skin, sweat or hair, they suggest that healthy individuals consuming a mixed diet are probably meeting their requirement for chromium. There are insufficient data, however, to establish a minimum requirement for adults.

Breast milk was found to contain 0.27 ± 0.10 ng Cr/mL and provided an average daily intake of 0.15 µg during the first month postpartum (Casey *et al.* 1985). Not enough information is available about the metabolism or requirement for chromium during infancy to make any recommendations.

References

Abraham, A.S., Sonneblick, M. and Eini, M. 1981. Serum chromium and aging. Gerontology 27:326-328.

Anderson, R.A. 1986. Chromium metabolism and its role in disease processes in man. Clin. Physiol. Biochem. 4:31-41.

Anderson, R.A. and Kozlovsky, A.S. 1985. Chromium intake, absorption and excretion of subjects consuming self-selected diets. Am. J. Clin. Nutr. 41:1177-1183.

Anderson, R.A., Polansky, M.M., Bryden, N.A., Roginski, E.E., Mertz, W. and Glinsmann, W. 1983. Chromium supplementation of human subjects: effects on glucose, insulin, and lipid variables. Metabolism 32:894-899.

Anderson, R.A., Polansky, M.M. and Bryden, N.A. 1984. Strenuous running. Acute effects on chromium, copper, zinc, and selected clinical variables in urine and serum of male runners. Biol. Trace Elem. Res. 6:327-336.

Borel, J.S. and Anderson, R.A. 1984. Chromium. *In* Biochemistry of the essential ultratrace elements. Frieden, E., ed. Plenum Press, New York, pp. 175-199.

Borel, J.S., Majerus, T.C., Polansky, M.M., Moser, P.B. and Anderson, R.A. 1984. Chromium intake and urinary chromium excretion of trauma patients. Biol. Trace Elem. Res. 6:317-326.

Brown, R.O., Forloines-Lynn, S., Cross, R.E. and Heizer, W.D. 1986. Chromium deficiency after long-term total parenteral nutrition. Dig. Dis. Sci. 31:661-664.

Bunker, V.W., Lawson, M.S., Delves, H.T. and Clayton, B.E. 1984. The uptake and excretion of chromium by the elderly. Am. J. Clin. Nutr. 39:797-802.

Casey, C.E., Hambidge, K.M. and Neville, M.C. 1985. Studies in human lactation: zinc, copper, manganese and chromium in human milk in the first month of lactation. Am. J. Clin. Nutr. 41:1193-1200.

Doisy, R.J., Streeten, D.H.P., Freiberg, J.M. and Schneider, A.J. 1976. Chromium metabolism in man and biochemical effects. *In* Trace elements in human health and disease. Vol. II. Essential and toxic elements. Prasad, A.S. and Oberleas, D., eds. Academic Press, New York, pp. 79-104.

Freund, H., Atamian, S. and Fischer, J.E. 1979. Chromium deficiency during total parenteral nutrition. J. Am. Med. Assoc. 241:496-498.

Gibson, R.S. and Scythes, C.A. 1984. Chromium, selenium, and other trace element intakes of a selected sample of Canadian premenopausal women. Biol. Trace Elem. Res. 6:105-116.

Gibson, R.S., MacDonald, A.C. and Martinez, O.B. 1985. Dietary chromium and manganese intakes of a selected sample of Canadian elderly women. Hum. Nutr.: Appl. Nutr. 39A:43-52.

Jeejeebhoy, K.N., Chu, R.C., Marliss, E.B., Greenberg, G.R. and Bruce-Robertson, A. 1977. Chromium deficiency, glucose intolerance, and neuropathy reversed by chromium supplementation, in a patient receiving long-term total parenteral nutrition. Am. J. Clin. Nutr. 30:531-538.

Kirkpatrick, D.C and Coffin, D.E. 1974. The trace metal content of representative Canadian diets in 1970 and 1971. Can. Inst. Food Sci. Technol. J. 7:56-58.

Meranger, J.C. and Smith, D.C. 1972. The heavy metal content of a typical Canadian diet. Can. J. Public Health 63:53-57.

Offenbacher, E.G., Spencer, H., Dowling, H.J. and Pi-Sunyer, F.X. 1986. Metabolic chromium balances in men. Am. J. Clin. Nutr. 44:77-82.

Peereboom, J.W.C. 1985. General aspects of trace elements and health. Sci. Total Environ. 42:1-27.

Rabinowitz, M.B., Gonick, H.C., Levin, S.R. and Davidson, M.B. 1983. Clinical trial of chromium and yeast supplements on carbohydrate and lipid metabolism in diabetic men. Biol. Trace Elem. Res. 5:449-466.

Schroeder, H.A., Nason, A.P. and Tipton, I.H. 1970. Chromium deficiency as a factor in atherosclerosis. J. Chronic Dis. 23:123-142.

Simonoff, M. 1984. Chromium deficiency and cardiovascular risk. Cardiovasc. Res. 18:591-596.

Underwood, E.J. 1977. Chromium. *In* Trace elements in human and animal nutrition. 4th ed. Academic Press, New York, pp. 258-270.

Vir, S.C. and Love, A.H.G. 1978. Chromium status of the aged. Int. J. Vitam. Nutr. Res. 48:402-404.

Wallach, S. 1985. Clinical and biochemical aspects of chromium deficiency. J. Am. Coll. Nutr. 4:107-120.

Other Trace Elements

The results of animal experiments, using purified diets and in some cases an ultra-clean environment, have indicated that trace elements such as cobalt, molybdenum, and silicon are essential for normal growth, reproduction or other bodily functions. Moreover, there is some evidence suggesting that arsenic, nickel, vanadium, lithium and boron may also be essential for animals (Underwood and Mertz 1987). In some cases, deficiencies were produced in animals by highly purified diets containing amino acids in place of protein or rigid reproductive and weaning conditions to prevent accumulation of the trace elements in the experimental animal. The significance of cobalt in the nutrition of man and other non-ruminants is confined to its presence in vitamin B_{12} (Smith 1987).

Although molybdenum deficiency in animals has long been known to cause a decrease in enzymes such as xanthine oxidase, aldehyde oxidase and sulphite oxidase, human cases of deficiency were only reported in this decade (Abumrad *et al.* 1981; Rajgopalan 1987). These involved a young man on long-term total parenteral nutrition with a preparation lacking molybdenum, and the latter was an inborn error of molybdenum metabolism. Deficiencies of the other previously mentioned trace elements in man have not been reported as yet (Underwood and Mertz 1987). It has been suggested that the requirements for these "ultratrace" elements are so low that frank deficiency may not be seen in man. The essentiality of them, however, may be demonstrated under various forms of nutritional, metabolic, hormonal or physiologic stress (Nielsen 1988).

Intake and Chronic Diseases

The trace element intakes from Western diets (µg/day) have been reported as follows: molybdenum, 50-200 (Mills and Davis 1987); silicon, 1000-1500 (Carlisle 1986); lithium, 100-2000 (Mertz 1986); boron, 2000-4000 (Nielsen 1986); nickel, 150-700 (Kirkpatrick and Coffin 1974; Nielsen 1987a); vanadium, 10-30 (Nielsen 1987b); arsenic, 20-100 (Anke 1986; Dabeka *et al.* 1987). These include data for nickel and arsenic in the Canadian diet. Foods of plant origin are major sources of molybdenum, silicon, lithium, boron and nickel, and those of animal origin, especially seafoods, provide the major proportion of dietary vanadium and arsenic. Some vegetables such as spinach, parsley and mushrooms are also high in vanadium, whereas cereals and starchy foods like rice, potatoes and yams contain appreciable amounts of arsenic (Anke 1986; Carlisle 1986; Mertz 1986; Nielsen 1986, 1987a,b; Mills and Davis 1987). Cow's milk has been reported to contain (µg/g): molybdenum, 0.05 (Mills and Davis 1987); boron, 0.5-1.0 (Nielsen 1986); nickel, less than 0.1 (Nielsen 1987a); vanadium, less than 0.03 (Nielsen 1987b); arsenic, 0.01-0.05 (Anke 1986). Mature human milk contains (µg/g): molybdenum, 0.01; nickel, 0.01; vanadium, 0.005 (Food composition and nutrition tables 1986/87, p.6,11). As more accurate methods for the determination of some of these elements are developed, some of the levels in milk may have to be revised. Since a dietary deficiency of any of these trace elements has not been reported in man under normal conditions (Underwood and Mertz 1987), the above intakes are presumed to be adequate. Nevertheless, epidemiological findings and some results of animal experiments have implicated inadequate or high intakes of trace elements such as vanadium, silicon or nickel in chronic cardiovascular disease (Mertz 1981). Recently an inadequate dietary intake of boron was suggested to be an important factor in the etiology of osteoporosis (Nielsen *et al.* 1987).

Toxicity

Although no cases of toxicity due to intake of any of these trace elements from normal diets have been reported, an excessive intake of molybdenum (10-15 mg/day) in some parts of the Soviet Union was associated with a gout-like syndrome (Underwood 1977; Mertz 1981). A high intake of cobalt from beer was incriminated in severe cardiac failure in heavy beer drinkers in Canada and the U.S. (Smith 1987). The toxic dietary levels (µg/g dry weight) of all these trace elements for animals are at least 25 times higher than the reported levels in the human diet. There is, therefore, a considerable margin of safety (Anke 1986; Mertz 1986; Nielsen 1986, 1987a,b; Mills and Davis 1987).

References

Abumrad, N.N., Schneider, A.J., Steel, D. and Rogers, L.S. 1981. Amino acid intolerence during prolonged total parenteral nutrition reversed by molybdate therapy. Am. J. Clin. Nutr. 34:2551-2559.

Anke, M. 1986. Arsenic. *In* Trace elements in human and animal nutrition. Vol. 2. 5th ed. Mertz, W., ed. Academic Press, Orlando, pp. 347-372.

Carlisle, E.M. 1986. Silicon. *In* Trace elements in human and animal nutrition. Vol. 2. 5th ed. Mertz, W., ed. Academic Press, Orlando, pp. 373-390.

Dabeka, R.W., McKenzie, A.D. and Lacroix, G.M.A. 1987. Dietary intakes of lead, cadmium, arsenic and fluoride by Canadian adults: a 24-hour duplicate diet study. Food Addit. Contam. 4:89-102.

Food composition and nutrition tables 1986/87. 3rd rev. ed. Wissenschaftliche Verlagsgesellschaft, Stuttgart.

Kirkpatrick, D.C. and Coffin, D.E. 1974. The trace metal content of representative Canadian diets in 1970 and 1971. Can. Inst. Food Sci. Technol. J. 7:56-58.

Mertz, W. 1981. The essential trace elements. Science 213:1332-1338.

Mertz, W. 1986. Lithium. *In* Trace elements in human and animal nutrition. Vol. 2. 5th ed. Mertz, W., ed. Academic Press, Orlando, pp. 391-397.

Mills, C.F. and Davis, G.K. 1987. Molybdenum. *In* Trace elements in human and animal nutrition. Vol. 1. 5th ed. Mertz, W., ed. Academic Press, San Diego, pp. 429-463.

Nielsen, F.H. 1986. Other elements: Sb, Ba, B, Cs, Ge, Rb, Ag, Sr, Sn, Ti, Zr, Be, Bi, Ga, Au, In, Nb, Sc, Te, Tl, W. *In* Trace elements in human and animal nutrition. Vol. 2. 5th ed. Mertz, W., ed. Academic Press, Orlando, pp. 415-463.

Nielsen, F.H. 1987a. Nickel. *In* Trace elements in human and animal nutrition. Vol. 1. 5th ed. Mertz, W., ed. Academic Press, San Diego, pp. 245-273.

Nielsen, F.H. 1987b. Vanadium. *In* Trace elements in human and animal nutrition. Vol. 1. 5th ed. Mertz, W., ed. Academic Press, San Diego, pp. 275-300.

Nielsen, F.H. 1988. Nutritional significance of the ultratrace elements. Nutr. Rev. 46:337-341.

Nielsen, F.H., Hunt, C.D., Mullen, L.M. and Hunt, J.R. 1987. Effect of dietary boron on mineral, estrogen, and testosterone metabolism in postmenopausal women. FASEB J. 1:394-397.

Rajgopalan, K.V. 1987. Molybdenum - an essential trace element. Nutr. Rev. 45:321-328.

Smith, R.M. 1987. Cobalt. *In* Trace elements in human and animal nutrition. Vol. 1. 5th ed. Mertz, W., ed. Academic Press, San Diego, pp. 143-183.

Underwood, E.J. 1977. Trace elements in human and animal nutrition. 4th ed. Academic Press, New York.

Underwood, E.J. and Mertz, W. 1987. Introduction. *In* Trace elements in human and animal nutrition. Vol 1. 5th ed. Mertz, W., ed. Academic Press, San Diego, pp. 1-19.

Electrolytes and Water

Sodium, potassium, and chloride are among the factors that are essential to maintain acid-base balance and osmotic equilibrium in the body. The major extracellular electrolytes are sodium and chloride, and the important intracellular cation is potassium. A membrane-bound enzyme, sodium-potassium adenosine triphosphatase (ATP-ase), facilitates the transport of sodium and potassium in opposite directions across cell membranes (Guyton 1981). Movements of sodium and potassium across cell membranes are also involved in nerve conduction and in muscle action.

Water is required for the transport of electrolytes and other nutrients, and is essential in metabolic reactions. It is also responsible for temperature regulation, lubrication of joints, cushioning of the nervous system and transmission of sound in the ear (Hays 1980).

Sodium and chloride are excreted in urine, feces and sweat. Loss of these electrolytes in the urine is controlled by hormonal mechanisms involving aldosterone, renin and angiotensin. Water excretion is also under the control of hormones, mostly the antidiuretic hormone secreted by the posterior pituitary. Water intake is controlled by thirst. Although a salt appetite is recognized in certain species, for example the rat, such an appetite has not been clearly demonstrated in humans during sodium deficiency (Stricker 1980). Humans, however, may acquire a taste for salt, and thus consume quantities far in excess of their needs (Bertino *et al.* 1982).

Salt is the most important source of sodium and chloride. Because salt is usually abundant in the food supply, and humans tend to like it, a dietary deficiency of sodium or chloride is unlikely. A dietary deficiency of potassium is also uncommon because of its presence in most foods. A deficiency of electrolytes may be caused by excessive losses from vomiting, diarrhea and sweating. Symptoms of sodium deficiency are loss of body weight, cramps, weakness, anorexia, mental apathy and coma. A deficiency of chloride leads to metabolic alkalosis. Deficiency of potassium is manifested by muscular weakness, abdominal bloating, cardiac arrythmias and weakness of respiratory muscles (Guthrie 1983).

Dehydration and its accompanying depletion of electrolytes results from negative balances of water and electrolytes. Such negative balances can be caused by a simple lack of intake in the presence of normal output, although that is uncommon. More often, the negative balances result from an intake inadequate to compensate for abnormal losses, as occur from vomiting or diarrhea. The deficits of electrolytes and water occur whenever total output by all routes exceeds total intake.

Chronic dehydration is characterized by a loss of appetite and an impaired capacity for work. The combination of increasing dehydration with high environmental temperatures may result in heat exhaustion, hallucination, and ultimately heat stroke. Prolonged exercise in the heat can induce profound changes in the distribution of water in the body. The loss of body fluid as sweat may impair ability to circulate the blood and control body temperature. Athletes can lose as much as six litres of fluid during an athletic event of significant duration (Consolazio 1983). Therefore, in hot weather, athletes must adjust their habits to deal with the additional water loss as sweat.

Large volumes of water should be ingested immediately after and during strenuous sports events, when the thirst response may be blunted (Canadian Paediatric Society 1983). Since a normal diet supplies enough electrolytes to meet an athlete's requirements, it is currently believed that dietary sodium, potassium, and chloride will easily replace those electrolytes lost with perspiration. Thus the replacement of water is more critical than that of electrolytes. In addition, proportionally more water than electrolytes is lost from body fluid as perspiration. After prolonged exercise in extreme heat, some sodium replacement may be advisable (Canadian Paediatric Society 1983). It is recommended that this be obtained from dilute sodium chloride solutions or a little extra salt on food.

Sodium is toxic when ingested in very high concentrations, producing internal hemorrhages, vomiting, peripheral circulatory failure, respiratory depression, and eventually death (Fregly 1984). This situation occurs when sodium is accidentally ingested in a concentrated form, such as when infants were given salt instead of sugar in their formula (Fregly 1984). Sodium toxicity does not occur in the normal range of dietary intakes.

Potassium can also be lethal when injected directly into the blood stream, causing the heart to stop beating (Fregly 1984). Its slow absorption from foods through the intestine does not normally lead to intoxication because urinary excretion and vomiting protect the body from its accumulation. Salt substitutes containing potassium chloride should be used with caution, especially by persons with impaired kidney function (Fregly 1984).

Sodium and Potassium Intakes

In Western countries, estimates of sodium intake vary from approximately 2.3 g (100 mmol) to 6.7 g (290 mmol) per day, the amount being generally proportional to the energy content of the diet (Altschul et al. 1984). One-fourth to one-third of this intake has been thought to be discretionary, but recent reports indicate that much lower percentages of total sodium come from salt added voluntarily (Altschul *et al.* 1984). Foods collected in four Canadian cities according to food consumption patterns, excluding fast foods, contained 1.1 g (48 mmol) sodium and 1.2 g (31 mmol) potassium per 1000 kcal (Shah and Belonje 1983). In this study, food was prepared as it would be in the home, but without adding salt. About 70% of the sodium and 50% of the potassium were provided by dairy products, meat, fish and poultry, and cereal products. In a Montreal study of diets consumed by adults, the sodium intake was estimated at 3.1 g (135 mmol) per day or 1.5 g (65 mmol) per 1000 kcal while that of potassium was 2.8 g per day (72 mmol) or 1.4 g (36 mmol) per 1000 kcal (Mongeau *et al.* 1989). Only about 5% of ingested sodium came from salt added at the table.

Water Intake and Output

Water used by the body comes from fluids ingested (1200 mL), moisture in foods (1000 mL) and that produced during metabolic oxidation (300 mL), totalling approximately 2.5 L per day in temperate climates. The daily output comprises urine (1300 mL), feces (60 mL), evaporation from the lungs (400 mL) and sweat (800 mL), but varies according to physical activity and temperature. The water requirement may increase by several litres per day to compensate for sweating and evaporation through the lungs (Murray 1987).

Sodium and High Blood Pressure

High blood pressure, defined as diastolic blood pressure equal to or greater than 90 mm mercury, is a major risk factor for cardiovascular disease, and occurs in approximately 10% of adults 20 years of age or older (Canada. Health and Welfare 1989).

The epidemiological relationship between sodium and blood pressure was reviewed by several authors (Gleibermann 1973; Froment *et al.* 1979; Houston 1986). Inter-population studies including a wide range of intakes generally showed a correlation between sodium intake and blood pressure, the prevalence of hypertension being almost nil at levels of less than 20 mmol per day, and up to 50% at levels of 400 mmol per day (Houston 1986). Comparisons within a country, however, yield inconsistent results and, in most cases, fail to show a relationship between dietary sodium and blood pressure (MacGregor 1985). This absence of a relationship has generally been ascribed to diverse problems. These included the difficulty of measuring habitual sodium intake. The multiplicity of factors, dietary and non-dietary, that are probably involved in the etiology of hypertension, the possibility that there is a threshold level of intake (probably around 100 mmol/day) above which there is no further increase in the prevalence of hypertension, and the existence in a segment of the population of a hereditary sensitivity to sodium are other factors that may obscure the relationship.

Two large studies, one conducted in several countries, the other in Scotland, addressed the question of whether sodium intake is related to blood pressure in the general population (Intersalt Cooperative Research Group 1988; Smith *et al.* 1988). The Intersalt Study, which examined the relationship across different countries, found significant positive relationships between 24-hour sodium excretion and systolic and diastolic blood pressure in individuals, and between the ratio of sodium to potassium and blood pressure. When the relationships were adjusted for age, sex, body mass index, alcohol consumption and urinary potassium excretion, systolic pressure continued to be positively but weakly linked to sodium. It was estimated that a reduction in sodium intake of 100 mmol (2.3 g) per day would correspond to a reduction in systolic blood pressure of 2.2 mm Hg and in diastolic blood pressure of 0.1 mm Hg. Of the two Canadian centres, Labrador but not St. John's showed a significant correlation between blood pressure and sodium intakes. From the results of all countries in the Intersalt Study it was concluded that the rise in blood pressure with age was related to sodium intake. Little hypertension occurred when the sodium intake was under 50 mmol per day. Only one (Kenya) of the 52 centres reported urinary sodium excretion in the threshold range of 50 to 100 mmol per day, and 48 centres reported higher values. In the range of sodium excretion of 100 to 400 mmol, the increase in blood pressure appeared to be too small for detection by methods used to study populations. Data are lacking in the critical range of 50 to 100 mmol (1.1 to 2.3 g) of sodium per day.

In the Scottish Heart Health Study (Smith *et al.* 1988), sodium excretion was weakly and positively correlated with blood pressure. The results of this study strongly suggest that the effect of sodium intake is overshadowed by other environmental factors such as body weight, alcohol consumption, and potassium intake. Furthermore, there are likely significant interactions between the effects of sodium and other dietary factors.

Several studies assessing the effects of sodium restriction to levels of 50 to 60 mmol per day for a period of two to six weeks in normotensive middle-aged individuals showed an average fall in systolic blood pressure of only 3.6 mm Hg (MacGregor *et al.* 1982; Grobbee and Hofman 1986). In addition, the administration of sodium loads within the range ingested by the average adult in western society for short intervals has little or no effect on blood pressure (Logan 1986). These findings do not, however, exclude the possibility that longer term alterations in sodium intake may have an effect on blood pressure, or that the threshold for a response has already been reached. Moreover, there may be subgroups within the general population, especially among newborns, older persons, American blacks and individuals with a family history of hypertension, whose blood pressure is responsive to sodium (Houston 1986; Weinberger *et al.* 1986; Mongeau 1987). This has been substantiated in the well designed Australian National Health and Medical Research Council Dietary Salt Study (1989).

In most industrialized societies, the average daily intake of sodium ranges from 150 to 200 mmol (3.5 to 4.6 g). Such levels of dietary sodium greatly exceed individual needs and may be reduced without harm to a level between 80 and 100 mmol (1.8 and 2.3 g) per day. It has been proposed from animal studies that sodium chloride may have a greater influence on blood pressure than sodium alone (Whitescarver *et al.* 1984; Kurtz and Morris 1985).

A controlled trial was conducted in two Belgian towns to investigate the feasibility and effects of a reduction in salt consumption at the community level (Staessen *et al.* 1988). The low-sodium intervention in one town was mainly directed at women, and implemented through mass media. The control town was merely observed. Cross-sectional random sampling at baseline and five years later revealed a significant decrease of 25 mmol per day in 24-hour urinary excretion in adult women but not in men, while blood pressure was not affected. This study and that of Thaler *et al.* (1982) indicate that a drastic reduction in salt intake is difficult to achieve in communities with an ubiquitous and generous use of sodium in prepared foods.

Potassium and Blood Pressure

Evidence from several sources suggests an inverse relationship between blood pressure and urinary 24-hour potassium excretion. The Intersalt Cooperative Research Group (1988) found a negative and significant pooled correlation for the relationships when adjustments were made for age, sex, body mass index, alcohol intake and sodium excretion. It was estimated that an increase of 100 mmol of potassium per day corresponded to a decrease in systolic blood pressure of 2.5 mm Hg and 1.7 mm Hg in diastolic blood pressure. Similarly, in the Scottish Heart Health Study, potassium excretion was weakly and negatively correlated with blood pressure, but unlike sodium, was significant in the stepwise regression models of systolic and diastolic pressure in men and in women (Smith *et al.* 1988).

Evidence of an association between dietary potassium and blood pressure is not consistent. Kesteloot and Joossens (1988) were unable to find a significant negative correlation between dietary potassium and blood pressure, although they were able to demonstrate a high degree of correlation between the dietary intake of potassium and its urinary excretion. Khaw and Barrett-Connor (1988), however, found a significant and negative relationship between dietary potassium and blood pressure before and after adjustment for age and dietary variables. It is unclear whether these discrepancies are related to confounding factors such as the high degree of collinearity between dietary potassium and calcium, and the inverse association with alcohol (Reed *et al.* 1985).

In a series of studies in experimental animals, Tobian (1986) demonstrated a protective effect, independent of blood pressure, of high potassium intake against stroke in stroke-prone spontaneously hypertensive rats. More recently Khaw and Barrett-Connor (1987) reported a significant inverse relationship between a 24-hour dietary potassium intake at baseline, and subsequent stroke-associated mortality in humans. It was estimated that a 10 mmol (0.4 g) increase in daily potassium intake was associated with a 40% reduction in the risk of stroke-associated mortality.

There is evidence from some short-term clinical trials on small numbers of subjects that potassium supplementation of 60 mmol (2.4 g) or more a day can lower blood pressure in untreated and treated hypertensive patients (Iimura *et al.* 1981; MacGregor *et al.* 1982; Kaplan *et al.* 1985). The effectiveness of potassium supplementation in lowering blood pressure is less apparent in normotensive individuals and in those who are concomitantly on a low sodium diet (Smith *et al.* 1985; Barden *et al.* 1986). Further studies are required to define the relationship between potassium intake and blood pressure.

Salt and Cancer

The evidence linking salt to gastric cancer is controversial. Some investigators found a positive correlation (Joossens and Geboers 1981; Tuomilehto *et al.* 1984) and others found no association (Walker 1982; Whelton and Goldblatt 1982). The association between salt and cancer is supported by the positive relationship between stroke mortality and stomach cancer mortality both between and within countries (Joossens and Geboers 1987).

A case control study in Newfoundland, Ontario and Manitoba showed no association between salt intake and gastric cancer (Risch *et al.* 1985). Other reports, however, noted a high incidence of gastric cancer and the consumption of salty foods in Colombia (Correa *et al.* 1983), in the blacks of Louisiana (Correa *et al.* 1985), and in Japan (Hara *et al.* 1985) and Hawaii (Haenszel *et al.* 1972).

Requirements

Sodium and Chloride

Adults

Requirements for these electrolytes have not been well defined but they can be estimated from the limited information available on the obligatory or minimal losses from the body, the amounts (based on body composition) required for fetal development and for growth, and the amounts secreted in milk during lactation.

From a review of various studies, Aitken (1976) has estimated the obligatory losses of sodium at 5.1 mmol (117 mg)/day per 100 kg body weight in sedentary adults not actively sweating. The loss in sweat, urine and feces accounted for 4.0, 1.0, and 0.1 mmol (92, 23 and 2.3 mg) respectively of the 5.1 mmol per 100 kg. The minimal requirement of sodium would therefore be around 3.5 mmol (80 mg) per day for a 70 kg man. This estimate is corroborated by the fact that primitive people have been reported to live on 2 to 10 mmol (46 to 230 mg) of sodium per day, and patients have been maintained on similar rations for many years without any problems (Dahl 1972).

Obligatory losses of potassium are estimated at 23.9 mmol (932 mg) per 100 kg body weight per day (Aitken 1976), the largest proportion coming from feces (12.4 mmol or 489 mg), then from sweat (6 mmol or 234 mg) and from urine (5.5 mmol or 214 mg). A 70 kg man would thus require a minimum of about 16 mmol (624 mg) per day. Since potassium is abundant in all types of diets, there are no reports of people habitually consuming diets containing such low quantities of potassium.

Salt (NaC1) is the predominant source of chloride in the diet; obligatory losses of this electrolyte are equivalent to those of sodium, i.e. about 5.1 mmol (178 mg) per 100 kg body weight per day, of which about 80% is excreted in sweat, and 20% in the urine, the amount in feces being negligible.

Given that it is difficult to measure obligatory losses, and that there are large variations in climate and levels of exercise that will affect the excretion of electrolytes, requirements for electrolytes cannot be defined. Intakes as low as 5 mmol per day each of sodium and chloride (115 mg and 175 mg), and 30 mmol of potassium (1170 mg) are sufficient to cover the needs of sedentary adults living in a temperate climate.

Infants and Children

The obligatory losses of sodium in infants have been estimated at 0.29 mmol (7 mg) per kilogram of body weight by Aitken (1976), and the daily needs for growth at 0.06 mmol per kilogram by the same author. Fomon (1974, pp. 268-9) estimated the requirement of infants up to four months at 2.5 mmol per day, and the advisable intake for the same age at 8 mmol per day. Human milk contains an average of 0.65 mmol (15 mg) per 100 mL (Aitken 1976). An infant taking 750 mL milk per day would receive 5 mmol (115 mg) of sodium per day. This would likely be sufficient at least for the first months of life. As soon as a child is fed solid foods, the intake surpasses the minimal needs several times so that risks of inadequate intake are practically non-existent except in cases of illness (fever, vomiting), where losses are important. As a practical requirement for normal children, an intake of 6 to 8 mmol (138 to 184 mg) per day, as suggested by Fomon (1974, pp. 268-9) for up to three years of age, appears adequate. Requirements of older children are not known but would not be likely to exceed 10 mmol (230 mg) per day, which is twice the minimal requirement for adults.

Pregnancy and Lactation

According to Fregly (1984), the total sodium required for pregnancy is about 750 mmol (17.25 g), based on a weight gain of 11 kg. The average need per day in addition to non-pregnant needs would be 3 mmol (69 mg). As mentioned, an average of about 5 mmol (115 mg) of sodium are secreted in 750 mL of human milk. An additional intake of 5 to 10 mmol (115 to 230 mg) of sodium per day should cover the extra needs of the lactating woman. The increased requirements for pregnancy and lactation are easily met from the mixed diet.

Potassium

There are no estimates of obligatory losses of potassium in infants, but growth needs have been estimated at 0.043 mmol (1.7 mg) per gram of weight gained (Aitken 1976). The loss in feces would be, however, higher than in adults, and is estimated at 14 mmol (546 mg) per day (Aitken 1976). In older children, requirements for growth would be around 60 mmol (2340 mg) per gram of weight gain in those under 30 kilograms of bodyweight, and around 30 mmol (1170 mg) per gram in those exceeding that weight. Fomon (1974) estimated the advisable intake of potassium for infants and children up to three years at 6 to 8 mmol (234 to 312 mg) per day. Requirements of potassium for pregnancy are estimated by Aitken (1976) at 320 mmol (12.48 g) or slightly over 1 mmol (39 mg) per day, and those for lactation at 12 mmol (468 mg) per day.

Recommendations

Intakes of sodium in Canada greatly exceed requirements. Comparisons of blood pressure in adults of different national populations tend to show that there is a positive correlation with sodium intake. Clinical studies on human adults with mild hypertension indicate that a reduction in sodium intake is associated with a decrease in blood pressure. On the basis of this evidence of potential benefit, and lack of evidence of potential risk, a decrease in the current intake of sodium by the Canadian population is recommended.

Consumers are advised to minimize their use of salt in cooking, to avoid its use at the table, and to select commercial foods low in added salt. To facilitate a reduction in sodium intake, food manufacturers are urged to reduce the addition of salt or other sources of sodium to processed and prepared foods.

In view of the potential beneficial effects of an increased intake of potassium on hypertension and stroke-related mortality rates, a potassium-rich diet which emphasizes fruits and vegetables is recommended.

Water intake, including that from food, is governed by thirst and should balance output.

References

Aitken, F.C. 1976. Sodium and potassium in nutrition of mammals. Commonwealth Agricultural Bureaux, Farnham Royal, England.

Altschul, A.M., McPherson, R.A. and Burris, J.F. 1984. Dietary sodium, the ratio Na+/K+ and essential hypertension. Nutr. Abstr. Rev. 54:823-844.

Australian National Health and Medical Research Council Dietary Salt Study Management Committee. 1989. Fall in blood pressure with modest reduction in dietary salt intake in mild hypertension. Lancet 1:399-402.

Barden, A.E., Vandongen, R., Beilin, L.J., Margetts, B. and Rogers, P. 1986. Potassium supplementation does not lower blood pressure in normotensive women. J. Hypertens. 4:339-343.

Bertino, M., Beauchamp, G.K., Engelman, K. and Kare, M.R. 1982. Dietary sodium and salt taste. *In* The role of salt in cardiovascular hypertension. Fregly, M.J. and Kare, M.R., eds. Academic Press, New York, pp. 145-154.

Canada. Health and Welfare. 1989. Main findings. Report of the Canadian Blood Pressure Survey. Ottawa.

Canadian Paediatric Society. Nutrition Committee. 1983. Adolescent nutrition: 4. Sports and diet. Can. Med. Assoc. J. 129:552-553.

Consolazio, C.F. 1983. Nutrition and performance. Johnson, R.E., ed. Pergamon Press, New York.

Correa, P., Cuello, C., Fajardo, L.F., Haenszel, W., Bolanos, O. and de Ramirez, B. 1983. Diet and gastric cancer: nutrition survey in a high risk area. J. Nat. Cancer Inst. 70:673-678.

Correa, P., Fontham, E., Pickle, L.W., Chen, V., Lin, Y. and Haenszel, W. 1985. Dietary determinants of gastric cancer in South Louisiana inhabitants. J. Nat. Cancer Inst. 75:645-654.

Dahl, L.K. 1972. Salt and hypertension. Am. J. Clin. Nutr. 25:231-244.

Fomon, S.J. 1974. Infant nutrition. 2nd ed. Saunders, Philadelphia, pp. 268-269.

Fregly, M.J. 1984. Sodium and potassium. *In* Nutrition Reviews' present knowledge in nutrition. 5th ed. Nutrition Foundation, Washington, D.C., pp. 439-458.

Froment, A., Milon, H. and Gravier, C. 1979. Relation entre consommation sodée et hypertension artérielle. Contribution de l'épidémiologie géographique. Rev. Epidemiol. Santé Publique 27:437-454.

Gleibermann, L. 1973. Blood pressure and dietary salt in human populations. Ecol. Food Nutr. 2:143-156.

Grobbee, D.E. and Hofman, A. 1986. Does sodium restriction lower blood pressure? Br. Med. J. 293:27-29.

Guthrie, H.A. 1983. Introductory nutrition. 5th ed. Mosby, St. Louis.

Guyton, A.C. 1981. Textbook of medical physiology. 6th ed. Saunders, Philadelphia.

Haenszel, W., Kurihara, M., Segi, M. and Lee, R.K.C. 1972. Stomach cancer among Japanese in Hawaii. J. Nat. Cancer Inst. 49:969-988.

Hara, N., Sakata, K., Nagai, M., Fujita, Y., Hashimoto, T. and Yanagawa, H. 1985. Statistical analyses on the pattern of food consumption and digestive-tract cancers in Japan. Nutr. Cancer 6:220-228.

Hays, R.M. 1980. Dynamics of body water and electrolytes. *In* Clinical disorders of fluid and electrolyte metabolism. Maxwell, M.H. and Kleeman, C.R., eds. McGraw-Hill, New York, pp. 1-36.

Houston, M.C. 1986. Sodium and hypertension: a review. Arch. Intern. Med. 146:179-185.

Iimura, O., Kijima, T., Kikuchi, K., Miyama, A., Ando, T., Nakao, T. and Takigami, Y. 1981. Studies on the hypotensive effect of high potassium intake in patients with essential hypertension. Clin. Sci. (Suppl.) 61:77s-80s.

Intersalt Cooperative Research Group. 1988. Intersalt: an international study of electrolyte excretion and blood pressure. Results for 24 hour urinary sodium and potassium excretion. Br. Med. J. 297:319-328.

Joossens, J.V. and Geboers, J. 1981. Nutrition and gastric cancer. Proc. Nutr. Soc. 40:37-46.

Joossens, J.V. and Geboers, J. 1987. Dietary salt and risks to health. Am. J. Clin. Nutr. 45:1277-1288.

Kaplan, N.M., Carnegie, A., Raskin, P., Heller, J.A. and Simmons, M. 1985. Potassium supplementation in hypertensive patients with diuretic-induced hypokalemia. N. Engl. J. Med. 312:746-749.

Kesteloot, H. and Joossens, J.V. 1988. Relationship of dietary sodium, potassium, calcium and magnesium with blood pressure. Belgian interuniversity research on nutrition and health. Hypertension 12:594-599.

Khaw, K.T. and Barrett-Connor, E. 1987. Dietary potassium and stroke associated mortality. N. Engl. J. Med. 316:235-240.

Khaw, K.T. and Barrett-Connor, E. 1988. The association between blood pressure, age and dietary sodium and potassium: a population study. Circulation 77:53-61.

Kurtz, T.W. and Morris, R.C., Jr. 1985. Hypertension and sodium salts. Science 228:352-353.

Logan, A.G. 1986. Sodium manipulation in the management of hypertension. The view against its general use. Can. J. Physiol. Pharmacol. 64:793-802.

MacGregor, G.A. 1985. Sodium is more important than calcium in essential hypertension. Hypertension 7:628-637.

MacGregor, G.A., Markandu, N.D., Best, F.E., Elder, D.M., Cam, J.M., Sagnella, G.A. and Squires, M. 1982. Double-blind randomised crossover trial of moderate sodium restriction in essential hypertension. Lancet 1:351-355.

MacGregor, G.A., Smith, S.J., Markandu, N.D., Banks, R.A. and Sagnella, G.A. 1982. Moderate potassium supplementation in essential hypertension. Lancet 2:567-570.

Mongeau, E., Cambiotti, L.W., Gelinas, M.D., Ledoux, M. and Lambert, J. 1989. Consommation de sodium dans une population adulte de Montréal. (unpublished report)

Mongeau, J.-G. 1987. Heredity and blood pressure in humans: an overview. Pediatr. Nephrol. 1:69-75.

Murray, R. 1987. The effects of consuming carbohydrate-electrolyte beverages on gastric emptying and fluid absorption during and following exercise. Sports Med. 4:322-351.

Reed, D., McGee, D., Yano, K. and Hankin, J. 1985. Diet, blood pressure and multicollinearity. Hypertension 7:405-410.

Risch, H.A., Jain, M., Choi, N.W., Fodor, J.G., Pfeiffer, C.J., Howe, G.R., Harrison, L.W., Craib, K.J.P. and Miller, A.B. 1985. Dietary factors and the incidence of cancer of the stomach. Am. J. Epidemiol. 122:947-957.

Shah, B.G. and Belonje, B. 1983. Calculated sodium and potassium in the Canadian diet if comprised of unprocessed ingredients. Nutr. Res. 3:629-633.

Smith, S.J., Markandu, N.D., Sagnella, G.A. and MacGregor, G.A. 1985. Moderate potassium chloride supplementation in essential hypertension: is it additive to moderate sodium restriction? Br. Med. J. 290:110-113.

Smith, W.C.S., Crombie, I.K., Tavendale, R.T., Gulland, S.K. and Tunstall-Pedoe, H.D. 1988. Urinary electrolyte excretion, alcohol consumption, and blood pressure in the Scottish Heart Health Study. Br. Med. J. 297:329-330.

Staessen, J., Bulpitt, C.J., Fagard, R., Joossens, J.V., Lijnen, P. and Amery, A. 1988. Salt intake and blood pressure in the general population: a controlled intervention trial in two towns. J. Hypertens. 6:965-973.

Stricker, E.M. 1980. The physiological basis of sodium appetite: a new look at the "depletion-repletion" model. *In* Biological and behavioral aspects of salt intake. Kare, M.R., Fregly, M.J. and Bernard, R.A. eds. Academic Press, New York, pp. 185-204.

Thaler, B.I., Paulin, J.M., Phelan, E.L. and Simpson, F.O. 1982. A pilot study to test the feasibility of salt restriction in a community. NZ Med. J. 95:839-842.

Tobian, L. 1986. High potassium diets markedly protect against stroke deaths and kidney disease in hypertensive rats, a possible legacy from prehistoric times. Can. J. Physiol. Pharmacol. 64:840-848.

Tuomilehto, J., Geboers, J., Joossens, J.V., Salonen, J.T. and Tanskanen, A. 1984. Trends in stomach cancer and stroke in Finland: comparison to northwest Europe and USA. Stroke 15:823-828.

Walker, A.R. 1982. Changing disease patterns in South Africa. S. Afr. Med. J. 61:126-129.

Weinberger, M.H., Miller, J.Z., Luft, F.C., Grim, C.E. and Fineberg, N.S. 1986. Sodium sensitivity and resistance of blood pressure in humans. Food Technol. 40:96-98.

Whelton, P.K. and Goldblatt, P. 1982. An investigation of the relationship between stomach cancer and cerebrovascular disease: evidence for and against the salt hypothesis. Am. J. Epidemiol. 115:418-427.

Whitescarver, S.A., Ott, C.E., Jackson, B.A., Guthrie, G.P., Jr. and Kotchen, T.A. 1984. Salt-sensitive hypertension: contribution of chloride. Science 223:1430-1432.

Part III

Some Non-Essential Dietary Components

Alcohol

Alcohol (ethanol) may be present in the diet as 5% by volume of beer, 12% of wine or 40% of spirits. Its average disappearance in Canada in 1986 was 28 mL (22g or 150 kcal or 630 kJ) per day per person fifteen years of age or older (Canada. Statistics Canada 1987). Alcohol provides 29 kJ or 6.93 kcal per gram, a level which is higher than that from carbohydrate or protein (Merrill and Watt 1973). The energy from high levels of alcohol, however, appears to be handled differently, with an increased consumption of oxygen and more heat production instead of the formation of high-energy phosphate bonds (Lieber 1984).

The view of Best *et al.* (1949) that the effects of high levels of alcohol result from the displacement of essential nutrients was altered by evidence of toxicity in the presence of adequate nutrient intakes (Lieber *et al.* 1963). Energy derived from alcohol, however, tends to replace energy derived from other sources (Thomson *et al.* 1988). Alcohol may also diminish the utilization of some nutrients (Lieber 1988).

Effects on Nutrients

The effect of occasional or moderate consumption of alcohol on nutritional status is not well documented. It is known that for many vitamins, single large doses and chronic ingestion of alcohol can impair absorption, metabolic conversions and utilization in peripheral tissues and enhance urinary excretion (Kalant 1987). Active absorption of thiamin, catalysed by Na^+, K^+-ATPase, decreases with alcohol; activation of this vitamin to thiamin pyrophosphate, the coenzyme of transketolase, also decreases with ethanol-induced liver injury (Hoyumpa 1980). In pyridoxine metabolism, acetaldehyde, which is produced by the degradation of alcohol, can displace pyridoxal phosphate from its binding protein and thereby enhance its degradation (Mezey 1985). Vitamin A is oxidized to its active form by liver alcohol dehydrogenase, a conversion that is impaired by excessive alcohol ingestion (Mezey 1985). There is considerable evidence that a high consumption of alcohol and diseases related to it have an adverse effect on vitamin status. Many reports of the effects of alcohol on mineral status are based on studies in alcoholics.

Amino acid uptake is also inhibited by the effect of alcohol on Na^+,K^+-ATPase activity as well as its depressing effect on gastrointestinal activity (Kalant 1987). Glucose tolerance tests are impaired by alcohol, which also depletes liver glycogen. Depending on the state of the glycogen stores, either hyperglycemia or hypoglycemia can ensue after alcohol ingestion. Administration of ethanol elevates the serum very low-density lipoprotein, a fraction that is particularly high in individuals with type IV hyperlipidemia (Shaw and Lieber 1988).

Chronic Diseases

Chronic ingestion of alcohol, at levels that the liver cannot readily metabolize, leads to disorders of the liver, heart muscle and particularly the nervous system. After alcohol enters the bloodstream, 5% to 10% is excreted in the urine and breath; the rest is metabolized mostly in the liver where alcohol dehydrogenase is the rate-limiting enzyme.

Chronic alcohol consumption is the main cause of cirrhosis in industrialized countries (Robbins and Kumar 1987).

A U-shaped curve for alcohol consumption and total mortality provided encouragement for a low level of intake, but was attributed to men with previously diagnosed cardiovascular disease becoming occasional or non-drinkers (Shaper *et al.* 1988). A negative association, however, between the prevalence of coronary heart disease and high-density lipoprotein (HDL) cholesterol was apparent in several epidemiological studies (Castelli *et al.* 1977; Gordon *et al.* 1977; Wilson *et al.* 1980). An increase in HDL-cholesterol correlated with a moderate intake of alcohol (Yano *et al.* 1977; Wilson *et al.* 1983; Criqui 1986). A subtype, HDL_3, enhanced by alcohol, differs from the protective HDL_2 (Lieber and Savolainen 1984). Hegsted and Ausman (1988) detected a negative association on an international basis between alcohol consumption and mortality from coronary heart disease. In a large prospective study on middle aged men, alcohol had no protective effect against ischaemic heart disease (Shaper *et al.* 1987). The situation became more complicated when a prospective study of middle-aged nurses indicated a decrease in coronary heart disease and stroke associated with a moderate intake of alcohol (Stampfer *et al.* 1988). On the other hand, consumption of alcohol in excess of 24 g, or two drinks daily, was associated with an increased risk of breast cancer (Longnecker *et al.* 1988).

From a review of many studies to determine if alcohol increases the risk of breast cancer, Byers (1988) found fairly consistent support that it does, but could not draw conclusions about doses that exert such an influence.

Others could not find evidence for alcohol in the genesis of breast cancer (Harris and Wynder 1988; Schatzkin *et al.* 1989). Positive correlations were recognized between high intakes of alcohol and oral, laryngeal and esophogeal cancers (U.S. N.R.C. 1982).

The association between alcohol consumption and hypertension is well established. In the Munich Blood Pressure Study, a significant factor for this condition in both men and women was alcohol consumption (Cairns *et al.* 1984). This was also the case for Japanese urban and rural men in whom both blood pressure and the prevalence of hypertension were related in a graded manner to alcohol intake (Ueshima *et al.* 1984). The Health and Nutrition Examination Survey in the United States also showed a contributory role of alcohol to hypertension (Gruchow *et al.* 1985). In New Zealand, men and women aged fifty years and older who consumed four drinks or more per day manifested increased systolic and diastolic blood pressure (Jackson *et al.* 1985). For most of the men in the Albany Study, the level of consumption was judged to be moderate, ranging from the equivalent of 0 to 90 oz. of spirits per month, but was still related to increased blood pressure when the rate exceeded 30 oz. per month (Gordon and Doyle 1986). Blood pressure in normotensive men fell in response to a reduction in alcohol consumption, and systolic blood pressure rose again upon the resumption of former drinking habits (Puddey *et al.* 1985). The direct pressor effect of alcohol has been attributed to arteriolar vasoconstriction (Potter *et al.* 1984). Alcohol is an important risk factor for hypertension, which is reversible when alcohol consumption is reduced (Saunders 1987).

Pregnancy

Fetal alcohol syndrome is the leading identified cause of mental retardation in the Western World (Abel 1988). The possibility of developing this condition, which is also characterized by growth retardation and congenital abnormalities, may be related to genetic factors, maternal age or parity and the pattern of alcohol ingestion (Abel and Sokol 1986). Binge drinking causes high blood alcohol concentrations in the fetus of experimental animals and can be particularly damaging (Webster *et al.* 1980). Whether moderate or social levels of alcohol consumption are part of a continuum of dose-related adverse effects on the fetus is a matter of controversy (Beattie 1988).

A history of antenatal alcohol abuse was readily associated with impaired mental and motor development in infants (Golden *et al.* 1982). On the basis of self-reported drinking patterns, women who consumed more than 30 mL absolute alcohol per day produced offspring with an enhanced frequency of fetal alcohol effects, and those who consumed four times that amount showed still more effects (Graham *et al.* 1988). The lowest amount of absolute alcohol implicated in fetal alcohol syndrome was 1 oz or 30 mL per day (Hingson *et al.* 1982), although a Canadian report indicated decreased infant muscle tone with intake of about 25 mL absolute alcohol per day (Staisy and Fried 1983). Rosett *et al.* (1983) found no difference between rare and moderate drinking, at the rate of 9 mL absolute alcohol per day, and reported a benefit to offspring of a reduction in alcohol consumption even at mid-pregnancy. Ingestion during late pregnancy of 30 mL absolute alcohol per day caused a greater decrease in birth weight than a similar amount consumed before pregnancy (Little 1977).

The toxicity of alcohol derives from the major oxidation product of ethyl alcohol, acetaldehyde, which is transferred by the placenta to the fetus (Karl *et al.* 1988). Although low levels of alcohol in two studies did not appear to be associated with congenital malformations, a grouping of results, from Northern California, according to organ systems showed that malformations in sex organs were related to alcohol consumption (Wyngaarden 1988). Since a safe level of alcohol consumption during pregnancy has not been defined, the most prudent measure is abstinence (Warren and Bast 1988).

Recommendations

In view of the adverse effect of alcohol on blood pressure and the possible replacement of foods that supply essential nutrients, adults consuming alcohol should limit their intake to less than 5% of total energy or two drinks per day, whichever is less. The most prudent course during pregnancy appears to be abstention from alcohol.

References

Abel, E.L. 1988. Fetal alcohol syndrome in families. Neurotoxicol. Teratology 10:1-2.

Abel, E.L. and Sokol, R.J. 1986. Maternal and fetal characteristics affecting alcohol's teratogenicity. Neurobehav. Toxicol. Teratol. 8:329-334.

Beattie, J. 1988. Alcohol and the child. Proc. Nutr. Soc. 47:121-127.

Best, C.H., Hartroft, W.S., Lucas, C.C. and Ridout, J.H. 1949. Liver damage produced by feeding alcohol or sugar and its prevention by choline. Br. Med. J. 2:1001-1006.

Byers, T. 1988. Diet and cancer. Any progress in the interim? Cancer 62 (Suppl.):1713-1724.

Canada. Statistics Canada. 1987. The control and sale of alcoholic beverages in Canada 1985. Ottawa.

Cairns, V., Keil, U., Kleinbaum, D., Doering, A. and Stieber, J. 1984. Alcohol consumption as a risk factor for high blood pressure. Munich Blood Pressure Study. Hypertension 6:124-131.

Castelli, W.P., Doyle, J.T., Gordon, T., Hames, C.G., Hjortland, M.C., Hulley, S.B., Kagan, A. and Zukel, W.J. 1977. HDL cholesterol and other lipids in coronary heart disease. The cooperative lipoprotein phenotyping study. Circulation 55:767-772.

Criqui, M.H. 1986. Alcohol consumption, blood pressure, lipids and cardiovascular mortality. Alcohol.: Clin. Exp. Res. 10:564-569.

Golden, N.L., Sokol, R.J., Kuhnert, B.R. and Bottoms, S. 1982. Maternal alcohol use and infant development. Pediatrics 70:931-934.

Gordon, T., Castelli, W.P., Hjortland, M.C., Kannel, W.B. and Dawber, T.R. 1977. High density lipoprotein as a protective factor against coronary heart disease. The Framingham Study. Am. J. Med. 62:707-714.

Gordon, T. and Doyle, J.T. 1986. Alcohol consumption and its relationship to smoking, weight, blood pressure, and blood lipids. Arch. Intern. Med. 146:262-265.

Graham, J.M., Jr., Hanson, J.W., Darby, B.L., Barr, H.M. and Streissguth, A.P. 1988. Independent dysmorphology evaluations at birth and four years of age for children exposed to varying amounts of alcohol in utero. Pediatrics 81:772-778.

Gruchow, H.W., Sobocinski, K.A. and Barboriak, J.J. 1985. Alcohol, nutrient intake, and hypertension in US adults. J. Am. Med. Assoc. 253:1567-1570.

Harris, R.E. and Wynder, E.L. 1988. Breast cancer and alcohol consumption. A study in weak associations. J. Am. Med. Assoc. 259:2867-2871.

Hegsted, D.M. and Ausman, L.M. 1988. Diet, alcohol and coronary heart disease in men. J. Nutr. 118:1184-1189.

Hingson, R., Alpert, J.J., Day, N., Dooling, E., Kayne, H., Morelock, S., Oppenheimer, E. and Zuckerman, B. 1982. Effects of maternal drinking and marijuana use on fetal growth and development. Pediatrics 70:539-546.

Hoyumpa, A.M. 1980. Mechanisms of thiamin deficiency in chronic alcoholism. Am. J. Clin. Nutr. 33:2750-2761.

Jackson, R., Stewart, A., Beaglehole, R. and Scragg, R. 1985. Alcohol consumption and blood pressure. Am. J. Epidemiol. 122:1037-1044.

Kalant, H. 1987. Alcohol use and nutrition. *In* Proceedings of symposium on diet, nutrition and health. Carroll, K.K., ed. McGill-Queen's University Press, Kingston, Ont.

Karl, P.I., Gordon, B.H.J., Lieber, C.S. and Fisher, S.E. 1988. Acetaldehyde production and transfer by the perfused human placental cotyledon. Science 242:273-275.

Lieber, C.S. 1984. Metabolism and metabolic effects of alcohol. Med. Clin. North Am. 68:3-31.

Lieber, C.S. 1988. The influence of alcohol on nutritional status. Nutr. Rev. 46:241-254.

Lieber, C.S. and Savolainen, M. 1984. Ethanol and lipids. Alcohol.: Clin. Exp. Res. 8:409-423.

Lieber, C.S., Jones, D.P., Mendelson, J. and DeCarli, L.M. 1963. Fatty liver, hyperlipemia and hyperuricemia produced by prolonged alcohol consumption despite adequate dietary intake. Trans. Assoc. Am. Physicians 76:289-300.

Little, R.E. 1977. Moderate alcohol use during pregnancy and decreased infant birth weight. Am. J. Public Health 67:1154-1156.

Longnecker, M.P., Berlin, J.A., Orza, M.J. and Chalmers, C. 1988. A meta-analysis of alcohol consumption in relation to risk of breast cancer. J. Am. Med. Assoc. 260:652-656.

Merrill, A.L. and Watt, B.K. 1973. Energy value of foods ... basis and derivation. Agricultural handbook no. 74. Human Nutrition Research Branch. Agricultural Research Service. United States Department of Agriculture, Washington, D.C.

Mezey, E. 1985. Metabolic effects of alcohol. Fed. Proc. 44:134-138.

Potter, J.F., Bannan, L.T. and Beevers, D.G. 1984. Alcohol and hypertension. Br. J. Addict. 79:365-372.

Puddey, I.B., Beilin, L.J., Vandongen, R., Rouse, I.L. and Rogers, P. 1985. Evidence for a direct effect of alcohol consumption on blood pressure in normotensive men, a randomized controlled trial. Hypertension 7:707-713.

Robbins, S.L. and Kumar, V. 1987. Basic pathology. 4th ed. Saunders, Philadelphia.

Rosett, H.L., Weiner, L., Lee, A., Zuckerman, B., Dooling, E. and Oppenheimer, E. 1983. Patterns of alcohol consumption and fetal development. J. Am. Coll. Obstet. Gynecol. 61:539-546.

Saunders, J.B. 1987. Alcohol: an important cause of hypertension. Br. Med. J. 294:1045-1046.

Schatzkin, A., Carter, C.L., Green, S.B., Kreger, B.E., Splansky, G.L., Anderson, K.M., Helsel, W.E. and Kannel, W.B. 1989. Is alcohol consumption related to breast cancer? Results from the Framingham Heart Study. J. Nat. Cancer Inst. 81:31-35.

Shaper, A.G., Phillips, A.N., Pocock, S.J. and Walker, M. 1987. Alcohol and ischaemic heart disease in middle-aged British men. Br. Med. J. 294:733-737.

Shaper, A.G., Wannamethee, G. and Walker, M. 1988. Alcohol and mortality in British men: explaining the U-shaped curve. Lancet 2:1267-1273.

Shaw, S. and Lieber, C.S. 1988. Nutrition and diet in alcoholism. *In* Modern nutrition in health and disease. 7th ed. Shils, M.E. and Young, V.R., eds. Lea & Febiger, Philadelphia, pp. 1423-1449.

Staisey, N.L. and Fried, P.A. 1983. Relationships between moderate maternal alcohol consumption during pregnancy and infant neurological development. J. Stud. Alcohol 44:262-270.

Stampfer, M.J., Colditz, G.A., Willett, W.C., Speizer, F.E. and Hennekens, C.H. 1988. A prospective study of moderate alcohol consumption and the risk of coronary disease and stroke in women. N. Engl. J. Med. 319:267-273.

Thomson, M., Fulton, M., Elton, R.A., Brown, S., Wood, D.A. and Oliver, M.F. 1988. Alcohol consumption and nutrient intake in middle-aged Scottish men. Am. J. Clin. Nutr. 47:139-145.

Ueshima, H., Shimamoto, T., Iida, M., Konishi, M., Tanigaki, M., Doi, M., Tsujioka, K., Nagano, E., Tsuda, C., Ozawa, H., Kojima, S. and Komachi, Y. 1984. Alcohol intake and hypertension among urban and rural Japanese populations. J. Chronic Dis. 37:585-592.

U.S. National Research Council. 1982. Diet, nutrition and cancer. Committee on Diet, Nutrition and Cancer. National Academy of Sciences, Washington, D.C.

Warren, K.R. and Bast, R.J. 1988. Alcohol-related birth defects: an update. Public Health Rep. 103:638-642.

Webster, W.S., Walsh, D.A., Lipson, A.H. and McEwen, S.E. 1980. Teratogenesis after acute alcohol exposure in inbred and outbred mice. Neurobehav. Toxicol. 2:227-234.

Wilson, P.W., Garrison, R.J., Castelli, W.P., Feinleib, M., McNamara, P.M. and Kannel, W.B. 1980. Prevalence of coronary heart disease in the Framingham Offspring Study: role of lipoprotein cholesterols. Am. J. Cardiol. 46:649-654.

Wilson, P.W.F., Garrison, R.J., Abbott, R.D. and Castelli, W.P. 1983. Factors associated with lipoprotein cholesterol levels. The Framingham Study. Arteriosclerosis 3:273-281.

Wyngaarden, J.B. 1988. Effects of moderate alcohol use during pregnancy. J. Am. Med. Assoc. 259:20.

Yano, K., Rhoads, G.G. and Kagan, A. 1977. Coffee, alcohol and risk of coronary heart disease among Japanese men living in Hawaii. N. Engl. J. Med. 297:405-409.

Aluminum

Aluminum, nonessential to humans, is one of the most common elements in our environment and comprises more than 8% of the earth's crust (Jones and Bennett 1986). While most aluminum is present in an insoluble and biologically unavailable form, the natural prevalence of aluminum in our environment ensures inevitable exposure to this ubiquitous element. Recently, there has been considerable interest in the toxicity of aluminum as a potential pathogenic factor in several human diseases. Aluminum has been implicated in diseases of the lungs, brain, blood and bone (Lione 1985; Crapper McLachlan and Farnell 1986). Current public health concerns regarding aluminum exposure have focussed on the possible role that aluminum may play in the etiology and pathogenesis of Alzheimer's disease. Epidemiological studies suggest that an environmental agent may be involved (Glenner 1982); aluminum has been implicated. In addition, certain biochemical changes associated with intracranial aluminum administration in experimental animals mimic those observed in senile dementias of the Alzheimer's type (Perl 1985; Crapper McLachlan and Van Berkum 1986; Crapper McLachlan *et al.* 1987). To address this concern, sources of exogenous aluminum and the metabolic handling of this common element must be explored, and the evidence implicating aluminum with the pathology of Alzheimer's disease examined, to discern if there is a need for concern over the ingestion of food sources of aluminum.

Sources of Aluminum

Aluminum is naturally present in trace amounts in water and most foods. Aluminum concentration of raw surface water varies depending upon geographical location. Acid rain may be a significant contributor to the aluminum content of water, since high acidity increases the solubility of aluminum and leaches large amounts of this element from the soil. Consequently, there is a resultant increase in the bioavailability of aluminum (Jones and Bennett 1986). Aside from the natural occurrence, further increases in the aluminum concentration in drinking water may be observed since aluminum sulphate is added in some instances as a flocculant during the purification process. Hence, the concentration of aluminum in drinking water may vary from 0.001-1.6 mg/L depending on the geographic location and water purification process used (Lione 1983). In general, concentrations of aluminum in various foods range from 0.02-5 mg/kg (wet weight), with higher amounts being observed in plant food (<.01-2.0 mg/kg) and some fish (0.70-1.40 mg/kg) and relatively lower amounts in most meat and dairy products (Sorenson *et al.* 1974). Certain fish (mackerel and tuna, 1-178 mg/kg) and shellfish (crab and crayfish, 35-45 mg/kg) can be especially high (Crapper McLachlan and Farnell 1986).

In addition to natural sources, aluminum may be added during the processing, preparation and storage of food. There are currently six aluminum salts approved for use as food additives which are used in various foods, such as processed cheese slices, to act as emulsifiers (50 mg aluminum/serving) and in preserving and pickling (5-15 mg/serving). Aluminum sulphate is used in several baking powders and leavening agents (5-15 mg/serving) and also as an anticaking agent in powdered soups and nondairy creamers (2% aluminum by weight) (Lione 1983). Storage of food in aluminum containers and cooking salty, acidic or alkaline food in aluminum cookware will further increase the levels of aluminum in food. New aluminum pots and utensils, along with foil wrap and aluminum cans, may contribute an additional 15% aluminum to the daily intake (Sorenson *et al.* 1974; Lione 1983).

Taking all dietary sources into consideration, it has been estimated that the average adult consumes between 1-30 mg aluminum/day (Sorenson *et al.* 1974), with a value of 20 mg/d accepted as representative (Underwood 1977; Lione *et al.* 1984). This implies that foods high in aluminum do not form a significant part of the diet for most people; however, consumption of such products can easily double or triple normal daily intake.

In contrast to foods, a number of nonprescription drugs such as antacids, buffered aspirin and antidiarrheals may contain considerable amounts of aluminum depending upon the specific formulation used. For example, possible daily aluminum doses resulting from the nonabusive use of antacids or buffered aspirins may be as high as 5000 mg or 730 mg, respectively (Lione 1985). Thus it can be seen that continued use of these products supplies aluminum far in excess of that provided in the diet. Unfortunately these direct comparisons of aluminum exposure are somewhat obscured by the fact that aluminum absorption is greatly influenced by the salt species present (Kaehny *et al.* 1977); hence relative bioavailability of water/food/pharmaceutical sources of aluminum cannot be addressed unless speciation of aluminum is taken into account.

Aluminum Metabolism

Although little is known about aluminum absorption, based on total body aluminum content of approximately 30 mg in man (Alfrey *et al.* 1980), it would appear that the lungs, skin and gastrointestinal tract all form effective barriers to aluminum under conditions of average exposure. However, when normal subjects are given oral loads of aluminum salts, increases in both plasma and urinary aluminum are observed. Absorption probably occurs in the acidic environment of the stomach and proximal duodenum (Greger and Baier 1983), and bioavailability is influenced by the aluminum salt species present (Kaehny *et al.* 1977). It has been suggested that the absorption of aluminum may involve an active process, perhaps related to calcium transport (Farnell *et al.* 1985). Availability of aluminum is influenced by such factors as nutritional deficiencies of divalent cations (Boegman and Bates 1984) and fluoride content of food and water supplies (Still and Kelley 1980). Overall, most ingested aluminum is unabsorbed and excreted in the feces (Underwood 1977).

Aluminum circulates in the bloodstream in both ultrafilterable and protein-bound fractions, with both albumin and transferrin serving this function. The unbound plasma aluminum has access to intracellular compartments, thus allowing for tissue accumulation with aluminum loading (Lione 1985). Although the precise handling of aluminum by the kidney is unknown, urinary excretion increases with aluminum intake. Presumably after saturation of plasma protein binding, the unbound aluminum is removed by the kidneys (Lione 1985). Biliary secretion of aluminum may also play an important role in elimination (Gorsky 1979), especially when smaller quantities of aluminum are involved.

In conclusion, it would appear that with low levels of exposure the body is well equipped to handle aluminum. This is accomplished through a combination of low GI absorption, plasma binding proteins and renal excretion of the free fraction, thus preventing accumulation of all but trace amounts of aluminum. However, when exposure to aluminum is high, such as that seen with the ingestion of antacids, tissue accumulations of aluminum may occur.

Human Diseases Associated with Aluminum Exposure

Cases of aluminum toxicity have been documented in conjunction with extremely high aluminum intakes as a consequence of therapeutic use of pharmaceuticals or in association with direct parenteral exposure (hemodialysis and total parenteral feeding) where the GI tract has been bypassed (Lione 1985; Crapper McLachlan and Farnell 1986). For example, hypophosphatemic osteomalacia, a syndrome of phosphate depletion with osteomalacia, can result from the intake of large amounts of aluminum-containing antacids. Some chronic renal failure patients on long-term hemodialysis exhibit a vitamin D resistant form of osteomalacia, brain encephalopathy associated with dementia, and/or dialysis-induced microcytic anemia. These disorders are all associated with very high aluminum intakes due to the ingestion of aluminum-containing phosphate binding gels to prevent hyperphosphatemia, and the use of non-deionized (aluminum-containing) water for hemodialysis treatment. The lung is also susceptible to aluminum toxicity; exposure to aluminum dust and flakes such as those produced from industrial exposure can produce pulmonary fibrosis. Aluminum is directly toxic to the GI tract, symptomized by general malaise, anorexia, vomiting and weight loss. Constipation is observed with antacids since aluminum directly inhibits smooth muscle contractility by an interference with calcium metabolism in the muscle cell (Lione 1985; Crapper McLachlan and Farnell 1986). These observations implicate aluminum as a pathogenic factor; however, they do not have a dietary component.

As stated earlier, of more public health concern is the possible role of aluminum in the pathogenesis of Alzheimer's disease. Much of this concern has arisen from two sources of epidemiological data. First, it was observed that aluminum concentrations were elevated in humans suffering from Alzheimer's disease when compared to age-matched controls (Crapper *et al.* 1973). This observation has subsequently been confirmed in several other laboratories. Furthermore, it appears that aluminum is concentrated in neurofibrillary tangle-bearing neurons (Crapper McLachlan 1986).

Second, supportive evidence linking aluminum with Alzheimer's disease emerged from studies in Guam and other areas which have a high incidence of neurofibrillary disease. Water and garden soil in these areas are high in aluminum and low in the divalent cations calcium and magnesium (Perl 1985). The incidence of amyotrophic lateral sclerosis and the dementia of Parkinson's disease has declined rapidly in Guam during the last two decades (Garruto *et al.* 1985), and Guamanians now have a risk that is only a few times higher than that observed in North America. Interestingly, this change in risk occurred concurrently with the introduction of Western commercial products, thus lending support to the hypothesis that an environmental factor is involved (Perl 1985). A direct association can not be drawn from these observations since aluminum is not the only environmental factor implicated. For example, the seed of the sago palm, which was used in food and traditional medicine on the island, contains a toxin which may also be a factor related to the high disease incidence observed in Guam (Kurland 1988). However, there are epidemiological reports from Norway (Vogt 1986; Flaten In Press) and Britain (Martyn *et al.* 1989) indicating that the risk of developing Alzheimer's disease is correlated with aluminum in drinking water.

Currently, aluminum is considered to be involved in the pathogenesis of the disease rather than the etiology (Crapper McLachlan 1986; Crapper McLachlan and Van Berkum 1986; Crapper McLachlan and Farnell 1986). Apparently, the normal brain has mechanisms which regulate aluminum metabolism. For instance, when the normal brain is exposed to high levels of aluminum, such as in renal failure, brain aluminum content may increase without signs of neurologic damage and aluminum appears to accumulate in the cytoplasm (Lione 1985; Crapper McLachlan and Farnell 1986), whereas in Alzheimer's disease, aluminum appears to concentrate in the nucleus of the cell (Perl 1985; Crapper McLachlan 1986). It is postulated that the healthy human brain has cytoplasmic binding ligands for aluminum which protect against nuclear aluminum accumulation. However, in the Alzheimer's brain a primary pathogenic event occurs which results in the loss of ligand and/or barrier which normally excludes aluminum from the nucleus (Crapper McLachlan *et al.* In Press); aluminum passes into the nucleus, possibly via calcium channels, where it penetrates the DNA-containing structures within the nucleus and alters nuclear function (Crapper McLachlan 1986; Crapper McLachlan and Farnell 1986; Crapper McLachlan and Van Berkum 1986).

Although it was originally hypothesized that aluminum could induce some of the histopathological changes observed in Alzheimer's disease, the neurofibrillary degeneration observed in Alzheimer's disease differs from that induced by aluminum injected into the brains of experimental animals (Munoz-Garcia *et al.* 1986). However, certain biochemical events appear to be similar in both human and experimental models of the disease. The neurons most susceptible are those having extensive dendritic trees with large diameter proximal roots and large volume somata. The large pyramidal-shaped neurons in the neocortex and hippocampus and large multipolar cells of thalamus, basal ganglia and brain stem are affected in both conditions (Crapper McLachlan and Farnell 1986). Neurons in these brain regions have a high density of transferrin receptors, suggesting that their selective vulnerability may be partly determined by aluminum entering the brain via the iron transport system (Candy *et al.* 1987). The four principal loci affected are the DNA-containing structures of the nucleus, the protein moieties of the neurofibrillary tangle, the amyloid cores of the senile plaque and cerebral ferritin (Crapper McLachlan 1986). That is, aluminum increases the binding of histones to DNA, which results in increased compaction of chromatin and reduced transcription. This reduction in transcription may in turn account for many of the disorders in neuronal metabolism, including the regulation of phosphorylation, calcium homeostasis, free radical metabolism, proteolysis and neurotransmitter metabolism (Crapper McLachlan In Press).

Despite the accumulating evidence that aluminum is an important factor in the pathogensis of Alzheimer's disease, at present there are two opposing views with regard to the functional significance of aluminum accumulation in Alzheimer's disease. One is that aluminum merely accumulates passively in neurons compromised by the degenerative process and has no physiological importance in the degenerative process *per se*. The other is that aluminum is an important environmental factor which can affect the rate of progression of the disease process (Crapper McLachlan 1986). Unfortunately this controversy will not be resolved until there is a greater understanding of the molecular disorders associated with Alzheimer's disease and the mechanism of action of aluminum at the molecular level.

Conclusion

A large amount of evidence implicates aluminum as a potential neurotoxic agent in the initiation or progression of neurofibrillary diseases, including Alzheimer's disease. Aluminum-induced encephalopathy in experimental animals may not exactly mimic the neuropathologic abnormalities observed with Alzheimer's disease, but the neurological effects are similar enough to indicate an association of aluminum with Alzheimer's disease. Of concern is the fact that animal models of encephalopathy use direct intracranial injections of aluminum and may not realistically mimic potential human exposure to this element. However, the prevalence of aluminum in our environment and the increase in bioavailability leads to concern with respect to the potential of aluminum toxicity, especially in light of the histopathological and biochemical evidence obtained from human autopsy material.

Evidence suggests that we are relatively well adapted to detoxify low environmental or natural levels of aluminum exposure and hence prevent accumulation of this potentially toxic metal. Many elderly people may be using high levels of aluminum-containing pharmaceuticals and are thus at risk for high levels of aluminum intake. In addition, changes in renal function with aging may compromise this important route of aluminum excretion from the body. When trying to determine if a slight increase in dietary sources of aluminum may be a risk factor, one has to remember that dietary intake is in the range of mg/d while intake from pharmaceuticals can be in the range of g/d. However, we currently have insufficient information about the forms of aluminum in food stuffs and hence its bioavailability and toxicity relative to that present in pharmaceuticals. Undoubtedly more research is necessary to establish the exact role aluminum may play in human diseases, including neurological disorders.

It must be recognized that at present this is a hotly debated field, thus making any specific recommendations unwarranted. However, in the interim it may be prudent to label aluminum-containing drugs and medications, and to begin addressing means by which environmental and food exposure to aluminum can be minimized.

References

Alfrey, A.C., Hegg, A. and Craswell, P. 1980. Metabolism and toxicity of aluminum in renal failure. Am. J. Clin. Nutr. 33:1509-1516.

Boegman, R.J. and Bates, L.A. 1984. Neurotoxicity of aluminum. Can. J. Physiol. Pharmacol. 62:1010-1014.

Candy, J., Edwardson, J., Faircloth, R., Keith, A., Morris, C. and Pullen, R. 1987. ^{67}Gallium as a potential marker for aluminum transport in rat brain. J. Physiol. 391:34P.

Crapper, D.R., Krishnan, S.S. and Dalton, A.J. 1973. Brain aluminum distribution in Alzheimer's disease and experimental neurofibrillary degeneration. Science 180:511-513.

Crapper McLachlan, D.R. 1986. Aluminum and Alzheimer's disease. Neurobiol. Aging 7:525-532.

Crapper McLachlan, D.R. and Farnell, B.J. 1986. Aluminum in human health. *In* Aluminum in the Canadian environment. NRCC No. 24759. Havas, M. and Jaworski, J.F., eds. National Research Council of Canada, Ottawa, pp. 153-173.

Crapper McLachlan, D.R. and Van Berkum, M.F.A. 1986. Aluminum: a role in degenerative brain disease associated with neurofibrillary degeneration. Prog. Brain Res. 70:399-410.

Crapper McLachlan, D.R., St. George-Hyslop, P.H. and Farnell, B.J. 1987. Memory, aluminum and Alzheimer's disease. *In* Neuroplasticity, learning and memory. Milgram, N.W., MacLeod, C.M. and Petit, T.L., eds. A.R. Liss, New York, pp 45-59.

Crapper McLachlan, D.R., Lukiw, W.J. and Kruck, T.P.A. In Press. Aluminum, altered transcription, and the pathogenesis of Alzheimer's disease. Environ. Geochem. Health.

Farnell, B.J., Crapper McLachlan, D.R., Baimbridge, K., DeBoni, U., Wong, L. and Wood, P.L. 1985. Calcium metabolism in aluminum encephalopathy. Exp. Neurol. 88:68-83.

Flaten, T.P. In Press. Geographical associations between aluminum and drinking water and registered death rates with dementia (including Alzheimer's disease) in Norway. Proceedings of the Second International Symposia on Geochemistry and Health, 1987. London.

Garruto, R.M., Yanagihara, R. and Gajdusek, D.C. 1985. Disappearance of high-incidence amyotrophic lateral sclerosis and parkinsonism-dementia on Guam. Neurol. 35:193-198.

Glenner, G.G. 1982. Alzheimer's disease (senile dementia): a research update and critique with recommendations. J. Am. Geriatr. Soc. 30:59-62.

Gorsky, J.E., Dietz, A.A., Spencer, H. and Osis, D. 1979. Metabolic balance of aluminum studied in six men. Clin. Chem. 25:1739-1743.

Greger, J.L. and Baier, M.J. 1983. Excretion and retention of low or moderate levels of aluminum by human subjects. Food Chem. Toxicol. 21:473-477.

Jones, K.C. and Bennett, B.G. 1986. Exposure of man to environmental aluminium — an exposure commitment assessment. Sci. Total Environ. 52:65-82.

Kaehny, W.D., Hegg, A.P. and Alfrey, A.C. 1977. Gastrointestinal absorption of aluminum from aluminum-containing antacids. N. Engl. J. Med. 296:1389-1390.

Katzman, R. 1986. Alzheimer's disease. N. Eng. J. Med. 314:964-973.

Kurland, L.T. 1988. Amyotrophic lateral sclerosis and Parkinson's disease complex on Guam linked to an environmental neurotoxin. Trends NeuroSci. 11:51-53.

Lione, A. 1983. The prophylactic reduction of aluminum intake. Food Chem. Toxicol. 21:103-109.

Lione, A. 1985. Aluminum toxicology and the aluminum-containing medications. Pharmacol. Ther. 29:255-285.

Lione, A., Allen, P.V. and Crispin Smith, J. 1984. Aluminum coffee percolators as a source of dietary aluminum. Food Chem. Toxicol. 22:265-268.

Martyn, C.N., Osmond, C., Edwardson, J.A., Barker, D.J.P., Harris, E.C. and Lacey, R.F. 1989. Geographical relation between Alzheimer's disease and aluminum in drinking water. Lancet 1:59-62.

Munoz-Garcia, D., Pendlebury, W.W., Kessler, J.B. and Perl, D.P. 1986. An immunocytochemical comparison of cytoskeletal proteins in aluminum-induced and Alzheimer-type neurofibrillary tangles. Acta Neuropathol. 70:243-248.

Perl, D.P. 1985. Relationship of aluminum to Alzheimer's disease. Environ. Health Perspect. 63:149-153.

Sorenson, J.R.J., Campbell, I.R., Tepper, L.B. and Lingg, R.D. 1974. Aluminum in the environment and human health. Environ. Health Perspect. 8:3-95.

Still, C.N. and Kelley, P. 1980. On the incidence of primary degenerative dementia vs. water fluoride content in South Carolina. Neurotoxicology 1:125-131.

Underwood, E.J. 1977. Trace elements in human and animal nutrition. 4th ed. Academic Press, New York.

Vogt, T. 1986. Water quality and health — study of a possible relationship between aluminium in drinking water and dementia. (Sosiale og Okonomiske Studier 61. Eng. Abstract). Central Bureau of Statistics of Norway, Oslo.

Aspartame

Despite the fact that no scientific evidence exists implicating sugar consumption per se in the etiology of chronic diseases, except dental caries (Glinsmann *et al.* 1986), health-conscious Canadians have turned to artificially sweetened products to satisfy their innate preference for sweet. Hence, the use of sugar substitutes is not confined to specific clinical populations such as diabetics or the obese, but rather is widespread, with approximately 50% of Canadian households (Heybach and Ross In Press) reporting the use of high-intensity sweeteners in either commercial food products or as tabletop sweeteners. This broad acceptance of high-intensity sweeteners is further supported by the fact that consumption is not confined to one segment of the population, but rather is observed across all age and socio-economic groups.

The use of high-intensity sweeteners in human diets is not new. For example, saccharin was first discovered in 1879 and came into widespread use in Europe in the 1920s. Saccharin dominated the market for nearly sixty years, with some competition from cyclamate in the 1950s and 1960s; however, it has now been almost entirely displaced by aspartame (Lecos 1981). This somewhat reflects concerns regarding the potential carcinogenicity of saccharin (Canada. Health and Welfare 1983) and cyclamates (Lecos 1981), resulting in restricted use of these sweeteners in either Canada or the U.S.A. Aspartame is currently the only high intensity sweetener approved for use as a food additive in both countries. However, aspartame's reputation is not unblemished, with concerns about its safety continuing to surface in both the scientific literature and lay press. To place these concerns in perspective, levels of aspartame consumption, the safety of aspartame and the role of artificially sweetened products in the marketplace must be evaluated.

Use of Aspartame

Aspartame first received approval for use as a sweetening ingredient in Canada in 1981, and is currently accepted for use in table-top sweeteners, ready-to-eat cereals, beverages, beverage concentrates and mixes, desserts, toppings, fillings and their mixes, chewing gum and breath fresheners (Canada. Health and Welfare 1981). The acceptable daily lifetime intake (ADI) was set at 40 mg/kg of body weight (Canada. Health and Welfare 1981), a level in concurrence with that established by the Joint FAO/WHO Expert Committee (1980). This value is substantially greater than predictions of daily adult consumption patterns calculated on the basis of replacing all sucrose (8.3 mg/kg of body weight) or all carbohydrate (approximately 25 mg/kg of body weight) in the diet (Horwitz and Bauer-Nehrling 1983). However, estimates of actual aspartame use in Canada have not been available until recently.

Patterns of aspartame use were estimated in a nationally representative survey of 10 413 Canadians in the late winter and late summer of 1987 (Heybach and Ross In Press). Seven-day dietary records in 15 (winter) or 17 (summer) food and beverage categories were evaluated. The food and beverage categories were chosen to represent all food and beverage products containing aspartame marketed in Canada at that time. Two time periods were used to reflect the predicted seasonal variation in consumption patterns, and to capture the predicted peak season for consumption of refreshment beverages, i.e. summer.

Of the total population surveyed, aspartame-containing products were consumed by 44% and 46% of the participants in winter and summer phases of the study, respectively (Heybach and Ross In Press). While not specifically reported, it appeared that a higher proportion of diabetics and those on sugar-avoiding or weight-loss diets consume aspartame-containing food products than the general population, a finding in agreement with a study on saccharin use by diabetics performed in the late 1970s (U.S. N.R.C. 1978), before aspartame was available. Thus, high-intensity sweeteners appear to provide a highly desired alternative to these groups of individuals.

To evaluate actual consumption levels, data were analyzed by a number of different criteria. The highest predicted exposure was derived from the 95th percentile intake data on eater-days. This represents the 95th percentile consumption levels only of those individuals who consume aspartame-containing products (i.e. eliminating non-users), only on those days in which aspartame was consumed (i.e. eliminating days in which aspartame intake was zero). This level of intake was well below the ADI (approximately 25% of ADI) at both time periods and across all subgroups studied (Table 18). Intake of aspartame was fairly constant, with average consumption ranging from 1.7 to 3.7 mg/kg of body weight and upper estimates of consumption being 5.8-16.8 mg/kg of body weight. Not surprisingly, intake of aspartame was slightly greater in the summer months than in the winter months. Interestingly, however, this presented itself as an increased intake at the 95th percentile, with little or no change in average daily intake or in the overall proportion of the population using aspartame-containing foods. This would suggest that little or no change in daily consumption patterns occurred in most individuals, with only a small proportion of people increasing their consumption during the summer months.

Table 18.
Aspartame Intake (mg/kg of body weight) in Individuals Using Sweetened Food Products[a]

	Winter		Summer	
	Average	95th[b]	Average	95th[b]
Total Eaters	2.0	7.5	2.1	8.3
Males	2.0	7.2	2.0	7.4
Females	2.1	7.6	2.1	8.9
Under 18 years	2.6	9.2	2.6	9.3
Under 2 years	4.6	16.8	3.3	10.4
2-5 years	3.7	15.6	3.6	13.1
6-12 years	2.7	7.1	2.6	7.3
13-17 years	1.8	5.8	1.7	8.1
Females aged 18-39	2.1	7.8	2.1	8.4
On sugar-reducing diets	2.3	9.1	2.4	10.4
On weight-loss diets	2.2	6.1	2.4	9.4
Diabetics	2.2	6.1	3.1	14.4

a. Reproduced from Heybach, J.P. and Ross, C. Aspartame intake was estimated in Canadians in the winter and summer of 1987. Values are for eater-days such that intake represents consumption only in individuals consuming aspartame products and excluding days on which no aspartame was consumed.

b. 95th Percentile.

Concerns regarding intakes of aspartame in young children have been raised. These concerns relate to the fact that children have the greatest caloric (food) intake relative to body size and hence the greatest potential for excessive intake. The data presented here support the contention that the highest intake of aspartame (relative to body size) is observed in children 2-5 years of age. However, more important is the observation that even in this subset of the population both average and 95th percentile intakes fall at least 60% below the ADI.

The findings of this study are in agreement with consumption patterns reported in the U.S. (Heybach and Allen 1986; International Food Information Council 1986). Therefore it would appear that with the present use of aspartame in food products it is unlikely that an individual, of any age group, would consume this sweetener in excess of the ADI. Concerns regarding the increasing number of food products containing aspartame cannot, at present, be substantiated since there is such a wide margin between actual intakes and the ADI. Furthermore, there are currently several new high-intensity sweeteners undergoing review with government agencies. If these new sweeteners enter the marketplace, aspartame intakes would be predicted to fall, not rise, as a consequence of competition.

Safety of Aspartame

General Population

Prior to its 1981 approval, aspartame underwent more testing than any other food additive in history. Aspartame, a dipeptide, is broken down in the gastrointestinal tract into its two constituent amino acids, phenylalanine and aspartic acid, and methanol; extensive safety testing was conducted on all three compounds (AMA 1985; Stegink 1987). However, there have recently been consumer and/or scientific complaints regarding the role of aspartame in seizure activity and adverse reactions, including headache, skin rashes and hives (Bradstock *et al.* 1986; International Food Information Council 1986). These complaints sparked renewed evaluation of aspartame's safety. With regard to adverse reactions, both the U.S. Centre for Disease Control (1984) and an FDA Advisory Committee on Hypersensitivity to Food Constituents (1986) concluded that while some individuals may have an unusual sensitivity to aspartame, there is no evidence that aspartame usage represents a significant health hazard to the general population. For example, placebo-controlled studies of dietary triggers of headache reported that headache incidence associated with all these compounds was similar to that reported for placebo itself (Lipton *et al.* 1988). Furthermore, it was concluded by a number of expert committees (Anon. 1986; Coelho 1986) that available data do not support the contention that aspartame, at current consumption levels, causes seizure. Thus, sensitive individuals should avoid aspartame-containing food products. These results, however, should not be extended to the general population. Clearly, with present usage patterns, aspartame is safe for the average individual.

Population Subgroups

Specific recommendations targeted to population subgroups relate to the safety of phenylalanine consumption, and the possible neurotoxic effects of highly elevated brain phenylalanine levels. High blood phenylalanine levels associated with phenylketonuria (PKU), a hereditary absence of the enzyme phenylalanine hydroxylase, produces a marked mental retardation as well as less dramatic effects on the developing central nervous system. The concern is that ingestion of aspartame may increase phenylalanine levels to those which will result in adverse effects to the brain. Obviously those individuals homozygous for PKU, especially while on phenylalanine restriction diets, should refrain from the use of aspartame.

The two subgroups of the population, however, which were initially targeted were those who were heterozygous for PKU, since they have a reduced capacity to metabolize phenylalanine and may be unaware of this, and pregnant women, as amino acids are concentrated by the placenta, exposing the fetus to higher amino acid levels than is observed in maternal blood.

With regards to the heterozygous PKU individual, studies have shown that blood phenylalanine levels, following a bolus dose of 34 mg/kg of body weight (close to the ADI), are higher than those of normal adults (Stegink 1984). However, the slightly higher plasma phenylalanine levels observed in the heterozygous PKU individual (20 µmol/dL versus 13 µmol/dL) would not be considered to be in the neurotoxic range.

In agreement with the Nutrition in Pregnancy National Guidelines (Canada. Health and Welfare 1987) aspartame intake should not exceed 40 mg/kg of body weight per day. A level of concern was based on experience with homozygous PKU infants and the determination of maternal blood phenylalanine levels which resulted in grossly manifested adverse central nervous system effects. Based on present consumption data, it would be unlikely that blood phenylalanine levels would reach this level in pregnant women. Furthermore, there is no evidence to suggest that aspartame consumption would affect the developing central nervous system. Thus, the only case for avoiding high-intensity sweeteners during pregnancy should be based on nutritional considerations, such as the overall nutrient content of the diet and nutrient-dense foods which may be displaced by the use of artificially sweetened products.

Role of Aspartame

One of the important questions to ask with regard to high-intensity sweeteners in general is the role that these products play in the marketplace. Most consumers are turning to artificially sweetened products due to their lower caloric density, in an attempt to reduce or maintain body weight and improve overall physical appearance. The increase in health and fitness consciousness of Canadians during the last decade has brought about an interest in both the quantity and quality of food consumed. Thus demand for low-calorie sweetened products is not confined to the obese attempting to lose weight, but is observed among body image-conscious individuals, independent of their present body weight status.

Interestingly, patterns of aspartame use do not show a gender bias (Heyback and Ross In Press), with males consuming equivalent intakes to that observed in females. The degree to which this reflects the fact that body image and weight control concerns are equally distributed across both sexes or that females, as the main food purchasers, influence eating patterns of the entire household cannot be discerned from this information. Nevertheless, it would appear that the perceived role of high-intensity sweeteners by the individual is in assisting with the achievement of reduced caloric intake.

Whether or not aspartame usage results in reduced caloric intake, however, is a subject of considerable debate. Recently there have been claims that high-intensity sweeteners do not aid in weight reduction and indeed may have appetite-stimulating properties. These concerns relate either to potential brain neurochemical changes associated specifically with aspartame intake (Wurtman 1983), or to mechanisms common to all high-intensity sweeteners where appetite mechanisms might be influenced through pre- or post-absorptive mechanisms functioning in conjunction with stimulation of the taste receptors (Blundell and Hill 1986). These hypotheses are by and large unsubstantiated. That is, most studies report either no change or a slight reduction in caloric intake associated with high-intensity sweeteners (Anderson and Leiter 1988; Calorie Control Council 1988). Thus aspartame does not appear to increase appetite; however, the reduction in total caloric intake, if it occurs, appears to be small and probably not physiologically relevant from a weight reduction perspective. Possibly the main benefit to high-intensity sweeteners is in their role in maintaining dietary compliance, as has been suggested for the diabetic (Crapo 1988), rather than in actual caloric restriction *per se*.

Conclusions

The demand for low-calorie sweetened food products has created a large market for food manufacturers; with aspartame being the high-intensity sweetener of choice at present. Current data suggests that consumption of aspartame is well below the ADI for all segments of the Canadian population.

References

American Medical Association. Council on Scientific Affairs. 1985. Aspartame. Review of safety issues. J. Am. Med. Assoc. 254:400-402.

Anderson, G.H. and Leiter, L.A. 1988. Effects of aspartame and phenylalanine on meal-time food intake of humans. Appetite 11 (Suppl. 1):48-53.

Anonymous. 1986. Safety of aspartame upheld again. Tufts Univ. Diet Nutr. Letter 4:2.

Blundell, J.E. and Hill, A.J. 1986. Paradoxical effects of an intense sweetener (aspartame) on appetite (letter). Lancet 1:1092-1093.

Bradstock, M.K., Serdula, M.K., Marks, J.S., Barnard, R.J., Crane, N.T., Remington, P.L. and Trowbridge, F.L. 1986. Evaluation of reactions to food additives: the aspartame experience. Am. J. Clin. Nutr. 43:464-469.

Calorie Control Council. 1988. A review of low-calorie sweetener benefits. Part 1. The Bariatrician. Spring:17-29.

Canada. Health and Welfare. Federal-Provincial Subcommittee on Nutrition. 1987. Nutrition in pregnancy. National guidelines. Ottawa.

Canada. Health and Welfare. Health Protection Branch. 1981. Aspartame. Information Letter No. 602, July 31, 1981. Ottawa.

Canada. Health and Welfare. Health Protection Branch. Educational Services. 1983. Sweeteners from A to X. Ottawa.

Coelho, Tony. 1986. Coelho discounts alleged link between aspartame and epilepsy seizures. Congressional Record, E 2206.

Crapo, P.A. 1988. Use of alternative sweeteners in diabetic diet. Diabetes Care 11:174-182.

FAO/WHO. 1980. Evaluation of certain food additives. Twenty-fourth report of the Joint FAO/WHO Expert Committee on Food Additives. W.H.O. Tech. Rep. Ser. 653:1-38.

FDA Advisory Committee on Hypersensitivity to Food Constituents. 1986. Conclusion on aspartame. Washington, D.C.

Glinsmann, W.H., Irausquin, H. and Park, Y.K. 1986. Evaluation of health aspects of sugars contained in carbohydrate sweeteners. Report of Sugars Task Force, 1986. J. Nutr. 116 (Suppl.): S1-S216.

Heybach, J.P. and Allen, S.S. 1986. Resources for inferential estimates of aspartame intake in the United States. *In* International Aspartame Workshop. Proceedings (ILSI/NF). International Life Sciences Institute — Nutrition Foundation. Marbella, Spain.

Heybach, J.P. and Ross, C. In Press. Consumption of aspartame in the Canadian population. J. Can. Diet. Assoc.

Horwitz, D.L. and Bauer-Nehrling, J.K. 1983. Can aspartame meet our expectations? J. Am. Diet. Assoc. 83:142-146.

International Food Information Council. 1986. Aspartame safety issues: a scientific update. Washington, D.C.

Lecos, C. 1981. The sweet and sour history of saccharin, cyclamate, aspartame. FDA Consumer 15:8-11.

Lipton, R.B., Newman, L.C. and Solomon, S. 1988. Aspartame and headache (letter). N. Engl. J. Med. 318:1200.

Stegink, L.D. 1984. Aspartame metabolism in humans: acute dosing studies. *In* Aspartame physiology and biochemistry. Stegink, L.D. and Filer, L.J., Jr., eds. Dekker, New York, pp. 509-553.

Stegink, L.D. 1987. The aspartame story: a model for the clinical testing of a food additive. Am. J. Clin. Nutr. 46:204-215.

[U.S.] Centre for Disease Control. 1984. Evaluation of consumer complaints related to aspartame use. MMWR Morbidity Mortality Weekly Rep. 33:605-607.

U.S. National Research Council. Committee for a Study on Saccharin and Food Safety Policy. 1978. Saccharin: technical assessment of risks and benefits. Washington, D.C.

Wurtman, R.J. 1983. Neurochemical changes following high-dose aspartame with dietary carbohydrates (letter). N. Engl. J. Med. 309:429-430.

Caffeine

Caffeine is consumed in coffee, tea, cola drinks, chocolate and a variety of drugs. It is estimated that in Canada 60% of ingested caffeine is from coffee, 30% from tea and 10% from cola drinks, chocolate and drugs (Gilbert 1981). The concentration of caffeine in coffee and tea and the volume consumed vary widely, but the mean intake of caffeine appears to be approximately 80 mg per cup (Stavric *et al.* 1988). Healthy adults absorb about 99% of ingested caffeine with peak blood levels reached within 15 to 45 minutes and they eliminate 50% of the dose in 3 to 7.5 hours (Bonati *et al.* 1982). In full-term infants the half-life of caffeine at birth is 82 hours but by five to six months of age it is somewhat below adult values at 2.6 hours (Aranda *et al.* 1979).

Species and individuals vary in their response to caffeine. Other influential factors include age, sex, pregnancy, body weight, disease, diet, exercise, stress, temperature, light, smoking and alcohol consumption. Even when confounding variables are taken into account, caffeine still increases the frequency and prevalence of headache, insomnia, palpitation and tremor (Shirlow and Mathers 1985). The equivalent of one cup of coffee has been shown to increase alertness during periods of fatigue (Dews 1982). Three cups of coffee consumed by an individual not accustomed to such an intake may produce mild anxiety, respiratory stimulation, cardiovascular effects, diuresis and increased gastric secretion (Robertson *et al.* 1978; Rall 1980). Intakes as low as 500 mg of caffeine (approximately six cups of coffee) per day have in some individuals led to insomnia, headache, anxiety, irritability and depression (Greden 1974). A dose of 450 mg caffeine on an empty stomach has induced tremors (Wharrad *et al.* 1985). At a level of 1 gram of caffeine per day, such symptoms as fever, agitation, trembling, rapid breathing, increased heart rate, cardiac palpitation, diuresis, nausea and anorexia may occur (Greden 1979).

An acute dosage of 5 to 10 g of caffeine (equivalent to 50 to 100 cups of coffee) caused tachycardia, convulsions, coma and even death due to shock, respiratory and heart failure (Eisele and Reay 1980). Similar symptoms, but no deaths, were reported in children at doses of 100 mg/kg body weight (Rowland and Mace 1976).

After several hours of abstinence by individuals accustomed to a high intake of caffeine, withdrawal symptoms of headaches, irritability, muscle tension and nervousness may be manifest and be reversed by caffeine (Greden 1979).

The level of habitual intake is a major predictor of individual differences in the response to caffeine. Consumers accustomed to large intakes of caffeine were more likely to react to 300 mg with increased alertness and decreased irritability, than were caffeine abstainers whose response was an upset stomach and "jitteriness" (Goldstein *et al.* 1965). Insomnia is a common side effect of large intakes of caffeine.

In behavioral studies, caffeine has been credited with reduced aggression (Cherek *et al.* 1983) and reduced academic performance (Gilliland and Andress 1981), but such findings are also disputed (Leviton 1983).

Chronic Disease

It appears that tolerance to cardiovascular effects of caffeine exists in some individuals and develops in others who regularly consume caffeine (Robertson *et al.* 1981; Robertson *et al.* 1984). A summary of recent studies indicated that caffeine does not produce a persistent increase in blood pressure (Myers 1988).

Views vary regarding the use of caffeine-containing beverages by individuals who have recently suffered a heart attack. In patients who received 300 mg of caffeine, as compared with placebo-treated patients, no appreciable alteration in heart rhythm occurred (Myers *et al.* 1987). In contrast, caffeine was considered to be a risk factor for heart attacks (Ashton 1987). Some early studies (Paul *et al.* 1963; Jick *et al.* 1973) concluded that there was a positive association between coffee consumption and increased risk of heart attack, while the Framingham study (Dawber *et al.* 1974; Wilson *et al.* 1989) and eight other studies reviewed in 1983 (Curatolo and Robertson 1983) found no such association. Later, two large prospective studies provided evidence for a positive association between caffeine use and cardiovascular disease. In a 25-year study of medical school graduates (La Croix *et al.* 1986) and in a 19-year study of employees (Le Grady *et al.* 1987), those drinking more than five or six cups of coffee per day doubled their risk of heart disease. Similarly, Rosenberg *et al.* (1988) found an increased risk of myocardial infarction with consumption of at least five cups of coffee per day. Serum cholesterol also rises with coffee consumption (Curb *et al.* 1986; Davis *et al.* 1988).

Epidemiological studies have failed to establish a causal relationship between caffeine and cancer of the bladder, pancreas, ovary or other organs (Grice 1984; Jacobsen *et al.* 1986; Nomura *et al.* 1986; Clavel *et al.* 1987). The chemical characteristics, metabolism, physiology and lack of mutagenicity of caffeine are not predictive of carcinogenicity. There is no evidence that caffeine consumption is associated with the development of fibrocystic breast disease, nor that a caffeine-restricted diet resolves signs and symptoms of disease (Ernster *et al.* 1982; Heyden and Muhlbaier 1984; Schairer *et al.* 1986).

Pregnancy and Lactation

In laboratory animals, very large intakes of caffeine led to birth defects, but human epidemiological studies did not find an association between caffeine consumption and low birthweight, preterm birth or birth defects (Leviton 1984; Wilson and Scott 1984).

Recommendation

The many studies conducted on the association between caffeine and health do not identify current levels of intake as contributing to undesirable behaviour, hypertension, cancer or birth defects. The evidence linking coffee consumption (not specifically caffeine) with heart disease, though not unanimous, provides a reason to limit intake to no more than the equivalent of four cups of coffee per day. The nutritional contribution of caffeine-containing foods does not argue for a greater intake. The reason for moderation in the consumption of caffeine is more compelling during pregnancy and lactation. Although caffeine is apparently not responsible for birth defects, it does cross the placenta, does appear in breast milk, does have undeniable physiological effects and is metabolized slowly by the infant.

References

Aranda, J.V., Collinge, J.M., Zinman, R. and Watters, G. 1979. Maturation of caffeine elimination in infancy. Arch. Dis. Child. 54:946-949.

Ashton, C.H. 1987. Caffeine and health. Br. Med. J. 295:1293-1294.

Bonati, M., Latini, R., Galletti, F., Young, J.F., Tognoni, G. and Garattini, S. 1982. Caffeine disposition after oral doses. Clin. Pharmacol. Ther. 32:98-106.

Cherek, D.R., Steinberg, J.L. and Brauchi, J.T. 1983. Effects of caffeine on human aggressive behavior. Psychiatry Res. 8:137-145.

Clavel, F., Benhamou, E., Tarayre, M. and Flamant, R. 1987. More on coffee and pancreatic cancer (letter). N. Engl. J. Med. 316:483-484.

Curatolo, P.W. and Robertson, D. 1983. The health consequences of caffeine. Ann. Intern. Med. 98:641-653.

Curb, J.D., Reed, D.M., Kautz, J.A. and Yano, K. 1986. Coffee, caffeine, and serum cholesterol in Japanese men in Hawaii. Am. J. Epidemiol. 123:648-655.

Davis, B.R., Curb, J.D., Borhani, N.O., Prineas, R.J. and Molteni, A. 1988. Coffee consumption and serum cholesterol in the hypertension detection and follow-up program. Am. J. Epidemiol. 128:124-136.

Dawber, T.R., Kannel, W.B. and Gordon, T. 1974. Coffee and cardiovascular disease: observations from the Framingham Study. N. Engl. J. Med. 291:871-874.

Dews, P.B. 1982. Caffeine. Annu. Rev. Nutr. 2:323-341.

Eisele, J.W. and Reay, D.T. 1980. Death related to coffee enemas. J. Am. Med. Assoc. 244:1608-1609.

Ernster, V.L., Mason, L., Goodson, W.H., III, Sickles, E.A., Sacks, S.T., Selvin, S., Dupuy, M.E., Hawkinson, J. and Hunt, T.K. 1982. Effects of caffeine-free diet on benign breast disease: a randomized trial. Surgery 91:263-267.

Gilbert, R.M. 1981. Caffeine: overview and anthology. *In* Nutrition and behavior. Miller S.A., ed. Franklin Institute Press, Philadelphia, pp. 145-166.

Gilliland, K. and Andress, D. 1981. Ad lib caffeine consumption, symptoms of caffeinism, and academic performance. Am. J. Psychiatry 138:512-514.

Goldstein, A., Warren, R. and Kaizer, S. 1965. Psychotropic effects of caffeine in man. I. Individual differences in sensitivity to caffeine-induced wakefulness. J. Pharmacol. Exp. Ther. 149:156-159.

Greden, J.F. 1974. Anxiety of caffeinism: a diagnostic dilemma. Am. J. Psychiatry 131:1089-1092.

Greden, J.F. 1979. Coffee, tea and you. The Science 19:6-11.

Grice, H.C. 1984. The carcinogenic potential of caffeine. *In* Caffeine: perspectives from recent research. Dews, P.B., ed. Springer-Verlag, New York, pp. 201-220.

Heyden, S. and Muhlbaier, L.H. 1984. Prospective study of fibrocystic breast disease and caffeine consumption. Surgery 96:479-484.

Jacobsen, B.K., Bjelke, E., Kvale, G. and Heuch, I. 1986. Coffee drinking, mortality, and cancer incidence: results from a Norwegian prospective study. J. Nat. Cancer Inst. 76:823-831.

Jick, H., Miettinen, O.S., Neff, R.K., Shapiro, S., Heinonen, O.P. and Slone, D. 1973. Coffee and myocardial infarction. N. Engl. J. Med. 289:63-67.

La Croix, A.Z., Mead, L.A., Liang, K.Y., Thomas, C.B. and Pearson, T.A. 1986. Coffee consumption and the incidence of coronary heart disease. N. Engl. J. Med. 315:977-982.

Le Grady, D., Dyer, A.R., Shekelle, R.B., Stamler, J., Liu, K., Paul, O., Lepper, M. and Shryock, A.M. 1987. Coffee consumption and mortality in the Chicago Western Electric Company Study. Am. J. Epidemiol. 126:803-812.

Leviton, A. 1983. Behavioral effects. Biological effects of caffeine. Food Technol. 37(9):44-47.

Leviton, A. 1984. Epidemiological studies of birth defects. *In* Caffeine: perspectives from recent research. Dews, P.B., ed. Springer-Verlag, New York, pp. 188-200.

Myers, M.G. 1988. Effects of caffeine on blood pressure. Arch. Intern. Med. 148:1189-1193.

Myers, M.G., Harris, L., Leenen, F.H.H. and Grant, D.M. 1987. Caffeine as a possible cause of ventricular arrhythmias during the healing phase of acute myocardial infarction. Am. J. Cardiol. 59:1024-1028.

Nomura, A., Heilbrun, L.K. and Stemmermann, G.N. 1986. Prospective study of coffee consumption and the risk of cancer. J. Nat. Cancer Inst. 76:587-590.

Paul, O., Lepper, M.H., Phelan, W.H., Dupertuis, G.W., MacMillan, A., McKean, H. and Park, H. 1963. A longitudinal study of coronary heart disease. Circulation 28:20-31.

Rall, T.W. 1980. The xanthines. *In* The pharmacological basis of therapeutics. Goodman, L.S., Gilman, A.G. and Gilman, A.Z., eds. MacMillan, New York, pp. 592-607.

Robertson, D., Frolich, J.C., Carr, R.K., Watson, J.T., Hollifield, J.W., Shand, D.G. and Oates, J.A. 1978. Effects of caffeine on plasma renin activity, catecholamines and blood pressure. N. Engl. J. Med. 298:181-186.

Robertson, D., Wade, D., Workman, R., Woosley, R.L. and Oates, J.A. 1981. Tolerance to the humoral and hemodynamic effects of caffeine in man. J. Clin. Invest. 67:1111-1117.

Robertson, D., Hollister, A.S., Kincaid, D., Workman, R., Goldberg, M.R., Tung, C. and Smith, B. 1984. Caffeine and hypertension. Am. J. Med. 77:54-60.

Rosenberg, L., Palmer, J.R., Kelly, J.P., Kaufman, D.W. and Shapiro, S. 1988. Coffee drinking and nonfatal myocardial infarction in men under 55 years of age. Am. J. Epidemiol. 128:570-578.

Rowland, D. and Mace, J. 1976. Caffeine (No-Doz) poisoning in childhood. West. J. Med. 124:52-53.

Schairer, C., Brinton, L.A. and Hoover, R.N. 1986. Methylxanthines and benign breast disease. Am. J. Epidemiol. 124:603-611.

Shirlow, M.J. and Mathers, C.D. 1985. A study of caffeine consumption and symptoms: indigestion, palpitations, tremor, headache and insomnia. Int. J. Epidemiol. 14:239-248.

Stavric, B., Klassen, R., Watkinson, B., Karpinski, K., Stapley, R. and Fried, P. 1988. Variability in caffeine consumption from coffee and tea: possible significance for epidemiological studies. Food Chem. Toxicol. 26:111-118.

Wharrad, H.J., Birmingham, A.T., Macdonald, I.A., Inch, P.J. and Mead, J.L. 1985. The influence of fasting and of caffeine intake on finger tremor. Eur. J. Clin. Pharmacol. 29:37-43.

Wilson, J.G. and Scott, W.J., Jr. 1984. The teratogenic potential of caffeine in laboratory animals. *In* Caffeine: perspectives from recent research. Dews, P.B., ed. Springer-Verlag, New York, pp. 165-187.

Wilson, P.W.F., Garrison, R.J., Kannel, W.B., McGee, D.L. and Castelli, W.P. 1989. Is coffee consumption a contributor to cardiovascular disease? Insights from the Framingham Study. Arch. Intern. Med. 149:1169-1172.

Part IV

Summary of Recommended Nutrient Intakes

Summary of Recommended Nutrient Intakes

Recommended Nutrient Intakes (RNIs) are expressed on a daily basis, but should be regarded as the average recommended intake over a period of time, such as a week.

Energy

Recommended energy intakes are those that will maintain categories of the population within the range of desirable body mass index (BMI) or attain this objective when the BMI falls outside this range.

A large number of Canadians are overweight, and because the risk of having an insufficient intake of essential nutrients increases as food consumption decreases, an increase in activity is a desirable alternative for many. It is particularly important that older people be encouraged to be physically active rather than control their weight solely by reduced energy intake.

Lipids

Lipids are an important source of energy and supply essential n-6 and n-3 polyunsaturated fatty acids. These acids should constitute at least 3% and 0.5% of energy (3.3 g/1000 kcal or 4.0 g/5000 kJ and 0.55 g/1000 kcal or 0.7 g/5000 kJ) respectively. The intake of total fat should be restricted to 30% of energy (33 g/1000 kcal or 40 g/5000 kJ) and the intake of saturated fatty acids to 10% of energy (11 g/1000 kcal or 13 g/5000 kJ). Cholesterol intake should be reduced and *trans* fatty acids in the food supply should not be increased.

Carbohydrates

A minimum amount of carbohydrate in the diet is necessary to prevent the formation of ketone bodies. The RNI for available carbohydrates is determined by the recommendations for fat and protein. It is recommended that 55% of energy (138 g/1000 kcal or 166 g/5000 kJ)) be derived from carbohydrates obtained from numerous sources, with an increase in complex carbohydrates.

Fibre

Though it is not possible to determine an RNI for dietary fibre, there is experimental evidence that insoluble fibre has a positive effect on bowel function, and epidemiological evidence that diets containing generous amounts of fibre are associated with a lower incidence of heart disease and certain cancers. An increased intake of complex carbohydrates will increase the intake of dietary fibre and should be obtained from a variety of sources.

Protein

The RNIs for protein were estimated by a modification of the factorial method (urinary, fecal and dermal losses during periods of little or no protein intake). It was assumed that maintenance requirements do not change throughout life. The estimated requirement for growth was based on average accretion values. The resulting safe level of protein intake, expressed in terms of an ideal protein, was adjusted for the quality and digestibility of protein in the habitual Canadian diet. The protein intake of typical Canadian diets is much greater than the RNI, but there is no evidence to suggest that current intakes should be reduced.

Vitamin A

Vitamin A has well-established roles in maintaining epithelial tissue, bone growth, vision and reproduction. The RNIs, expressed as retinol equivalents, are based on the maintenance of adequate liver stores. Evidence relating ß-carotene intake to the risk of certain types of cancer is insufficient to support a specific recommendation with respect to this nutrient. It is sufficient to support, in general terms, a greater reliance on fruit and vegetables as sources of vitamin A activity.

Vitamin D

The role of the biologically active vitamin D metabolites is to maintain serum calcium and phosphorus at concentrations which will support bone mineralization and other cellular processes. Although vitamin D requirements can be met entirely from solar radiation, requirements must be estimated because of those who receive little or no direct sunlight. Thus the RNI for infants assumes no exposure to sunlight; the elderly are assumed to absorb vitamin D less efficiently and to have less exposure to sunlight. It is emphasized that the margin of safety for vitamin D taken orally is unusually narrow, and oral consumption should never exceed twice the recommended amounts.

Vitamin E

The biological role of vitamin E is based on its antioxidant properties. Activity is expressed in international units or in d-γ-tocopherol equivalents. Requirement is determined primarily by the concentration and composition of polyunsaturated fatty acids in the tissues, and hence in the diet. Nevertheless, it is not possible to define requirement in terms of a fixed ratio to dietary polyunsaturated fatty acids, and reliance is placed on the observed efficacy of current intakes. The proposed effect of vitamin E on risk reduction for cancer was not found to be substantive.

Vitamin K

Vitamin K is comprised of members of a family of compounds derived from 2-methyl-1,4-napthoquinone. Members of the family are found in plant and animal tissues and are synthesized by intestinal bacteria. Its most important function is in blood coagulation. Recent advances in the determination of circulating levels of abnormal prothrombin have made possible an estimate of requirement.

Vitamin C

Vitamin C is involved in a wide range of biological processes, many of which depend on the reducing activity of the vitamin. The 1983 recommended intake was related to the attainment of a maximum conversion of vitamin C to its metabolites. Current evidence indicates that the metabolites are not themselves biologically active, and no health benefits are to be had from stimulating their production at the maximum rate. An intake estimated to provide a reserve for at least one month is the basis for the recommendation in this report. No additional intake could be justified on the basis of reducing the risk of chronic diseases, but persons who smoke need a greater intake.

Thiamin

Thiamin is involved in two types of reactions in carbohydrate metabolism. Its requirement is thus related to energy expenditure and is expressed as 0.4 mg/1000 kcal or 0.48 mg/5000 kJ. A minimum daily intake of 0.8 mg is advocated when energy intake falls below 2000 kcal.

Riboflavin

Riboflavin is a constituent of two coenzymes involved in tissue respiration and the direct oxidation of substrates. The RNI is 0.5 mg/1000 kcal or 0.6/5000 kJ with a minimum based on an energy intake of 2000 kcal.

Niacin

Niacin occurs in two coenzymes which remove hydrogen from substrates during glycolysis and respiration. A niacin equivalent (NE) is 1 mg niacin or 60 mg tryptophan. About 3% of ingested tryptophan is oxidized to niacin. The RNI is 7.2 NE/1000 kcal or 8.6 NE/5000 kJ with a minimum based on an energy intake of 2000 kcal or 8.4 MJ/day.

Vitamin B_6

Vitamin B_6 acts as a co-factor for enzymes involved in protein metabolism. The requirement is related to protein intake and is expressed as 15 µg pyridoxine per gram of protein.

Folate

Folate occurs in a group of coenzymes involved in purine synthesis, in DNA synthesis and many other biochemical reactions. Recommended intakes are based on the prevention of deficiency and the maintenance of stores. The recommendation for pregnancy is one of the rare instances that may require the use of supplements.

Vitamin B_{12}

Vitamin B_{12} functions in the metabolism of amino acids and some fatty acids and amino acids for energy. Deficiency leads to megaloblastic anemia and neurological disorders. Recommended intakes are based on the prevention of deficiency symptoms and the maintenance of body stores.

Biotin

Biotin performs its metabolic role as the prosthetic group of several carboxylases. No definite estimate of requirement can be made, but the usual intake of Canadians is thought to be sufficient.

Pantothenic Acid

Pantothenic acid is a component of two coenzymes, coenzyme A and acyl carrier protein. Requirement is related to energy intake but no definite estimates can be made. Because there is no evidence of deficiency it is assumed that the Canadian diet provides sufficient amounts of the vitamin.

Calcium

Ninety-nine percent of the calcium in the body is located in the bones and teeth, but the remaining 1% has a pervasive involvement in metabolic processes, including enzyme activation, nerve transmission, membrane transport, blood clotting, muscle contraction and hormone function. It is particularly difficult to establish the RNI for calcium because of the body's ability to adapt to a wide range of intakes. It would be risky to assume, however, that the low calcium intake typical in countries with a cereal-based diet would be adequate for those consuming the Canadian diet. On the other hand, the efficacy of providing very large intakes of calcium to prevent post-menopausal bone loss was discounted.

Phosphorus

Phosphorus is a major structural element of the bones and teeth but 20% is present in major classes of macromolecules, including proteins, nucleic acids and phospholipids. The high energy bonds in adenosine triphosphate and other phosphate compounds provide the energy to drive most metabolic processes. Requirement is believed to parallel that for calcium.

Magnesium

Magnesium is the fourth most abundant cation in the human body; bone contains 60% of the total and only 1% is extracellular. Magnesium plays a key role in many fundamental enzymatic reactions, including the transfer of phosphate groups, the initiation of fatty acid oxidation, the synthesis and degradation of DNA and many others. The kidney has a remarkable ability to conserve magnesium, and symptomatic deficiency has been observed only in the case of predisposing or complicating disease states.

Iron

Iron is involved in the transport and storage of oxygen, mitochondrial electron transport, catecholamine metabolism and DNA synthesis. Requirement is estimated from consideration of obligatory losses, growth (where appropriate), the maintenance of stores and efficiency of absorption from the Canadian diet. Mean values were used because it is recognized that the efficiency of absorption changes markedly in response to iron status.

Iodine

Iodine functions in thyroid hormones which are involved in thermoregulation, intermediary metabolism, protein synthesis, reproduction, growth and development, erythropoiesis and neuromuscular function. The RNI is based on the maintenance of a normal plasma concentration.

Zinc

Zinc is present in a wide range of metalloenzymes which play an important part in the metabolism of proteins, carbohydrates, lipids and nucleic acids. The recommended intake is based on the replacement of average obligatory losses, plus a factor for individual variability and an average absorption rate. Although zinc deficient diets may lead to growth retardation and an impaired immune response, intakes in excess of the RNI provide no advantage and may adversely influence copper metabolism.

Copper

The main function of copper is its role in the cuproenzymes that catalyze oxido-reduction reactions involved in erythropoiesis, connective tissue formation, oxidative phosphorylation and catecholamine synthesis. There is evidence that low copper intakes are associated with heart abnormalities; an RNI has not been estimated because of inadequate data.

Fluoride

Fluoride essentiality seems to be confined to the integrity of tooth enamel, and the RNI is based on the reduction in the incidence of dental caries in children. Fluoridation of water supplies is recommended when natural levels are below 1 mg/L. Evidence of the value of fluoride in the prevention of osteoporosis is weak.

Manganese

Manganese functions as both a non-specific activator and specifically as a constituent of a number of enzymes such as arginase, pyruvate carboxylase and superoxide dismutase. Blood manganese concentrations appear to be lower in epileptics but there is no evidence that manganese deficiency is causative. Estimates of requirement have been based on balance studies but for the present must be considered tentative.

Selenium

Selenium functions in glutathione peroxidase. This enzyme catalyzes the reduction by glutathione of hydrogen peroxide and fatty acid hydroperoxides, thus preventing the generation of oxygen free radicals which cause decomposition of polyunsaturated fatty acids. This function is related to that of vitamin E. Selenium requirement has not been firmly established. There is some evidence that selenium exerts a protective effect against cancer, but since Canadian intake is already in what is believed to be the effective range, no increase is indicated and indeed is counter-indicated by the narrow margin of safety for this element.

Chromium

The primary physiological function of chromium is to potentiate the action of insulin. Although chromium supplementation has been shown to improve glucose tolerance in diabetic individuals, there is little evidence that chromium deficiency is involved in the etiology of diabetes. Balance studies do not provide sufficient evidence upon which to base an RNI but there is no evidence that present intakes are inadequate.

Other Trace Elements

Animal experiments using purified diets and specialized equipment have indicated the essentiality of cobalt, molybdenum, silicon, lithium and boron. Of this group, only molybdenum has been shown to be essential for humans. There is some evidence of toxicity from these elements but there is a safety factor of at least 25 times attached to present intakes.

Electrolytes and Water

Sodium and potassium are essential, but sodium is consumed at excessively high levels and present intakes should be reduced. Potassium intake will be increased in diets that place increased emphasis on fruits and vegetables. Water intake, including that from food, should balance output.

Alcohol

Alcohol has been shown to have an adverse influence on blood pressure and may dilute the nutrient density of the diet. It is recommended that intake not exceed 5% of total energy or two drinks per day, whichever is less. During pregnancy, abstention from alcohol is prudent.

Aluminum

The intake of aluminum from foods is low compared to that from drugs.

Aspartame

The consumption of aspartame appears to be within acceptable levels for all segments of the population.

Caffeine

Caffeine occurs in various beverages, chocolate and drugs and can cause adverse reactions at excessive levels. The recommendation is to limit caffeine intake from all sources to no more than the equivalent of four cups of coffee per day.

Table 19
Summary of Examples of Recommended Nutrients Based on Energy Expressed as Daily Rates

Age	Sex	Energy kcal	Thiamin mg	Riboflavin mg	Niacin NE[b]	n-3 PUFA[a] g	n-6 PUFA g
Months							
0-4	Both	600	0.3	0.3	4	0.5	3
5-12	Both	900	0.4	0.5	7	0.5	3
Years							
1	Both	1100	0.5	0.6	8	0.6	4
2-3	Both	1300	0.6	0.7	9	0.7	4
4-6	Both	1800	0.7	0.9	13	1.0	6
7-9	M	2200	0.9	1.1	16	1.2	7
	F	1900	0.8	1.0	14	1.0	6
10-12	M	2500	1.0	1.3	18	1.4	8
	F	2200	0.9	1.1	16	1.1	7
13-15	M	2800	1.1	1.4	20	1.4	9
	F	2200	0.9	1.1	16	1.2	7
16-18	M	3200	1.3	1.6	23	1.8	11
	F	2100	0.8	1.1	15	1.2	7
19-24	M	3000	1.2	1.5	22	1.6	10
	F	2100	0.8	1.1	15	1.2	7
25-49	M	2700	1.1	1.4	19	1.5	9
	F	2000	0.8	1.0	14	1.1	7
50-74	M	2300	0.9	1.3	16	1.3	8
	F	1800	0.8[c]	1.0[c]	14[c]	1.1[c]	7[c]
75 +	M	2000	0.8	1.0	14	1.0	7
	F[d]	1700	0.8[c]	1.0[c]	14[c]	1.1[c]	7[c]
Pregnancy (additional)							
1st Trimester		100	0.1	0.1	0.1	0.05	0.3
2nd Trimester		300	0.1	0.3	0.2	0.16	0.9
3rd Trimester		300	0.1	0.3	0.2	0.16	0.9
Lactation (additional)		450	0.2	0.4	0.3	0.25	1.5

a. PUFA, polyunsaturated fatty acids

b. Niacin Equivalents

c. Level below which intake should not fall

d. Assumes moderate physical activity

Table 20.
Summary Examples of Recommended Nutrient Intake Based on Age and Body Weight Expressed as Daily Rates

Age	Sex	Weight kg	Protein g	Vit. A RE[a]	Vit. D µg	Vit. E mg	Vit. C mg	Folate µg	Vit. B_{12} µg	Cal-cium mg	Phos-phorus mg	Mag-nesium mg	Iron mg	Iodine µg	Zinc mg
Months															
0-4	Both	6.0	12[b]	400	10	3	20	50	0.3	250[c]	150	20	0.3[d]	30	2[d]
5-12	Both	9.0	12	400	10	3	20	50	0.3	400	200	32	7	40	3
Years															
1	Both	11	19	400	10	3	20	65	0.3	500	300	40	6	55	4
2-3	Both	14	22	400	5	4	20	80	0.4	550	350	50	6	65	4
4-6	Both	18	26	500	5	5	25	90	0.5	600	400	65	8	85	5
7-9	M	25	30	700	2.5	7	25	125	0.8	700	500	100	8	110	7
	F	25	30	700	2.5	6	25	125	0.8	700	500	100	8	95	7
10-12	M	34	38	800	2.5	8	25	170	1.0	900	700	130	8	125	9
	F	36	40	800	5	7	25	180	1.0	1100	800	135	8	110	9
13-15	M	50	50	900	5	9	30	150	1.5	1100	900	185	10	160	12
	F	48	42	800	5	7	30	145	1.5	1000	850	180	13	160	9
16-18	M	62	55	1000	5	10	40[e]	185	1.9	900	1000	230	10	160	12
	F	53	43	800	2.5	7	30[e]	160	1.9	700	850	200	12	160	9
19-24	M	71	58	1000	2.5	10	40[e]	210	2.0	800	1000	240	9	160	12
	F	58	43	800	2.5	7	30[e]	175	2.0	700	850	200	13	160	9
25-49	M	74	61	1000	2.5	9	40[e]	220	2.0	800	1000	250	9	160	12
	F	59	44	800	2.5	6	30[e]	175	2.0	700	850	200	13	160	9
50-74	M	73	60	1000	5	7	40[e]	220	2.0	800	1000	250	9	160	12
	F	63	47	800	5	6	30[e]	190	2.0	800	850	210	8	160	9
75+	M	69	57	1000	5	6	40[e]	205	2.0	800	1000	230	9	160	12
	F	64	47	800	5	5	30[e]	190	2.0	800	850	210	8	160	9
Pregnancy(additional) 1st Trimester			5	100	2.5	2	0	300	1.0	500	200	15	0	25	6
2nd Trimester			20	100	2.5	2	10	300	1.0	500	200	45	5	25	6
3rd Trimester			24	100	2.5	2	10	300	1.0	500	200	45	10	25	6
Lactation (additional)			20	400	2.5	3	25	100	0.5	500	200	65	0	50	6

a. Retinol Equivalents

b. Protein is assumed to be from breast milk and must be adjusted for infant formula.

c. Infant formula with high phosphorus should contain 375 mg calcium

d. Breast milk is assumed to be the source of the mineral.

e. Smokers should increase vitamin C by 50%.

Notes